EFFECTIVE COUNSELING IN AUDIOLOGY

Perspectives and Practice

Edited by

John Greer Clark
and
Frederick N. Martin

Prentice Hall, Englewood Cliffs, New Jersey 07632

Library of Congress Cataloging-in-Publication Data

Effective counseling in audiology: perspectives and practice/edited
  by John Greer Clark and Frederick N. Martin.
        p.   cm.

    Includes bibliographical references and index.
    ISBN 0-13-181348-X
      1. Hearing impaired—Counseling of.   2. Audiologist and patient.
  I. Clark, John Greer.   II. Martin, Frederick N.
      [DNLM: 1. Hearing Disorders—psychology.   2. Counseling—methods.
  3. Professional-Patient Relations.   WV 270   E274 1994]
  RF291.E34   1994
  617.8'9—dc20
  DNLM/DLC
  for Library of Congress   93-1240
                                                                CIP

Acquisitions editor: Julie Berrisford
Editorial/production supervision
  and interior design: Mary Anne Shahidi
Cover design: Bruce Kenselaar
Prepress buyer: Kelly Behr
Manufacturing buyer: Mary Ann Gloriande

©1994 by Prentice-Hall, Inc.
A Simon & Schuster Company
Englewood Cliffs, New Jersey 07632

Printed in the United States of America
10 9 8 7 6 5 4 3 2 1

ISBN 0-13-181348-X

Prentice-Hall International (UK) Limited, *London*
Prentice-Hall of Australia Pty. Limited, *Sydney*
Prentice-Hall Canada Inc., *Toronto*
Prentice-Hall Hispanoamericana, S.A., *Mexico*
Prentice-Hall of India Private Limited, *New Delhi*
Prentice-Hall of Japan, Inc., *Tokyo*
Simon & Schuster Asia Pte. Ltd., *Singapore*
Editora Prentice-Hall do Brasil, Ltda., *Rio de Janeiro*

To our wives, Suzanne and Cathy,
for their support and patience
during the many hours required
to complete this book.

Contents

Foreword

In a world of ever-increasing technological sophistication audiologists may become so immersed in the tools of measurement of hearing impairment that they lose sight of the human being suffering the hearing loss and the impact of that loss on family and friends. A good example is the fitting of a tiny canal aid to an elderly person who lacks the fine motor control necessary to insert and remove the instrument. Or spending an hour carrying out an ABR on a baby to verify the presence of a severe loss, but only a few minutes conveying the significance of this finding to the distraught parents.

Counseling is the *sine qua non* of aural rehabilitation. It is the important process of telling people what you found, what it means, and what needs to be done, and doing so with tact and sensitivity.

In this important volume John Clark and Fred Martin have assembled a group of authors well qualified to remind us of the important role of counseling in the total rehabilitative process. Topics range from identification in children, to conveying diagnostic information, to acceptance of hearing aids.

Thoughtful clinicians are ever concerned that their counseling skills are adequate, appropriate, and informed. A careful reading of this book will certainly assist all of us in such an evaluation.

James Jerger
Houston, TX

Preface

It is not certain exactly when the profession of audiology had its beginnings. It is even debatable how the profession got its name. There is little doubt, however, that the major impetus for the advancement of this field began at the close of World War II, when many veterans with varying degrees of service-connected hearing loss returned to civilian life, facing an uncertain future complicated by the unexpected adjustments and problems presented by their new disability. Audiology, as a separate profession, evolved in response to the challenge of providing aural rehabilitation for these returning veterans, buttressed by professionals with backgrounds in otology, speech-language pathology, psychology, and education.

Some suggest that over the years the medical aspects of hearing loss may have overshadowed the profession's original rehabilitative goals. Despite the many technological advances in hearing instrumentation and fitting procedures, some may further argue that audiologists have not provided full service within the management process because of a tendency to minimize the importance of a humanistic approach to counseling.

It is of great importance to the success of audiology as a profession, and to the success of those whom the profession serves, that we continue to expand our knowledge and capabilities in both the diagnosis and rehabilitation of hearing disorders. However, it is of equal importance that we not lose sight of the humanistic side of our professional endeavors, regardless of the particular niche within audiology that we may find ourselves.

It is toward the encouragement and further development of this important humanistic aspect of our profession that we have directed this book. Counseling, as viewed and practiced by many audiologists, is no more than a content transfer between the audiologist and patient. Although such content counseling is of great importance in both diagnostic and rehabilitative procedures, we must never underestimate the impact of our personal communications with patients and their families. We must know how to deliver our messages effectively and how to develop an effective alliance with our patients if we are to help them to help themselves toward improved communication. In this text we have striven to blend useful content counseling topics with a counseling approach that recognizes and confronts the strong affect base that inevitably permeates our dialogue with patients.

The personal attributes that must be cultivated in the on-going context of clinical experience can develop only over time. However, this development is paramount if we are to become more effective in our clinical interactions with patients. Obviously, a book of this kind can only partially address counseling attributes and skills appropriate to our profession. It is offered as a supplement to the exposures that all of us are afforded through clinical practice and continuing education.

We have asked each contributor to attempt to maintain a consistent writing style that we hope will enhance continuity among the chapters of this book. We have, however, allowed the contributors to refer to those we serve in the manner they feel most comfortable: that is *patients* in some chapters and *clients* in others. We have closely monitored content to avoid unnecessary duplication of material. However, since this book is not necessarily designed to be read straight through from cover to cover, restating of some important principles or concepts has been necessary so that each chapter can be read independently, depending on the needs of the reader. Where appropriate, authors have referred to other chapters within the text for further explanation of a topic, or for related discussion. Readers will find a number of appendices throughout the text that we hope may prove useful to their patient interactions. Many of these have been designed for ease of photocopying for distribution to patients. Indeed, we encourage this.

As a result of the nontechnical nature of the subject matter within this book, the material should be easily digested by undergraduate and graduate students as well as practicing audiologists. Although audiologists will undoubtedly be the primary readers of this book, its content should prove useful to anyone who works with those with impaired hearing, including otolaryngologists, speech-language pathologists, hearing aid dispensers, and educators of the deaf and hearing impaired.

We are indebted to the authors of this text, all of them well known in their respective fields, for their generous sharing of experiences and ideas. We believe the variety of their backgrounds has made possible this multidimensional approach to the subject of audiological counseling. We must also acknowledge Katherine Clark's editorial expertise in the review of portions of this text.

JOHN GREER CLARK
FREDERICK N. MARTIN

Contributors

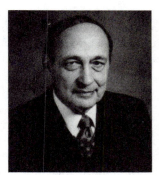

Jerome G. Alpiner (Ph.D., Ohio University) is Coordinator of Audiology at the Veterans Administration Medical Center in Denver, Colorado. His extensive publications and presentations cover a wide range of audiological concerns with an emphasis on adult audiological rehabilitation. He has chaired numerous committees for state and national associations including the American Speech-Language-Hearing Association Committee on Rehabilitative Audiology. Dr. Alpiner is co-editor of the widely used text *Rehabilitative Audiology: Children and Adults*, a Fellow of the American Speech-Language-Hearing Association and the American Academy of Audiology, and a past president of the Academy of Rehabilitative Audiology.

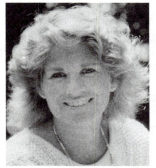

Dale V. Atkins (Ph.D., University of California at Los Angeles) is a family communications specialist with a private practice in New York City. Her areas of expertise are in the emotional adjustment of families with hearing-impaired children, sibling relationships, intergenerational communication, interfaith marriages, and the prevention of sexual molestation of children.

Dr. Atkins is the author of *Sisters: A Practical, Helpful Exploration of the Intimate and Complex Bond between Female Siblings*, co-author of "NO!-GO!-TELL!" a child protection curriculum, co-author and host of "Confronting Antisemitism," a Family Awareness Film Project, and editor of *Families and Their Hearing-Impaired Children*. Dr. Atkins has authored five book chapters, several journal and magazine articles, and numerous conference/convention papers. Dr. Atkins is a popular public speaker and a frequent guest and guest host in the media. Within the field of hearing impairment, she is a member of the Alexander Graham Bell Association of the Deaf, the National Association for the Deaf, and Auditory-Verbal International.

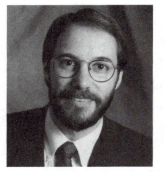

John Greer Clark (Ph.D., University of Cincinnati) has been in an independent private practice since 1982. His primary interests in audiological rehabilitation are in hearing instrumentation and patient counseling. A Fellow of the American Academy of Audiology, he is a recipient of the Honors of the Ohio Speech and Hearing Association and the Prominent Alumni Award from the Communication Sciences and Disorders Department at the University of Cincinnati. In addition to more than 35 publications on various topics related to communication disorders, Dr. Clark is the author of *Audiology for the School Speech-Language Clinician* and *The ABC's to Better Hearing*. He is co-editor of *Tinnitus and Its Management* and, as associate editor of *Hearsay*, he has served as journal issue editor for "Counseling Considerations in Communication Disorders" and "Geriatric Issues in Audiology and Speech-Language Pathology," and co-editor of "Assistive Listening Devices and Augmentative Communication." Dr. Clark is certified by the American Speech-Language-Hearing Association in both audiology and speech-language pathology.

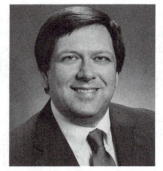

Dean C. Garstecki (Ph.D., University of Illinois at Urbana-Champaign) is professor of audiology, hearing science, and otolaryngology, head of the Audiology and Hearing Science Program, and director of the Hugh Knowles Center for Clinical and Basic Science in Hearing and Its Disorders at Northwestern University. His research focuses on study of the habits, attitudes, and speech-processing abilities of hearing-impaired aging adults and on measurement of electroacoustic characteristics of assistive listening devices. He has authored 16 book chapters, 35 journal articles and 160 convention or conference papers, largely on topics related to rehabilitative audiology. Dr. Garstecki has edited a National Student Speech-Language Hearing Association monograph on report writing in audiology and has codeveloped computer software for selection of assistive devices for hearing-impaired adults. He is a Fellow of the American Academy of Audiology, Northwestern University's Buehler Medical Center on Aging, and the American Speech-Language-Hearing Association (ASHA). He is a Founding Fellow of the Hugh Knowles Center, a member of the Chicago Hearing Society's Board of Directors, past president of the Academy of Rehabilitative Audiology and of the Chicago Speech-Language-Hearing Association. Dr. Garstecki is a former chair of the ASHA Committee on Rehabilitative Audiology and vice chair of the ASHA Council on Professional Standards. He has received the Honors of the Chicago Speech-Language-Hearing Association, was named Marquette University's Alumnus of the Year, and was appointed as an Honorable Kentucky Colonel by the governor of Kentucky in recognition of his service to individuals with hearing loss.

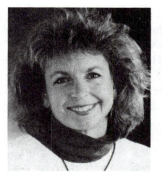

Cheryl DeConde Johnson (Ed.D., University of Northern Colorado) has been an educational audiologist and hearing consultant since 1976. She is also the parent of a daughter who is hard of hearing. She currently works part time with Greeley School District 6, in Greeley, Colorado, and as the audiology consultant for the Colorado Department of Education. In addition, Dr. Johnson is a regional coordinator for both the Department of Education and the Department of Health for services for children birth through 21 years, including the Home Intervention Program for newborns to 3-year-olds. She has taught classes and supervised graduate students for the University of Northern Colorado, lectured extensively, and authored numerous articles and chapters. Her special interests are in educational and pediatric audiology, with particular emphasis in habilitation and services for hard-of-hearing children, and infants and their families. Dr. Johnson is a Fellow of the American Academy of Audiology and a past president of the Educational Audiology Association.

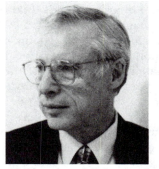

Frederick N. Martin (Ph.D., City University of New York) holds the Lillie Hage Jamail Centennial Professorship in Communication Sciences and Disorders at The University of Texas at Austin. His specialty is clinical audiology, and he has particular interests in the areas of pediatric diagnosis and patient–parent counseling. The author of *Introduction to Audiology*, now in its fourth edition, *Introduction to Audiology: A Study Guide*, *Principles of Audiology*, *Clinical Audiometry and Masking*, and *Basic Audiometry*, Dr. Martin has edited *Pediatric Audiology*, *Medical Audiology*, and *Hearing Disorders in Children* in addition to the 10-volume series entitled *Remediation of Communication Disorders*. He has also authored 14 book chapters, over 100 journal articles, and more than 75 convention or conference papers. Dr. Martin is a Fellow of the American Speech-Language-Hearing Association and the American Academy of Audiology. He has won the Teaching Excellence Award of the College of Communication, and the Graduate Teaching Award of The University of Texas.

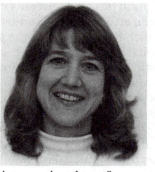

Shelley D. Smith (Ph.D., Medical Genetics, Indiana University) is an associate professor of otolaryngology and human communication at the Boys Town National Research Hospital. Her research interests have been in the phenotypic and genetic characterization of communication disorders, particularly localization of genes causing reading disability and deafness syndromes. She is the editor of a book entitled *Genetics and Learning Disabilities* and has authored or co-authored over 35 journal articles and book chapters on these topics, along with over 30 presentations at national and international conferences. She is certified as a Ph.D. Medical Geneticist by the American Board of Medical Genetics, and provides genetic services to families through the Boys Town National Research Hospital and the University of Nebraska Medical Center.

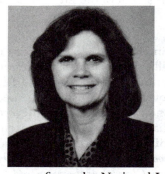

Linda M. Thibodeau (Ph.D., University of Minnesota) is an associate professor in the Program of Communication Sciences and Disorders at The University of Texas at Austin. Dr. Thibodeau holds dual certification in Speech-Language Pathology and Audiology and has worked as a speech-language pathologist and audiologist in a major medical center and as a language/learning disabilities teacher in the public schools. She presently serves as project director of the Interdisciplinary Aural Habilitation Training Program at The University of Texas and has a current grant from the National Institute on Deafness and Other Communication Disorders to study the relationship between psychoacoustic processing and speech reception deficits as a function of aging and hearing loss. Further research interests include the use and evaluation of frequency-modulated (FM) amplification systems. Her research has been published in a number of refereed journals.

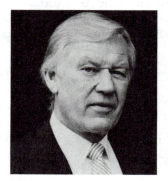

Samuel Trychin (Ph.D., George Washington University) is professor of psychology at Gallaudet University, Washington, DC. His speciality is application of psychological concepts, principles, and procedures to problems experienced by hard-of-hearing people and their families, friends, and co-workers. He has developed a program titled Living with Hearing Loss under the joint sponsorship of Gallaudet University and Self Help for Hard of Hearing People (SHHH) organization. As part of this program, he has written numerous books and articles and produced several videotapes on topics related to the psychosocial aspects of hearing loss. Dr. Trychin has also conducted more than 150 workshops and classes nationally on topics related to coping with hearing loss and has worked closely with more than 1,000 hard-of-hearing people and their family members. He is a member of the American Psychological Association and is listed in the National Register of Health Service Providers in Psychology. A licensed psychologist in the District of Columbia and Maryland, Dr. Trychin is hard of hearing and has been wearing hearings aids since 1953.

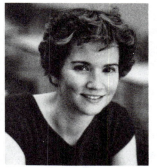 Madeleine L. Van Hecke (Ph.D., DePaul University) is a professor of psychology at North Central College in Naperville, Illinois, where she teaches courses in developmental and clinical psychology. She has received the Clarence F. Dissinger Award for Excellence in Teaching and the Sears-Roebuck Award for Educational Leadership and Teaching Excellence. Dr. Van Hecke is active in faculty development, presenting workshops at various institutions, and acting as faculty development coordinator at her own college under a grant from the Lilly Endowment. She is particularly interested in how to encourage students' critical and creative thinking and has written numerous papers related to this topic. A registered psychologist in the state of Illinois, Dr. Van Hecke received her clinical internship training at Illinois Masonic Medical Center in Chicago. Her special clinical research interest is in helping people cope with illness and disability.

chapter one

Audiologists' Counseling Purview

John Greer Clark

As the reader will discover in this and subsequent chapters, research frequently challenges audiologists to reexamine the effectiveness of their own counseling procedures. In this first chapter, Dr. Clark introduces the counseling philosophies this book addresses and the responsibility audiologists share in providing sensitive and caring support for their patients. Discussions provided in this chapter and throughout this book are designed to facilitate a high and admittedly difficult goal: to make coping with hearing loss easier for patients and families alike and to suggest strategies for life adjustments that will be as successful and fulfilling as possible.

> People exist by virtue of the help they give to one another. That's what I believe. Helping people improves the helped person's life and keeps the helping person human.
>
> Chaim Potok
> *In the Beginning*

INTRODUCTION

Despite audiology's origins in aural rehabilitation, the evolution of our field has decisively drifted toward diagnostic evaluations within the medical setting. Indeed, over the years, medical settings have, by far, become the most prevalent place of employment for audiologists (American Speech-Language-Hearing Association, 1992). Diagnostic evaluations in audiology have become increasingly advanced through continued research in differential assessment and technological advances in computerized instrumentation. Behavioral and electrophysiological diagnostic procedures have allowed us through the years to pair ourselves with our otolaryngology colleagues through the provision of detailed evaluations beneficial to the physician in determining medical management.

Within the medical environment, in-depth patient counseling frequently is overshadowed by the often *perceived* more intriguing realm of diagnostic testing. As Robinson (1991) points out, the drift in audiology toward technical management instead of human management is unmistakable. However, as Hawkins (1990) has stated, the many technological advances in our field may only be of minor importance to our final success with patients when compared to the counseling and rehabilitative aspects of our care.

As audiologists' professional autonomy increases within expanding private practice settings, as well as within more traditional employment settings, we begin to embrace an increasingly active role in hearing care. When not working within the confines of the more technical aspects of a medical practice, patient contact time becomes more personal. We begin to assume the mantle originally intended by our professional forebears.

When audiology eventually becomes a truly autonomous profession, it will evolve within our role as hearing *care* professionals. To be sure, diagnosis is an integral part of that role, as our rehabilitative strategies clearly cannot be designed nor implemented apart from a complete understanding of the patient's hearing status. However, as audiologists, we come into our own when we begin to face the challenge of caring for our patients and their families through an ongoing interpersonal dialogue, the kind of dialogue that can only emerge within a positive, well-developed relationship with our patients. Thus, recent and continuing changes within the profession that will lead to greater autonomy are presenting us with precisely those opportunities for patient care that pioneers in the field knew well. We are finally returning home.

The purpose of this chapter is to examine the role of audiologists in meeting their patients' counseling needs. In this chapter, I will discuss the difference between psychotherapy and support counseling and address some of the counseling uncertainties that cause audiologists to bias their counseling efforts toward content or information transfer counseling. In addition, this chapter will provide an overview of counseling theories and explore some of the personal attributes that lead to successful patient management in a humanistic manner. Finally, our own limitations as counselors will be explored along with the need to recognize when referral for more in-depth counseling may be needed.

UNDERSTANDING OUR COUNSELING RESPONSIBILITIES

The Need to Counsel

Counseling is a recognized and vital component to the intervention services that we provide to our patients (see Appendix 1–1). To be most effective in serving patients and their families, audiologists must become adept not only in the diagnosis of auditory disorders and the rehabilitative management of these disorders, but also in the more elusive area of successful patient–professional relationships that may be built and maintained through the art of counseling. Unfortunately, the counseling provided during time allotted for patient contact does not always address the patients' concerns or meet their counseling needs (Bernstein, Bernstein, & Dana, 1974). Even more unfortunately, we do not always recognize the deficiencies in the counseling we provide.

Audiologists often feel uncomfortable in their role as patient counselor. We sometimes feel uncertain as to how far our counseling should go, just as do many other health care professionals (Bernstein et al., 1974). Nevertheless, regardless of our uncertainties, the need for counseling may be a crucial part of the management process, particularly for parents or adult patients whose reactions to what we tell them are often complex. They may be confused over the diagnosis itself, uncertain about recommended rehabilitative measures, and worried over prognostic limitations. In addition, they will certainly be suffering disappointment and emotional pain for the loss or diminution of hearing abilities and the accompanying change adult patients envision in lifestyle or the altered developmental potentials parents perceive for their child.

Mr. Gallegos finally gave in to his wife's "nagging." In an effort to reestablish peace in his home, he agreed to get his hearing tested. He was sure the results would be normal. Now after failing his hearing test, he realizes he had been denying his hearing problems for several years. He was surprised when he was told that it was a "nerve" loss and that only hearing aids would help. "Hearing aids! And for God's sake, why two of them?" He finds he resents the ease with which others communicate and the fact that they don't seem to appreciate or understand his difficulties.

Over the past 3 years, Holly Virginia has experienced a decrease in hearing from normal levels to her present severe bilateral sensorineural hearing loss. This young woman, who had only recently begun juggling the demands of career and family responsibilities, is trying hard to cope with the sudden changes in her life. Her frustrations at home and work seem to fuel her anger and grief.

Last month, Mrs. French gave birth to the son she and her husband had been eagerly awaiting. Their lives had seemed perfect to them; after 10 years of marriage, they had felt the time was right to begin a family. The enormity of their shock was surpassed only by the grief and guilt they felt as their profoundly hearing-impaired son became a part of their lives.

Mrs. Duchesne is frustrated and angry. Her 5-year-old son has been in speech-language therapy for 2 years. Progress continues in Ian's language development, and most of his articulation errors have been corrected. Now the audiologist says Ian has another case of otitis media. Mrs. Duchesne fears he may need a fourth set of ventilating tubes. The problem keeps coming back, and each time Ian's progress in therapy slows. Why can't they fix it right?

Clearly, for these patients counseling is crucial. But who has the responsibility of helping Mr. Gallegos adjust to what has happened in his life—or Holly, whose world has turned upside down so suddenly— or parents like Mrs. French or Mrs. Duchesne, who are frightened of the future and frustrated with the present—or the many others who must somehow learn to cope successfully and positively with the real trauma associated with auditory disorders? These are examples of people who come into any of our offices on any of our workdays. An accurate diagnosis alone does not provide the help these people need or lessen the pain they are experiencing. Are audiologists stepping beyond the boundaries of their profession when they provide more than content counseling?

As discussed by Dr. Van Hecke in Chapter 5, professionals in service fields, including audiologists, are in a unique position to provide counseling "naturally" as part of the dialogue that evolves between the professional and the patient. It is within this dialogue that it is quite appropriate for audiologists to extend their professional responsibilities to encompass the emotional–support needs of their patients. This counseling is precisely within our domain.

Some of our reservations about counseling stem from the differences we recognize between ourselves and our patients: age, life experiences, physical handicap, and so on. To diminish this natural barrier, we perhaps need to restructure our thinking before we consult with patients. In the counseling role, it may be helpful not to dwell on the differences that obviously exist between us. Instead, we need to identify with those aspects that we do have in common with those we serve.

Suzanne is a young audiologist who only recently graduated from the university. As she approaches the geriatric patient in the waiting room, she fears she may have difficulty relating to him. She believes he may not accept recommendations and guidance from someone who is probably not any older than his oldest grandchild.

Dave is an audiologist who plans to get married next summer. He has no children and has never had the experience of rearing children. He feels unprepared to talk with the parents of an infant newly diagnosed as hearing impaired. How will the parents of this child accept consultation from one who has not been through the route of pain and disappointment upon which they have just embarked?

The perceived gap between audiologist and patient can be bridged, and it is on making this bridge that the professional must concentrate. We have all experienced the emotions of disappointment, pain, confusion, uncertainty, and fear. The emotions of our patients are human, not unique. Although the intensity of emotional experience may vary— as does the cause—we can, nevertheless, empathize with that experience. This empathy becomes the bridge across the gap, regardless of how wide the gap may seem. Once we recognize the similarities we share with our patients, we can begin to develop the close rapport we need if we are to assist them in addressing their concerns.

Audiologists, like other health care professionals, are not immune to the natural tendency to avoid unpleasant confrontations and situations. Much of this insecurity with the counseling process stems from insufficiencies in academic preparation (McCarthy, Culpepper, & Lucks, 1986). Unfortunately, in an effort to provide clinical competence to audiologists in training, universities often give the development of effective counseling and listening skills an inappropriately low priority. However, while academic programs clearly need a greater emphasis on the counseling process, audiologists cannot hide behind a lack of preparation. We remain responsible for accepting our counseling role.

In an early publication, Ross (1964) notes that professionals may reduce their own anxieties simply by ignoring their patient's difficulties in coping. Knowing that the patient will also be seeing other professionals in the course of diagnosis and treatment, audiologists may rationalize that somebody else will undoubtedly counsel the patient or family about any problems or matters of concern. However, as Ross points out, the "somebody else" may have similar anxieties and defenses with the result that the patient receives help from no one.

Many emotions may surface as the relationship progresses between audiologists and their patients. It is important to be aware of these emotions as they begin to evolve. The emotions within the grieving process (see Chapter 5 for a discussion of grieving) are not unique to the parents of a recently diagnosed handicapped child. These emotions are also common among adults who experience a diminution of one of their major senses or functions (Tanner, 1980).

Even after early grieving, adult patients and parents may experience further emotional stress throughout the management process (Clark, 1990). Confusion and frustration may develop when patients or parents do not fully understand management strategies. Disappointment, or even anger, may accompany the patient's own ineffectual attempts at communication. And many adult patients and parents may become hostile or negative when trying to cope with a management process that, to them, may appear only minimally effective or excessively protracted. Patients and families have the right to express these emotions. Audiologists have the responsibility to recognize these emotions for what they are and to accept them without trying to deny or minimize them. Emotions must be worked through from within before they can be channeled along productive avenues.

The Audiologist as a Nonprofessional Counselor

When working with patients facing emotional crises, audiologists frequently take on the role of "nonprofessional" counselor. Certainly, professional counselors are not the only ones in a position to counsel. Counseling is often provided by professionals who are not trained counselors such as educators, lawyers, clergy, family physicians, and even friends. Rarely do those in need of counseling seek out social workers, psychologists, or psychiatrists.

Kennedy (1977, 1981) has discussed the role of the nonprofessional counselor. Within this role, audiologists, like professionals in other service fields, are not trained as professional counselors. Often the feeling that they must fill a counseling void by assuming the responsibilities of a professional counselor makes them even more insecure. However, audiologists, as nonprofessional counselors, need not perceive themselves as long-term therapists. *Our mission is not to identify and resolve all the conflicts that may be present within our patients.* To paraphrase Kennedy (1981), we must retain our primary identity as audiologists who are responding sensitively to needs and experiences that go beyond our usual management endeavors. No one, not even mental health professionals, can be effective counselors when they hold forth an impossibly high standard for themselves.

Nonprofessional counselors cannot be expected to provide the perfect response in each counseling encounter. As Kennedy states, only by scaling down expectations can nonprofessional and professional counselors decrease their own guilt when they fall short of meeting their expectations. Audiologists should not feel, realistically, that their efforts can ever successfully compensate for the trauma that has happened in their patients' lives. They cannot expect to make up for the loss in communication function as experienced by an adult patient, the patient's adult children or spouse, or by the parents of a hearing-impaired child. In the absence of this realistic approach, the stress audiologists may feel in their counseling endeavors can often become self-defeating.

Nonprofessional counselors must at all times be themselves. The straightforward empathic human response is the best approach. As Kennedy states, it allows nonprofessional counselors to concentrate on the crisis at hand, not on all that has preceded, nor on everything that may follow. Only when audiologists can define their role as counselors for those with impaired hearing can they become comfortable within that role, and in turn provide an effective adjunct to their management endeavors.

OUR COUNSELING ROLE DEFINED

Ongoing and effective support counseling is an important and highly necessary adjunct to the content–educational counseling audiologists provide their patients (Stone & Olswang, 1989). The difference between content counseling and emotional support counseling is easily recognized by most of us. However, the demarcation between emotional support counseling and psychotherapy is often more clouded. It is partially because of this uncertainty in counseling definitions that our counseling attempts remain largely within the content realm.

The goal of psychotherapy is to reorganize or reinterpret the personal conflicts patients may have within themselves. These intrapersonal conflicts may have little basis in subjective reality and may manifest themselves as anxiety, depression, persistent guilt, confusion, or ambivalence.

As contrasted with psychotherapy, counseling is based upon a well-patient model. The majority of the patients and families that we see for audiological services are psychologically normal people who are presently confronting and trying to cope with one or more major disruptions in their lives. The counseling we provide within our practices is a supportive counseling that builds upon renewed perceptions of the difficulties encountered. This form of support counseling is usually short term and does not necessitate a reorganization or reinterpretation of personality. Its goal is to help patients and families to make practical changes in their lives that will help them develop a more positive approach to their own handicaps, the technological assistance available to them, and the residual communication difficulties they may still experience.

COUNSELING THEORIES

Support counseling provided by audiologists as nonprofessional counselors may certainly take a form less structured than that provided by social workers, psychologists, and psychiatrists. Audiologists' counseling usually evolves naturally as part of the dialogue that arises within the clinic visit. Through this dialogue, a "therapeutic alliance" can develop in which the audiologist and patient see their relationship as an opportunity to work together to help the patient achieve a goal (Van Hecke, 1990). To achieve this alliance effectively, audiologists should familiarize themselves with basic counseling theory. Three counseling theories within the well-patient model of support counseling that audiologists should be acquainted with are the person-centered theory of counseling (Rogers, 1959, 1979), the behavioral theory (Skinner, 1953), and the cognitive (rational-emotive) theory (Ellis & Grieger, 1977).

A practical counseling text for audiologists cannot include a comprehensive study of these counseling theories. However, the interested reader is encouraged to seek out the original references cited or more detailed discussions within communicative disorders literature as may be found in the writings of Luterman (1984, 1991) or Rollin (1987). We might begin a review of these theories by considering Rogers's person-centered approach to counseling and some of the personal attributes he believes to be important.

Rogers's Person-Centered Counseling

A central tenet of person-centered counseling theory is that the patient knows best. Through this nondirective approach to counseling, the audiologist helps patients tap their own inner resources to reach solutions to their problems. The audiologist avoids the persona of the appointed expert who will recommend clear solutions or offer authoritarian guidance. Instead, the person-centered approach challenges patients to accept responsibility for their own lives and to trust their inner resources as they build greater self-awareness and self-acceptance (Mearns & Thorne, 1988).

Some people with hearing loss may fixate on their disability to the extent that the disability becomes the reality of their self-image. The lowered self-concept that results can greatly impede progress toward resolution of their communication problems. Through the audiologist's nonjudgmental acceptance of patients' behaviors and attitudes, as expressed within person-centered counseling, patients can begin to perceive their assets, not their disabilities, as the reality. As assets are placed above disabilities, self-worth increases, a process that in turn makes it more likely that improved communication through residual hearing can be moved in a positive direction.

To practice Rogers's person-centered counseling, a variety of personal attributes are necessary that we as audiologists may want to cultivate to enhance our own counseling efforts.

Congruence with self. Audiologists who allow themselves to be themselves, without hiding behind an air of inflated professionalism and unnecessary jargon, permit the greatest opportunity for positive and constructive patient change and development. Audiologists who are congruent with themselves will not portray themselves as all-knowing and thereby will decrease patients' expectations that answers will always be provided for them. Instead, the behavior of such audiologists will help patients find resources within themselves for needed behavioral or cognitive changes. Further, this trait will enable them to maintain a relaxed and friendly manner and an ability to accept both suggestions and criticisms from patients.

Unconditional positive regard.

> He did not treat the rich foreign merchant differently from the servant who shaved him and the peddlers from whom he bought bananas and let himself be robbed of small coins.
>
> Hermann Hesse
> *Siddhartha*

Unconditional positive regard refers to a professional's ability to accept patients as human beings of importance in their own right. Whether a private, fee-paying patient of professional stature or a welfare recipient whose bill is covered through third-party reimbursement, each patient clearly has the right to self-direction and to the same measure of respect.

Empathic understanding. Empathic understanding refers to audiologists' ability to appreciate how specific problems are perceived by their patients, thus requiring careful listening to patients' explanations of their concerns and feelings. As Sanders (1980) has stated, empathy permits the audiologist to "absorb the emotionally laden, poorly defined problem" as expressed by the patient and then to reflect the problem back to the patient in the objective manner necessary to facilitate the search for a solution.

During Mr. Farrell's first post-fitting consultation, he states, "These hearing aids are not giving me the benefit I had hoped for." The audiologist responds, "Certainly expectations are sometimes higher than hearing aids can attain. However, for your particular hearing loss, Mr. Farrell, I can assure you this is the most appropriate fitting."

At this point what Mr. Farrell needs most is not assurance that the fitting is correct, but reassurance that speaks to the frustration he is feeling. While the audiologist's statements may be true, a more empathic response might have been, "I know your hearing problem can be quite annoying and that your hearing aids don't provide normal hearing. Tell me what you've been experiencing lately and whether you've noted any improvement in your hearing since you first started wearing your hearing aids. I'd like to help you."

The second response reveals a higher level of empathy that may help Mr. Farrell to explore his feelings and expectations more fully. The ensuing discussion may even reveal additional areas in which the audiologist may be of assistance. Further discussion of active listening, which is the foundation of empathic listening, may be found in Chapter 2.

The Blending of Counseling Theories

It is the clinical interrelationship and not the representative technique of the various schools of thought that contributes most to the effectiveness of counseling (Avila, Combs, & Purkey, 1977, cited in Rollin, 1987). This may especially be true for support counseling provided within the framework of auditory disorders management. In practice, many find their best approach is an eclectic approach, rather than being closely tied to a single counseling method (Arbuckle, 1970). The approach we take, and the way we blend portions of varying counseling theories, will largely depend upon the individual circumstances of a given relationship we have with a patient.

Using the precepts of Rogers's approach to counseling as a primary foundation, we may wish to blend in aspects of other counseling methods as individual circumstances dictate. Certainly a number of different counseling theories could be successfully used with the person-centered approach. Two such theories that I have found particularly useful in audiology practice are the behavioral counseling theory (Skinner, 1953) and the cognitive (rational-emotive) approach to counseling (Ellis & Grieger, 1977).

Behavioral Counseling Theory

Behavioral counseling theory is familiar to those who have employed the principles of operant conditioning in pediatric hearing evaluations. According to Skinner (1953), a behavior is learned when followed by a circumstance that brings satisfaction to the individual. For example, an isolationist behavior may be positively reinforced when a person with a hearing loss discovers anxiety is decreased by avoiding interactions with others. The satisfaction of this positive reinforcement increases the probability that this isolationist behavior will be increased.

The audiologist who employs the conditioning methods of behavioral counseling serves as a supportive advisor to a counterconditioning program, gradually guiding the patient through a series of successive approximations to a desired goal. As such, behavioral counseling is a directive approach, with the patient working in concert with the audiologist to achieve environmental conditions that may help to produce positive behavioral change. Although this is a directive approach, the supportive aspects of Rogers's person-centered counseling can be effectively blended with behavioral counseling theory.

Like many adults, Mr. Lampe has developed a hearing loss slowly over a number of years. As time has progressed, he has gradually drawn away from many of the activities he once enjoyed as they began to create an increasing number of opportunities for frustration and embarrassment because of his hearing loss.

Many of the activities that Mr. Lampe has withdrawn from were once enjoyed in the company of his wife. Mrs. Lampe used to derive a large measure of her own enjoyment from these activities because they were done with her husband. She had hoped that Mr. Lampe's new hearing aids would allow the two of them to enjoy some of their former outlets together once again. She is disappointed at Mr. Lampe's reluctance to reenter those aspects of life that had previously brought them both much enjoyment.

Certainly Mr. and Mrs. Lampe should be encouraged to explore joint activities once again. Mr. Lampe may be reluctant to pursue some of these activities because he now views them as inappropriate for reasons other than his hearing loss. Some may indeed be inappropriate given his residual hearing deficits, even with amplification and assistive devices. However, activities that may be appropriate should be considered as a viable source of enjoyment for Mr. and Mrs. Lampe as a couple.

The audiologist can be helpful in guiding this couple as they investigate these activities so they are aware of difficult areas and possible solutions to these difficulties before they are encountered. By helping to eliminate some of the negatives that may be encountered when pursuing an activity with decreased hearing, and stressing the positives of involvement, Mr. Lampe's avoidance behavior may be reduced through the positive reinforcement he receives through participation. Some of the coping strategies discussed by Dr. Trychin in Chapter 10 may be useful when working with couples like the Lampes.

Cognitive (Rational-Emotive) Counseling Theory

In the first century A.D., the philosopher Epictetus stated, "Men are disturbed not by things, but by views which they take of them" (Trower, Casey, & Dryden, 1988). This statement fairly closely sums up the underlying thesis of cognitive or rational-emotive counseling theory. This approach to client counseling holds that forward movement in counseling is impeded by basic irrational beliefs that yield self-defeating thoughts and behaviors.

Emilie has a severe hearing impairment with poor speech discrimination bilaterally. Ear-level amplification only slightly augments her speechreading abilities. She has found that through the use of a direct audio-input microphone extended near a talker's mouth she can converse much more effectively. However, she believes this form of assistance to verbal communication is cumbersome and therefore offensive to those she encounters. Because of this belief, she avoids speaking with anyone but close acquaintances.

The goal of cognitive counseling is not to change Emilie's belief for her, but to teach her the skills needed to identify and modify her own self-defeating thoughts or beliefs.

The audiologist's display of empathy and understanding while helping patients place their life experiences in a realistic perspective can be a powerful combination. Toward this end, we may dispute patients' negative views through direct questioning of their stated assumptions. In the example with Emilie, the audiologist may ask questions such as: "What is the worst thing that could happen if you did use your microphone with a casual acquaintance?" "How do you know that it would be offensive to those you talk with?" "What is it that makes that so terrible?" Or "What would it take to convince you that the effectiveness of your microphone outweighs any of the disadvantages you foresee?"

Cognitive therapy may also be used to point out the irrational constraints ordinary linguistic structures may place on our lives. For example, when a patient insists he or she cannot wear hearing aids at the office, the audiologist may want to point out that anything is possible. What the patient has done is choose not to wear hearing aids at the office. Once this is accepted, it is possible to explore the reasons behind the choice.

Another constricting language structure is the use of "but" instead of "and." ("I want to wear my new hearing aids, but they are so noticeable" changes to "I want to wear my new hearing aids, and they are so noticeable." These two thoughts can exist together. One does not have to preclude the other.) Similarly, the use of "I am" changes to "I did" or "I have done" ("I am so stupid when it comes to mechanical devices" changes to "I have done stupid things before with mechanical devices"); the use of "I should" changes to "I want to" or "I don't want to" ("I should wear a second hearing aid" becomes "I want to—or do not want to—wear a second hearing aid"). Each of these linguistic changes places the responsibility for action or outlook with the patient. However, before attempting to make linguistic changes with patients, the audiologist should already have established a strong relationship with the patient. Otherwise, these attempts may seem intrusive and highly annoying (Luterman, 1991).

Cognitive counseling techniques may also include the use of role-playing as a means of demonstrating the irrationality of a patient's beliefs or modeling more rational beliefs or behaviors. Analogies are also useful, as well as humor and a full acceptance of the patient despite the presence of beliefs that may appear absurd or irrational (Rollin, 1987; Trower et al., 1988). Through these means, the audiologist helps patients to recognize the absurdity of their beliefs, to relinquish these beliefs, and to adopt new or more adaptive beliefs (Ellis & Grieger, 1977).

COUNSELING REFERRALS

Of course, on occasion, a patient may require more counseling than audiologists can provide within their nonprofessional counseling role. As discussed throughout this text, our patients may experience a variety of emotions during the course of hearing care management. Through the emotional support counseling we can provide, we can usually assist our patients and their family members to confront these emotions effectively and to move forward in improving their communication problems. Our own supportive efforts can be greatly enhanced by exposing our patients to others who have learned to cope with similarly difficult experiences. The value of support groups in the successful management of those with hearing loss and their families is discussed in detail for our work with parents and children in Chapter 6 and with adults in Chapter 10.

However, when forward movement stops due to patient or family inability or unwillingness to confront the emotions of hearing loss, it is time for referral to a more skilled counselor. In addition, we may see parents or adults with hearing loss in need of family therapy that is outside our area of expertise. And, of course, just as there are emotionally disturbed individuals within the hearing population, we will at times see a hearing-impaired individual suffering from an emotional disturbance who will need more help than we can provide.

To be prepared if the need for referral arises, audiologists should have a full awareness of local resources for psychological and social intervention. According to Kennedy (1981), awareness of these resources borders on being an ethical requirement of nonprofessional counselors. Indeed, the Code of Ethics statements of the American Academy of Audiology and of the American Speech-Language-Hearing Association specifically state that we must use every resource available, including referral to other specialists as the need arises, to provide the best service possible.

When considering a referral, it is important to select mental health professionals who are familiar with hearing impairment. Psychologists in school programs for hearing-impaired children or schools for the deaf can often serve as a referral source or provide valuable referral information. These professionals can also provide an invaluable service to those audiologists who do not possess the sign language fluency required to adequately counsel the manual deaf population. As suggested by Vernon and Ottinger (1989), when counselors familiar with hearing loss are not available, an audiologist's time may be well spent providing needed orientation to community mental health professionals.

Some audiologists may feel they are abandoning patients if they turn them over to another professional. However, as Kennedy (1977) states, an appropriate referral is not an abandonment of the individual but a recommendation made in the patient's best interest. And certainly the audiologist will continue the relationship with the patient as the hearing care professional. But the question remains: How do we as audiologists, acting within our role as nonprofessional counselors, know when a referral for more in-depth counseling is advisable?

Determining the Need for Referral

A number of circumstances may signal the need for referral. A parent who experiences a sense of guilt over a child's handicap may seek to assuage this guilt through an immersion within advocacy roles for those with impaired hearing. While this action can be admirable, if unremitting guilt leads to the parent's abandoning other family, professional, or personal responsibilities, that parent may need professional counseling in order to place things in perspective. Parents or spouses of adult patients are also in need of referral if they remain persistently intolerant of residual communication difficulties within the family. Similarly, parents or spouses of adults with hearing loss who may become emotionally withdrawn from the hearing-impaired family member may need more assistance in coping with a handicap within the family than we, as audiologists, are prepared to offer. Parents who repeatedly put off purchasing hearing aids for their child obviously have some unresolved issues that the audiologist has not been able to help them resolve.

Parents may have unrealistically high expectations that clearly do not match their child's abilities, or unrealistically low expectations that may create an overly dependent child with low self-esteem. Parents with persistently unrealistic expectation levels may need more counseling than the audiologist can provide. The same may be true for parents who have grown to place excessive pressure on the siblings of a child with impaired hearing.

Some spouses of adult patients may also continue to hold unrealistic communication expectations for their mates. If the audiologist's attempts to mold expectations to be congruent with hearing abilities have repeatedly failed, there may exist underlying issues that will be better addressed through referral.

These are only a few examples of unresolved conflicts continuing within a family. Certainly when feelings of guilt, denial, anger, or depression continue unabated, a referral for further counseling is necessary. But how do audiologists effectively broach this subject that for many bears such negative connotations?

Phrasing the Recommendation

It is important for us not to be uncertain about referrals we are making. If we exhibit uncertainties over the referral, our patients will undoubtedly feel the same uncertainty. The referral should not come as a total surprise to the patient but should come naturally out of the growing relationship the audiologist and patient have shared. If we suspect a referral may need to be made at some point, this concern can be shared with the patient early within discussions.

It is also important that we be honest with our patients about the need for referral. As Kennedy (1977) states, the reason may be simple and straightforward. We may feel that certain patients' needs are beyond our level of competence at the time, or that the patient needs assistance on a more regular or long-term basis than we can provide.

Our honest approach in counseling referrals requires that we be willing to answer any questions about the referral and to explore the patient's feelings about this change. It is helpful to talk about the person or clinic a patient is being referred to. The patient, however, should be given the responsibility of setting up any actual appointments.

When discussing referrals with our patients, it is also helpful to be conscious of referral semantics. "Counselor" sounds better to many than does "therapist." Similarly, "social worker" may bring to mind images of child protection agencies, and "psychiatrist" and "psychologist" both may cause patients to think of mental illness. It is appropriate to remind patients that we believe that their need for help is like that of many others in their position. The problems they must learn to cope with are very real and very stressful aspects of their lives.

Finally, when referral is made, the audiologist should arrange a follow-up contact with the patient. It is imperative that we determine if the patient followed through on the referral and, if not, that some help is forthcoming.

CONCLUSION

While audiologists often lack academic training in counseling, we retain a responsibility to provide our patients with more than the direct mechanics of hearing care. The purpose of this chapter was to heighten understanding of the counseling responsibilities audiologists share, and to consider the approach we may take toward meeting these responsibilities through our role as nonprofessional counselors. In addition, when providing counseling services to patients, audiologists must remain aware of their own counseling limitations and the need to refer patients for more in-depth counseling when required.

In order to provide effective counseling within audiological management, audiologists must develop a strong interpersonal relationship with their patients. The development and maintenance of this relationship will be explored in depth in Chapter 2.

REFERENCES

AMERICAN SPEECH-LANGUAGE-HEARING ASSOCIATION, Demographics Department. (1992). Demographic Profile of the ASHA Membership. Rockville, MD: Authors.

AMERICAN SPEECH-LANGUAGE-HEARING ASSOCIATION. (1993). Preferred practice patterns for the professions of speech-language pathology and audiology. *Asha, 35,* Supplement 11.

ARBUCKLE, D. S. (1970). *Counseling: Philosophy, theory and practice* (2nd ed.). Boston: Allyn & Bacon.

AVILA, D. L., COMBS, A. W., & PURKEY, W. W. (Eds.). (1977). *The helping relationship source book* (2nd ed.). Boston: Allyn & Bacon.

BERNSTEIN, L., BERNSTEIN, R. S., & DANA, R. (1974). *Interviewing: A guide for health professionals.* New York: Appleton-Century-Crofts.

CLARK, J. G. (1990). Counseling in communicative disorders: A responsibility to be met. *Hearsay,* Spring/Summer, 4–7.

ELLIS, A., & GRIEGER, R. (1977). *Handbook of rational-emotive therapy.* New York: Springer-Verlag.

HAWKINS, D. (1990). Technology and hearing aids: How does the audiologist fit in? *Asha, 32,* 42–43.

KENNEDY, E. (1977). *On becoming a counselor: A basic guide for nonprofessional counselors.* New York: Continuum.

KENNEDY, E. (1981). *Crisis counseling: The essential guide for nonprofessional counselors.* New York: Continuum.

LUTERMAN, D. (1984). *Counseling the communicatively disordered and their families.* Boston: Little, Brown.

LUTERMAN, D. (1991). *Counseling the communicatively disordered and their families* (2nd ed.). Boston: Little, Brown.

MCCARTHY, P. A., CULPEPPER, N. B., & LUCKS, L. (1986). Variability in counseling experiences and training among ESB accredited programs. *Asha, 28,* 49–52.

MEARNS, D., & THORNE, B. (1988). *Person centered counseling in action.* London: Page Publications.

ROBINSON, D. O. (1991). Universities and aural rehabilitation: In search of tigers. *Audiology Today, 3*(1), 22–23.

ROGERS, C. R. (1959). A theory of therapy personality and interpersonal relationships. In S. Koch (Ed.), *Psychology: A study of science* (Vol. 3, pp. 184–256). New York: McGraw-Hill.

ROGERS, C. R. (1979). Foundations of the person-centered approach. *Education, 100*(2), 98–107.

ROLLIN, W. J. (1987). *The psychology of communication disorders in individuals and their families.* Englewood Cliffs, NJ: Prentice Hall.

ROSS, A. O. (1964). *The exceptional child in the family.* New York: Grune & Stratton.

SANDERS, D. A. (1980). Hearing aid orientation and counseling. In M. C. Pollack (Ed.), *Amplification for the hearing-impaired* (2nd ed., pp. 343–391). New York: Grune & Stratton.

SKINNER, B. F. (1953). *Science and human behavior.* New York: Free Press.

STONE, J. R., & OLSWANG, L. B. (1989). The hidden challenge in counseling. *Asha, 31,* 27–31.

TANNER, D. C. (1980). Loss and grief: Implications for the speech-language pathologist and audiologist. *Asha, 22,* 916–928.

TROWER, P., CASEY, A., & DRYDEN, W. (1988). *Cognitive-behavioral counseling in action.* London: Page Publications.

VAN HECKE, M. L. (1990). Listening with your heart: Counseling parents of children with speech and hearing impairments. *Hearsay,* Spring/Summer, 8–14.

VERNON, M., & OTTINGER, P. J. (1989). Psychosocial aspects of hearing impairment. In Schow, R., & Nerbonne, M. A. (Eds.), *Introduction to Aural Rehabilitation,* 241–270.

APPENDIX 1–1

COUNSELING

Procedures to facilitate the patient's/client's recovery from or adjustment to a communication disorder. Specific purposes of counseling may be to provide the patient/client and his/her family/caregiver with information and support, make appropriate referrals to other professionals, and help the patient/client to develop problem-solving strategies to enhance the (re)habilitation process.

Professionals Who Perform the Procedure(s)

Speech-language pathologists and audiologists.

Expected Outcome(s)

- Professionals assist patient/client to develop appropriate goals for recovery from, adjustment to, or prevention of a communication or related disorder by facilitating change and growth in which patients/clients become more autonomous, more self-directing, and more responsible for achieving their potential and realizing their goals to communicate more effectively.

Clinical Indications

- Counseling services are offered as part of speech, language, hearing, or swallowing screenings, assessments, or intervention procedures; or upon request or referral.
- Counseling services may include:
- —Assessment of counseling needs.
- —Provision of information.
- —Use of strategies to modify behavior and/or the patient's/client's environment.
- —Development of coping mechanisms and systems for emotional support.
- Counseling is conducted in the patient's/client's chosen communication mode and linguistic system.
- Professionals are responsible for ensuring that the patient/client receives adequate emotional/support counseling. To this end, referrals to and consultation with mental health professionals may be an integral component of counseling in speech-language pathology and audiology.

Setting/Equipment Specifications

Counseling is conducted in a setting conducive to patient/client comfort, confidentiality, and uninterrupted privacy.

Safety and Health Precautions

Counseling procedures must ensure the safety of the patient/client and clinician and adhere to universal health precautions (e.g., prevention of bodily injury and transmission of infectious disease).

Documentation

- Speech-language pathologists and audiologists prepare, sign, and maintain, within an established time frame, documentation that reflects the nature of the professional service. When appropriate and with written consent, reports are distributed.
- Documentation includes a statement of results and recommendations, including the need for further counseling or referral.
- Documentation includes results of previous related screenings, assessments, and interventions, if available.

chapter two

Understanding, Building, and Maintaining Relationships with Patients

John Greer Clark

Fundamental to a productive relationship, as this book stresses throughout, is the ability of audiologists to listen carefully to what their patients are saying and to respond to the need that often lies beyond their words. In this chapter, Dr. Clark presents some of the primary underpinnings in the development of a solid and positive relationship between audiologists and their patients and so provides a foundation for the chapters that follow. In the effort to attain the highest level of competency in diagnostic procedures, audiologists may sometimes risk slighting the development of important interpersonal skills. The technological advances in this field can rarely ensure maximum gain for patients apart from a degree of skill and effort in counseling and rehabilitation.

> He did not await anything with impatience and gave neither praise nor blame—he only listened.
>
> Hermann Hesse
> *Siddhartha*

INTRODUCTION

Paramount to effective hearing care management is the successful development and maintenance of a healthy professional–patient relationship. Without this relationship, patients cannot begin to receive the full measure of audiological care and attention that their hearing disorders deserve.

The purpose of this chapter is to explore some of the considerations that lie at the core of a positive relationship with patients. Within the context of this relationship, this chapter includes discussion of the types of questions patients and parents may ask as well as the types of responses we, as audiologists, should attempt to embrace or, conversely, try to avoid. It is through the counseling interactions that take place between audiologists and their patients that the human aspects of hearing care truly evolve.

THE PROFESSIONAL–PATIENT RELATIONSHIP

As discussed by Bernstein, Bernstein, and Dana (1974), every relationship has the potential of tapping a vast range of emotions, both positive and negative, as well as clear ambivalence. The relationship that evolves does so through verbal and nonverbal communication, and the quality of this communication directly influences the quality of the relationship.

Unlike social relationships, which possess a degree of mutual exchange, the professional–patient relationship inevitably tends to become more one-sided with the professional in control (Bernstein et al., 1974), particularly when the patient views the professional as "the expert" who holds all the answers. This unbalanced relationship, if allowed to develop, can be detrimental to successful hearing care.

The audiologist's goal is to have patients achieve independence and an ability to define and solve their own difficulties. When the audiologist is placed in control as the expert, patients become more dependent and continue to seek only those solutions that can be provided to them. Sanders (1980) points out two immediate problems with this perspective. First, when we, as the professionals, are perceived as having all the answers, the burden of responsibility for success or failure necessarily falls upon our shoulders. Second, the solutions we propose are based on our concept of the patient's difficulties and may, in fact, only approximate the patient's own perception of the problem.

Certainly, the "expert" approach is viable, for example, in situations that can be resolved through direct electroacoustic modification of hearing instrumentation. In many other situations, however, solutions may not be so easily attained. Most often in the interactions we have with patients, we must help them realize that we can only help them find the solutions they are seeking, not provide these solutions ourselves. In the last analysis, directions and ultimate solutions can come only from within patients themselves: Our job is simply to set the stage for this to happen.

Mrs. Christopherson reports that she is having increasing difficulty taking her 3-year-old profoundly hearing-impaired son on excursions outside of the home. "He screams loudly sometimes and everyone stares at us. And the hearing aids seem to invite so many unwanted questions from strangers. Now when I take him with me, I leave his hearing aids at home—they're always just short outings anyway."

Parents need to be able to describe their feelings within a nonjudgmental environment. Rather than attempting to provide direction for Mrs. Christopherson, the audiologist might respond with a question, thereby creating a safe atmosphere for further exploration of this mother's feelings. "What do you say to people when they ask about the hearing aids?"

This mother's apparent intolerance of her son's hearing aids may have its roots within some unresolved denial of the hearing loss or residual grieving for the handicap. The audiologist's question opens the arena for discussion of possible underlying issues as well as an exploration of possible responses that could be given to curious strangers. This questioning response helps to place the locus of control within the parent's court where it belongs. Exposing parents, like the mother in this example, to positive role models within the deaf community can also help them to explore resolutions to unresolved issues.

Throughout our interactions with patients and families, we must remain supportive and understanding while moving toward an interaction based on mutual participation. It is mutual participation that makes possible the kind of an open and responsible alliance that enables patients to begin to help themselves. This alliance is aimed at increasing self-sufficiency and self-guidance so that patients will develop enough confidence to continue the management plan without frequent consultation with the audiologist. Without development of this self-sufficiency, patients continue to seek guidance from their audiologist and so increase their own level of dependence on others.

RECOGNIZING SOCIAL STYLES

Each of us has our own social style that comes into play when interacting with others within both professional and nonprofessional settings. As Wilson (1978) states, our individual social style develops as we learn to cope with life while simultaneously attempting to keep our tensions at a manageable level.

One view of social style provides a division of people's personalities into four basic styles of operation: the Driving, the Expressive, the Amiable, and the Analytic (Wilson, 1978). Table 2–1 provides descriptions of these four social styles. While each of us carries within our personalities components from more than one of these styles, one style is usually dominant.

Subdividing Social Styles

Each social style may be subdivided along the lines of a person's degree of assertiveness and responsiveness. People considered as "high-assertive" are those who speak out, take charge, make strong statements, and are forward and demanding. Their behavior is often characterized as "telling." In contrast, a low-assertive person's behavior is characterized as "asking." These people may be

TABLE 2–1 Social Style Descriptors

The Driving Style

   Drivers are task-oriented individuals who seem to know what they want in life and where they are headed. They are high-assertive, self-controlled people who often get their way through their assertiveness while keeping the open display of their emotions and feelings in check. Their behavior is characterized by *telling* and *controlling* their feelings.

The Expressive Style

   Like Drivers, Expressives are highly assertive people. However, they do not hesitate to display their positive and negative feelings openly. They are people-people, placing more importance on relationships than on tasks. Expressives are very intuitive and rely more heavily on their "gut" reactions than on objective data. Their behavior is characterized by *telling* and *emoting*.

The Amiable Style

   Like the Expressives, the Amiables display their feelings openly, but appear less aggressive and assertive. They appear agreeable and interested in establishing relationships. Their behavior is characterized by *asking* and *emoting*.

The Analytic Style

   The Analytics *ask* and *control*. Their assertiveness level is low, but they are in high control of their emotions. These are the people who ask questions and gather information so they may examine an issue from all sides.

Source: Wilson Learning Corporation (1978).

viewed as quiet, unassuming, and cooperative, and are good listeners. They tend to let others take charge. Wilson places assertiveness on a continuum and points out that there is no best place to be on the assertiveness scale, with each position having its own unique strengths and weaknesses.

   Responsiveness is defined as the perceived effort individuals may make to control their own emotions when relating to others. As with assertiveness, one's responsiveness is placed on a continuum, and again each place within the continuum has its merits. We may think of high-responsive people as those who openly display their feelings, emotions, and impressions. Highly responsive people are enthusiastic, friendly, and informal. People at the high-responsiveness end of the continuum are characterized as "emoting." In contrast, low-responsive people are characterized as "controlling," as they keep their emotions in check. They may be described as cool, unemotional, and businesslike.

   Applying the responsiveness and assertiveness continuums to each of the social styles described in Table 2–1 results in a social style profile grid (Table 2–2) into which we can place ourselves and the patients who seek our assistance. Most people's social styles fall into one of the 16 boxes of the profile grid.

Making the Most of Social Style Recognition

As mentioned earlier, each social style has its own strengths and weaknesses. (See Table 2–3.) By attempting to build on our strengths while trying to minimize recognized weaknesses, we can become more effective in our relationships with patients. Further, by taking note of a patient's social style, we can modify our own responses to be more in tune with the responses of our patients. Such modification

TABLE 2–2 The Social Style Profile Grid

Responsiveness (High ↓ — ↑ Low)				
Low	Analytic Analytic	Driving Analytic	Analytic Driver	Driving Driver
	Amiable Analytic	Expressive Analytic	Amiable Driver	Expressive Driver
	Analytic Amiable	Driving Amiable	Analytic Expressive	Driving Expressive
High	Amiable Amiable	Expressive Amiable	Amiable Expressive	Expressive Expressive

Low ← Assertiveness → High

Source: Wilson Learning Corporation (1978). Used with permission.

can help to bolster the rapport that, for some patients, may remain somewhat elusive.

Finally, when we can recognize the social style of others, we can begin to anticipate how people are likely to behave in many situations and how they may respond to us. As Wilson (1978) points out, social-style recognition is vital to our understanding that the manner in which a given patient treats us is less a reaction to us than we might have thought. It is more often a function of the other person's own ingrained social style.

Early within the initial office visit it became obvious that Mr. Vincent was a storyteller. He was upbeat on life, and almost everything reminded him of something or someone. He was fun to be around, and the audiologist found that this day, which had begun like so many Mondays, was beginning to be more tolerable.

Mr. and Mrs. Alexander arrived promptly at the scheduled time for their son's appointment. Earlier in the week, 4-year-old Robbie had been diagnosed with a severe high-frequency sensorineural hearing loss. The audiologist had requested a return visit to allow more time to discuss further the ramifications of the hearing loss and the rehabilitative recommendations. Mrs. Alexander had arrived prepared with many well-conceived questions. She presented a formal air as she persisted in a steady quest for more details.

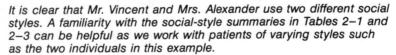

It is clear that Mr. Vincent and Mrs. Alexander use two different social styles. A familiarity with the social-style summaries in Tables 2–1 and 2–3 can be helpful as we work with patients of varying styles such as the two individuals in this example.

Recognizing Mr. Vincent as an expressive, the audiologist in the first example will do well to take time to develop a personal relationship with Mr. Vincent. An impersonal, clinical facade will not help Mr. Vincent in his search for recommendations he can implement. The audiologist may need to probe for factual data within this patient's effusiveness. Opinionated objections to rehabili-

TABLE 2–3 Social Style Identifiers

SOCIAL STYLE	STRENGTHS	WEAKNESSES
Amiable	Supportive	Conforming
	Cooperative	Retiring
	Dependable	Noncommittal
	Personable	Emotional
Analytic	Industrious	Uncommunicative
	Persistent	Avoiding
	Accurate	Exacting
	Systematic	Impersonal
Driver	Determined	Controlling
	Thorough	Tough-minded
	Decisive	Dominating
	Efficient	Impersonal
Expressive	Personable	Opinionated
	Enthusiastic	Excitable
	Dramatic	Attacking
	Energizing	Promotional

Source: Wilson Learning Corporation (1978).

tative suggestions will be best countered by supportive third-party stories. As expressives tend to be excitable, the audiologist should be careful not to overwhelm Mr. Vincent with details.

In the second example, Mrs. Alexander is an analytic individual and will appreciate details. Excessive small talk will be seen as intrusive to the appointment's mission. Emotional appeals should be avoided with this mother. Instead, the audiologist will relate best by displaying some expertise in problem solving and analysis. However, as analytic personalities are often indecisive, progress may be enhanced if specific examples are provided and a specific course of action is recommended.

As stated earlier, the relationship that evolves throughout the course of our relationships with patients evolves throughout the course of management and must be based on mutual respect and cooperation. Recognizing our own social style, and that of others, can aid in reaching this level with our patients. The success of the ensuing relationship largely begins with the audiologist's first appointment with the patient (Clark, 1982, 1987).

INITIAL PATIENT CONTACT

The contact provided during the first appointment gives us the opportunity to evaluate how our patients view their problems and why they have sought a hearing evaluation. If a case-history questionnaire has not been filled out before the initial interview, this is the time to obtain background information.

Stream and Stream (1978) and Goodwin (1984) stress the prudence of asking why this consultation has been sought. If there has been a previous evaluation of the hearing, we need to find out how the patient felt at that time about the findings and recommendations. The answers to these questions reveal the patient's awareness and understanding of the present situation and provide the audiologist with some insight into the problem as the patient perceives it. Finally, the audiologist should ask what the patient hopes will be gained from the present evaluation.

The initial contact time serves us not only as a time for gathering pertinent case-history information, but also allows us the opportunity to build a rapport that will at least partially allay the patient's apprehensions. We must remember that this is also the time when patients form their first impressions of the audiologist. When addressing adult patients or parents, it is always preferred to use the title "Mr.," "Mrs.," or some other appropriate title if known. It is presumptuous and can diminish the patient's sense of dignity to assume we are on a first-name basis without having been asked to take on such informality. It is especially wise to adhere to this general rule when working with the elderly.

In our clinical interactions if we can display an air of professional confidence, tempered with respect for the patients who are seeking our advice and an appreciation for their feelings, a more open exchange will be possible. Through our own attentiveness, we must convey the impression that the patient is our sole concern and will remain so throughout the appointment. Only interruptions of great importance should be tolerated.

Bernstein et al. (1974) point out that many health professionals operate under the misconception that rapport and a positive relationship with patients are established by continuing friendly or neighborly small talk about current news, local sports teams, weather, and so on. However, to delay the real business at hand can be burdensome to patients and may imply that we are not taking their concerns seriously. Rapport is established by demonstrating a genuine interest in and attentiveness to the patient.

It is often held that the initial interview process should have three main goals: to establish a positive relationship with the patient, to elicit pertinent information, and to observe the patient's behavior. An interview approach composed of direct questions and answers may be successful in accomplishing the second goal. However, this approach may reveal little about the patient, and thus the other two goals are not approximated, let alone attained.

I believe an open, conversational-style interview may be significantly more productive than the more restrictive direct question, medical-style approach. Through a conversational approach we can guide patients through the telling of their difficulties and concerns and those factors associated with them. During the interview it is least distracting if we take only a few pertinent notes, relying more heavily on our memory to write out specific information after the patient has left. Once patients have started talking, they should be permitted to continue without interruption. Pauses within a patient's discourse should serve as an opportunity to express interest, request clarification, or offer encouragement, but not as a juncture for changing course. Detailed questions can be safely postponed, thereby demonstrating the audiologist's regard for the importance of what the patient has to say.

> Following introductions, the audiologist makes clear eye contact with Mrs. Hill and asks, "What is it that brought you in to see me?" Thus, the interview has begun in a nonrestrictive manner with all avenues open for discussion.
>
> *An opening such as this may be more productive than the more restricted or narrow question "What is your primary complaint?" or "Tell me about your hearing loss."*

A good working format for obtaining case-history information is the open interview preceded by a paper-and-pencil direct-question history form and self-assessment questionnaire completed by the patient. Reviewing these completed questionnaires before seeing the patient allows the audiologist to recognize what areas need further expansion before the interview closes. Placed near the end of the interview, direct questions achieve clarification rather than interference. Audiologists should give consideration to the value of mailing a case-history questionnaire and an information packet to patients prior to their appointment time as discussed by Dr. Martin in Chapter 3.

The initial interview provides information regarding the problem and the patient's perception of the problem. For this reason, the first interview may be of equal importance to the subsequent evaluation. The information obtained in conjunction with the test findings will help in the decisions the audiologist and the patient or parent will have to make jointly for the patient's welfare.

QUESTIONS PATIENTS ASK

Questions that patients ask generally fall into one of three categories (Luterman, 1979). The first of these is the content question, which seeks further information or explanation. For example, "Does my child hear all sounds equally, or can she hear some sounds better than others?" A straightforward, concise answer, void of jargon, is best here. The second type of question, the confirmation question, is usually asked in hope that the audiologist will confirm an opinion or position the asker has already formed on a given issue, such as educational placement, or communication mode, and so on. When such questions are posed it is often best to determine the asker's position or opinion before beginning an exposition on the topic of interest.

> Recently, Mr. and Mrs. DeBoer's 3-year-old son, Eric, was found to have a bilaterally severe sensorineural hearing loss. During a follow-up visit with the audiologist, Mrs. DeBoer asked, "Would sign language training be a good approach with Eric?"
>
> Mr. Rhind recently returned from service in the marines. He came to the audiology clinic with a complaint of a persistent "high-pitched whine that's driving me crazy." He says he has read several magazine articles on tinnitus and asks, "Are those masker things I've read about any good for helping ear noises like mine?"
>
> *To avoid a content response to Mrs. DeBoer, the audiologist might respond, "How do you feel Eric would do with a visual form of communicating such as signing?" This allows the parents an opportunity to voice concerns and opinions about signing that they may have developed from talking with others about signing. A similar response can be given to Mr. Rhind's inquiry about tinnitus maskers, or to other confirmation questions posed by parents and patients.*

In both of the preceding examples, a simple content-oriented answer to a confirmation question may not address the more pertinent issues underlying the patient's inquiry. A content answer also tends to distance the asker from the management process at the very time a management bond needs to be formed.

The third type of question, a question with an affective base, is rooted in an underlying emotional need that may not be met if responded to through a direct content response. Unfortunately, it is a content response that is usually given to these questions.

> Finding it difficult to ask her question, Mrs. DeBoer asks as the consultation seems to be coming to a close, "Could taking a lot of antihistamines during my pregnancy have caused Eric's hearing loss?" The audiologist begins the ensuing dialogue with a sympathetic response: "It is natural to want to know the reasons behind things when so much is unknown."
>
> Mr. Gallegos has successfully adjusted to his new hearing aids. He and his wife are pleased with his improved hearing abilities. His wife says, "I wish Ron hadn't been so stubborn. We should have done this years ago." After a moment's reflection, Mr. Gallegos inquires, "Would my hearing be better today if I had gotten these things sooner?"
>
> The audiologist opens a dialogue on the topic of Mr. Gallegos's procrastination by stating, "We often wonder what we could have done differently to change things."
>
> *Through her inquiry, Mrs. DeBoer reveals a glimpse of her underlying feelings of guilt about the origin of her child's impairment. Similarly, Mr. Gallegos is expressing an unstated concern or perceived guilt over his own procrastination. The issues underlying both of these questions are not addressed through a simple negative content response. Yes, such a response may be available and if available will need to be given. However, the true feelings of guilt also need to be addressed here, and the nonjudgmental statements by the audiologist serve as good openers to begin a dialogue.*

Questions like Mrs. DeBoer's, Mr. Rhind's, and Mr. Gallegos's may be answered under differing circumstances through statements rooted within a content, confirmation, or affective base. However, it is important for the intention of the question to be understood correctly. Concerns that are expressed and questions that are asked are too often viewed by professionals as no more than the patient's need for further information. This view precludes the audiologist's ability to adequately address the emotions and needs underlying parent and patient inquiries.

Audiologists, as most health care professionals, tend to gravitate toward content or informational counseling when, because of their own insecurities or lack of counseling experiences, they subconsciously avoid communicating with their patients on a personal level. Content counseling is clearly appropriate in patient management and often appropriately comprises the larger portion of our counseling interactions. However, we must make sure that we do not allow our possible misperceptions of the patient's request for further information to preclude an adequate response to the emotions and needs underlying patient inquiries (Clark, 1984, 1985).

RESPONSES TO PATIENTS' STATEMENTS, QUESTIONS, AND CONCERNS

Direct Honesty

When patients or family members ask questions that clearly seek a content response, we must provide a direct and honest answer. The information requested should not be provided in partial answers or with "silver linings" simply as a means of sparing feelings. This, of course, is not to say that objectivity must lack empathy. However, when patients or families are in need of emotional support, they must not be given false hopes that will only have to be reconciled at some later date.

In cases of severe to profound hearing loss, the realization that unfounded dreams of normalcy will not come true has often been delayed until the child reaches adolescence (Cohen, 1978). As discussed by Dr. Martin in Chapter 3 and Dr. Johnson in Chapter 8, information on the realistic implications of hearing impairment needs to be provided to parents as early as possible. However, we must guard against making prognostications without sufficient data. The anticipated impact of extrinsic variables—such as socioeconomic level, family support and intactness, or financial responsibilities and burdens—may not be available during the early stages of hearing care management. Similarly, the impact of intrinsic variables—including the child's intellectual level, central auditory intactness, visual abilities, and projected learning potential through a manual/visual versus an aural/oral approach to language—may not be known (Clark, 1983).

From Chapter 1 you may recall Mrs. French who had just given birth to a son with profound hearing loss. In the midst of the parents' grief when fitting their child with his first hearing instruments the audiologist sought to reassure the parents. "It's amazing to me how well children with hearing loss learn with today's hearing aids and auditory trainers. Sammy will probably be able to attend school in your neighborhood in regular classes. I even know kids with hearing losses like Sammy's who are doing well in college."

 We all share the quite normal desire to make things better in the midst of tragedy or grief. However, the audiologist's statements here are clearly inappropriate, as neither supporting nor refuting data are yet available.

To provide an honest answer to questions or an accurate depiction of things to come we often must admit to our own limitations. If needed information is not available, this fact should be explained openly. If the information is available through another source, or through further or future evaluation, as with Sammy French in the preceding example, the audiologist is obligated to obtain the requested information or to make whatever referral is necessary for the patient to receive a more complete answer to questions. As Ross (1964) points out, frankly admitting that we do not have the answer to a specific question will increase the patient's confidence in our services more than an attempt to cover ignorance with an authoritarian attitude that suggests the patient does not have the right to ask that question at this time.

Certainly honesty must undergird all of the responses we make to our patients. The types of responses we may give to our patients can be categorized and discussed within a variety of frameworks. However, when we depart from the security of responses with a directive or content-oriented base, our responses to questions or comments may be categorized as either hostile, evaluative, probing, or understanding. As discussed by Bernstein et al. (1974), the first of these response forms should obviously be avoided, and the second two should be used with caution. It is the final response, understanding, that makes effective counseling possible.

The Hostile Response

The hostile response emerges when audiologists perceive certain statements or actions as an affront to their professionalism or training. The stress and aggravation that may accompany a patient's ineffectual attempts at communication, combined with difficulty in accepting a management program that may at times appear only minimally effective or excessively protracted, may result in hostilities or the expression of negative attitudes. While this frustration may appear to be directed at the professional, it is most often an expression of the patient's inner stress. Hostility must not confront hostility. Instead, if we can resist feeling professionally threatened or challenged, we can diffuse the patient's hostility by showing that we respect and understand the patient's feelings and by helping the patient recognize the universality of those feelings. The goal of every confrontation should be to increase the patient's confidence and inner security, not the audiologist's (Clark, 1989).

The Evaluative Response

The evaluative response comes into practice when we pass judgment on our patients' feelings, actions, or concerns or when we project to our patients how we believe they should feel or act. Obviously, such a response is detrimental to the relationship we are building with our patients and, in the long run, can only decrease the effectiveness of hearing care services.

When patient contact time is limited, professionals often evaluate the situation quickly and then give advice or direction. While this kind of decisive response may leave us with the impression that we have helped, our patients may, in fact, leave the office with advice they poorly comprehend and may even believe that their own assessment of their difficulties has been wrong. As a result, after consultation with the audiologist, patients may actually feel less sure of themselves than before.

Evaluation of a situation, followed by a concise, directive, and nonjudgmental content response, is many times appropriate in hearing care management. However, if audiologists allow patients to talk out their feelings and attitudes during their limited time together, patients may find their problems more clearly defined and alternatives clarified. If patients leave feeling that they have been better understood and accepted as individuals, the session will have fostered increased self-esteem and nurtured confidence and readiness to tackle the problems ahead.

The Probing Response

The probing response encourages further information, expansion, or clarification and, therefore, can be very useful in hearing care management. However, we should be cautious that such probing is not interpreted by a patient to mean that we will be able to provide solutions if we are given enough detail. As discussed earlier, solutions provided directly by the audiologist can remove the sense of control from the patient and therefore often do not achieve the audiologist's intended goal.

While direct probes are often necessary during patient contact, the audiologist should be wary of the direction that these questions may lead. Too often they can lead into a content-based session with the audiologist doing most of the talking, thereby possibly sidetracking the real root of a given concern—or the patient's perception of it.

The Understanding Response

The understanding response, which demonstrates the audiologist's interested concern, is a powerful and effective response mode for building and maintaining strong relationships with patients. This form of response comes most easily for the professional who has developed a high degree of empathy.

The understanding response can be beneficial to patient management during content counseling, as well as counseling with more emotionally laden issues. The immediate gain from this form of response is that it reduces patients' fear that we may pass judgment on what they may say, and thus opens the session for further discussion and exploration. This response can be developed only through practice and the determined effort to combine the best aspects of active or reflective listening, reassurance, and probing with a sincere respect for the individuality and dignity of each patient.

The success of the understanding response depends on an unconditional acceptance of patients as human beings of importance in their own right. As Rogers (1961) has stated, this acceptance implies respect or regard for the patient's attitudes of the moment, regardless of how negative or positive these attitudes may be or how greatly they may vary from attitudes the patient has expressed in the past.

Active listening, as shown through the audiologist's ability to reflect the expressed feelings of the patient, is a further key to the understanding response. Reflection is the attempt to understand our patients' viewpoint and to communicate that understanding in a way that permits patients to examine their feelings or beliefs from another perspective, thus allowing for a continued and perhaps broader consideration of their problems. A major pitfall of counselor reflections occurs when the content of patient statements is reflected rather than the feelings or underlying attitudes.

Reflections of feelings, while simple in principle, are often difficult in practice, as they differ greatly from our long and more familiar experience of responding to content. When attempting to develop an understanding response through this reflection of feelings, the audiologist might try to select the one word that best describes the patient's feelings underlying a given statement. While reflecting patient statements, the audiologist should remain cognizant of the impact the reflection can have on the direction of dialogue and, in turn, on the progress of the session with the patient.

An elderly hearing-impaired patient with severe manual dexterity limitations relates to her audiologist, "I try my best at home, but my husband is never satisfied with my efforts." The audiologist, perceiving a sense of exasperation in the patient's words and tone, reflects, "You are angry that your husband doesn't see how hard you are trying."

Certainly the audiologist should try to reflect the patient's feelings accurately. However, even inaccurate reflections (the patient in this example may not have been expressing anger, but perhaps only frustration or disappointment) demonstrate the audiologist's attempt to understand, thereby fostering continued discussion.

As discussed earlier in connection with the hostile response, when patients speak negatively of what they perceive as lack of progress in management, the audiologist will make greater headway by openly recognizing this dissatisfaction than by becoming defensive. A reflection such as "You don't feel you are hearing significantly better in many environments" can help the patient view the professional as accepting and understanding, a perception that in turn may foster greater patience and cooperation throughout the course of management. When patients' negative feelings are consistently recognized and reflected, more positive feelings tend to follow.

In addition to statement reflection, the understanding response also may be conveyed through expressions of acceptance. Simply stating that we understand or appreciate a person's feelings may be especially useful when the patient is disclosing information that might reveal feelings of shame or guilt. Acceptance should not be equated with either agreement or approval. In fact, agreement and approval are more suggestive of an evaluative response than of understanding.

REASSURANCE HAS ITS LIMITS

Effective support during emotional crises, and later during ongoing hearing rehabilitation, is often vital to the success of continued hearing care. This support can be effectively provided through an understanding, accepting, and nonjudgmental attitude on the part of the audiologist. Contrary to common practice, effective support is not always best provided through the easy reassurance offered by most professionals (Clark, 1990a).

Unfortunately, one of the more common ways of attempting to give support, in both personal and professional encounters, is through the verbal reassurance that everything will be all right, or will work out for the best, or is not as bad as it currently seems. While such reassurance avoids or minimizes emotional encounters, it does not resolve communication difficulties.

Reassurance implies that a patient's anxieties do not—or should not—really exist to the extent expressed. By denying the patient's emotions in this way, the audiologist makes it more difficult to recognize the patient's feelings and concerns. This, in turn, hampers rather than facilitates resolution of emotions that must be confronted and resolved before rehabilitation can take place. By precluding further discussion of underlying concerns, the audiologist often assumes that assistance has been successfully proffered. Instead, those verbal reassurances have all too often protected the audiologist's own feelings, not the patient's.

A common example of inappropriate reassurance occurs when patients being fitted with hearing aids express annoyance at the loud sounds they hear through their hearing aids or the "barrel effect" they might perceive from their own voices when speaking while wearing amplification. These complaints, which signal excessive low frequency amplification or inappropriate or insufficient venting, are often met with reassurances such as, "This is still new for you and you are still adapting to the sounds you hear." Although such reassurances might be appropriate in many instances, they frequently are overused, to the detriment of successful hearing aid fittings (Hawkins, 1986; Killion, 1988). And, again, when these reassurances are used inappropriately, they create an effective denial of patients' concerns that may preclude further discussion. As a result, the audiologist is left with the misimpression that a little reassurance was all the situation required: The patient is left with the problem still unresolved.

Similarly, reassurance may be even more inappropriate when confronting emotionally charged issues. "Pep talks" do not always foster the kind of reassurance and inner security a patient is seeking. For example, adult patients who express shock, surprise, disbelief, or dismay when told unexpectedly that their hearing impairment is permanent do not need reassurance that the loss is not as bad as it seems, or that the audiologist has seen patients with more serious hearing disorders, or even with coexisting disabilities, who adjusted successfully to amplification. Parents of a child with a similar problem do not need such verbal solace either.

During their brief time with us, if patients are given the opportunity to express their concerns freely, they have a better chance of achieving the kind of lasting reassurance that arises from within than they might otherwise be able to attain. When we take the time to listen to our patients, we also convey an openness to further questions that might otherwise remain unasked. This openness of the understanding response permits an honest confrontation with underlying concerns and so results in a positive effect that reassurance alone cannot achieve.

Effective counseling requires a delicate balance. Verbal reassurance is not always inappropriate. In fact, in some instances, verbal reassurance from the audiologist is highly desirable, particularly reassurance that a given hearing disorder is fairly common, that there is a known cause (when etiology is identifiable), that symptoms are annoying but not dangerous or necessarily indicative of impending deafness or insanity (as in idiopathic tinnitus), and that a course of management is available.

However, it is also important for audiologists to foster a climate in which patients can express themselves freely. Only when patients can recognize and deal with their real concerns can they develop the inner assurance they will ultimately need if hearing management is to be successful. It is impossible to overestimate this kind of reassurance, which comes from being listened to by an empathetic listener who shows respect for patients and a desire to understand their concerns, rather than being quick to overwhelm them with advice or empty solace. Only after underlying concerns have been addressed can audiologists successfully meet the needs of those with hearing loss.

Following what appeared to be a successful hearing aid fitting and postfitting consultation, Mrs. Collier, an 85-year-old woman who attends her appointments alone, comments, "I just hope I can learn to adjust to everything."

Sensing Mrs. Collier's lingering insecurities, the audiologist reassures her, "I think you are going to do quite well. In a very short time you have successfully mastered putting the hearing aids in and taking them out. You have told me of the improvements amplification has provided you at church and in talking with your neighbors. From our discussions and your comments, I believe you have very realistic expectations regarding the benefits and some of the limitations of your new hearing aids. With a little time you'll feel even more confident. But I do want you to feel free to call me if any problems develop. Just to make sure you're doing well, we're going to send you a notice to come back in six months to thoroughly check your new hearing aids."

Later, in the waiting room while waiting for a taxi, Mrs. Collier again voices her concern regarding her ability to adjust to everything, this time to the receptionist. Rather than reassuring the patient as the audiologist had done, the receptionist unknowingly reflects her own perception of Mrs. Collier's statement, "Are you concerned that you may have difficulties with your new hearing aids?"

"Actually, I think I'll do well with that. But so many things have changed. My husband died three years ago, and now my niece, the only relative I have in town, is moving to Seattle because of her husband's promotion."

The receptionist's reflection has allowed Mrs. Collier the opportunity to express her real concerns. The receptionist was then able to give Mrs. Collier the name of an agency that works to assist able-bodied elderly citizens to continue living independently. In this instance, the receptionist was clearly the more effective counselor. We, as audiologists, need to be on guard against working with hearing loss to the exclusion of the entire individual.

EMOTIONAL RESPONSE TRANSFORMATIONS

Life would be easier for all of us if emotions could be dealt with more openly. Unfortunately, in our clinical interactions, the emotions of both patients and professionals are often transformed as they come to the surface. This lack of emotional honesty can be further compounded by the fact that most of us are not even aware that the alteration has happened.

It is not the intention of the support–educational counseling employed by audiologists to uncover unconscious patterns (Stone & Olswang, 1989). Nevertheless, to work effectively with the persons we serve, audiologists must learn to recognize signs of emotional metamorphoses. This recognition enables us to respond more effectively to concerns that may lie beneath the surface of clinical exchanges (Clark, 1990b).

Emotional Redirections

Reaction formation. Occasionally the emotions of an adult client or a parent may be unconsciously redirected in an effort to avoid confrontation with a diagnosed handicap. One of these redirections, reaction formation, manifests itself when the person attempts to avoid a feared response to a situation by strongly endorsing or adopting a conflicting attitude that may be perceived as socially more palatable or personally more advantageous. For example, parents whose initial reaction to their child's handicap may be to turn from increased responsibilities and emotional heartbreak by rejecting the initial diagnosis of their child's handicap may, instead, exhibit a reaction formation: often overprotecting the child or overaccepting the handicap (Mitchell, 1988).

Although reaction formation can affect management negatively, it can also have a positive influence. In avoiding the initial urge to deny the diagnosis, some parents may become strong advocates for services to the hearing impaired or may become service providers themselves (Mitchell, 1988). However, it certainly would be within the audiologist's purview to help direct parents appropriately so that during this period their other family responsibilities do not fall along the wayside.

Reaction formation is also present in varying degrees among adult patients. For example, adults who adamantly refuse even a no-risk trial of amplification may reject the potential benefits of hearing instruments because they fear the cost involved or, more likely, because of an unwillingness to confront the personal perception of handicap associated with hearing aids. The patient may de-emphasize listening difficulties and blame others for communication problems. In much the same way, when considering binaural amplification, some patients may overstress the benefit presently derived from a single hearing instrument and convince themselves that the second instrument would provide no additional assistance.

Intellectualization.   Intellectualization emerges when adult patients or parents of handicapped children have difficulty expressing their sadness or grief over a diagnosis. Instead, they may attempt to make the session abstract, impersonal, theoretical, and thus unemotional. Mitchell (1988) points out that through intellectualization, patients may question the accuracy of testing, the examiner's credentials, or the efficacy of the recommendations provided. Intellectualization may be employed more by fathers than by mothers of handicapped children (Mitchell, 1988). Similarly, with adult patients this means of emotional redirection seems to occur more often among males.

A nondefensive attitude is the best approach to intellectualization. The audiologist must resist feeling professionally threatened or challenged and be prepared to demonstrate repeatedly a respect and understanding for the emotions that may underlie whatever form of intellectualization is emerging. In this situation, as always, the goal of every clinical encounter must be to increase the patient's or family's confidence and inner security, not the audiologist's.

Emotional Projections

Projections.   Another transformation of emotional response is the transference or projection of past feelings into a current situation (Bernstein et al., 1974; Webster, 1977). Within their relationships with patients, audiologists are often viewed as authority figures by the patients they serve. For this reason, patients may transfer or project onto the audiologist feelings from interactions with past authority figures. Depending on the nature of their previous relationships with parents, teachers, physicians, and/or law enforcement officials, patients may project feelings of trust, distrust, dislike, or admiration. These projections can significantly color clinical interactions in ways that the professional would be sometimes unaware.

Positive projections may lead to highly compliant patients who are reluctant to voice concern about their own belabored rehabilitative progress or admit lack of understanding of the information the audiologist provides. When the patient appears too accepting, we must be especially alert to unexpressed problems or anxieties that may lie just beneath the smiling facade such a patient often presents. The use of such open-ended questions as "In what ways do you see improvement in your hearing?" or "What listening areas are still difficult for you?" may help the patient to be more candid than simply asking "Do you feel you are doing better than you were?" or "Are you pleased with the improvement you have seen?"

On the other hand, negative projections arising from past circumstances may manifest themselves in repeated criticisms of the treatment process or unrealistic expectations for improvement. Only when we choose not to respond defensively or angrily can we begin to break the hostility–counterhostility cycle that may evolve from these encounters. If we can remember that present negative responses may have been aroused by a patient's own past rather than our efforts at intervention, then we may be able to react more empathetically when these feelings are expressed.

Counterprojections. Unfortunately, projections are not one-sided. Just as the client may project feelings and attitudes from the past onto the audiologist, audiologists also may bring their own past emotions into a present interaction. Obviously, this counterprojection of emotions works to the detriment of the kind of relationship we hope to achieve with patients.

> Don't resent what may be uncongenial to you in him. He may not deserve it, for we know no certain ill of him.
>
> Charles Dickens
> *David Copperfield*

All of us carry certain prejudices and immaturities from the past. Through the course of ordinary human experience it is easy to develop attitudes and negative feelings that certain patients may all too quickly arouse. For example, some of us may find it difficult to work with the elderly, the infirm, the multihandicapped, the unwashed, or the obese.

It is important that we recognize our own feelings so that we may begin to guard against those stimuli that may arouse negative emotions. Such self-monitoring is not always possible. But if feelings can be recognized for what they are, we can take steps to ensure that patients receive the understanding and patience they deserve. Accomplishing this goal may sometimes necessitate referral to another provider. If referral is not made and our own lack of self-awareness persists, the relationship with the patient and any therapeutic effectiveness are inevitably jeopardized.

NONVERBAL PATIENT BEHAVIOR

Professionals who have fully incorporated an understanding response in their interactions with patients will display a vigilance for nonverbal patient behavior. Often patients' nonverbal behavior belies something they have not been able to verbalize.

The audiologist may wish to bring these behaviors (gestures, tone of voice, posture, facial expression) to patients' attention, allowing them to draw their own conclusions about its meaning. While patients may deny the validity of the audiologist's observations, such observations will frequently permit unexpressed feelings to surface for a more open discussion.

AWARENESS OF AMBIVALENCE

A state of ambivalence arises when both positive and negative feelings regarding a given issue exist simultaneously. Prospective candidates for biofeedback to alleviate tinnitus, for example, might desire the benefits outlined within the proposed biofeedback therapy program while simultaneously fearing or harboring reservations about what they view as "electronic hypnosis." Other patients might recognize the increased communication abilities through assistive listening devices while remaining hesitant to make their hearing handicap more visible.

Feelings of ambivalence are normal, and audiologists can best deal with these feelings when they recognize and understand the nature and concept of ambivalence. We must realize that the treatment plans that are most successfully followed are those that our patients view as reasonable for themselves.

RESPECTING CLINICAL SILENCE

Within social contexts, silences often are viewed as uncomfortable gaps that we are prone to fill with a question, remark, or even at times a completely irrelevant comment. These conventions may serve our needs well within a social context. However, within professional contexts silence can, itself, serve as a form of response by providing temporal space for reflection and an opportunity for our patients to assume responsibility for their own progress (Clark, 1989). When we fill the silent pauses within exchanges, we reinforce the patient's perception that the audiologist is responsible for initiating and maintaining the discussion. Our natural desire to fill the silent voids often works to the detriment of our management endeavors. Our questions or comments may be inappropriately timed, disrupt the patient's thought processes, or sidetrack an issue that may not have been fully explored. We must always strive to enhance our patient's ability toward self-direction, not impede it. Silence can often be effective in achieving this goal.

As a general rule, it may be advantageous to honor silences in clinical exchanges when they are initiated by the patient. There are times, however, when silence may be inappropriate. Silences with patients who tend to be distrustful or evasive can increase the distance between our patients and us and so, in turn, decrease the rapport we are striving to establish. Knowing when to remain silent often requires the same sensitivity as needed for interjecting the appropriate remark (Bernstein et al., 1974).

CONCLUSION

To ensure effective hearing care, audiologists must appreciate the importance of the counseling process and accept responsibility for it. We have a responsibility to understand our patients and to respond openly, honestly, and compassionately to their questions and to the need behind those questions. Toward this end, audiologists need to be aware of a variety of response modes and the impact of these responses on patient encounters.

REFERENCES

BERNSTEIN, L., BERNSTEIN, R. S., & DANA, R. H. (1974). *Interviewing: A guide for health professionals*. New York: Appleton-Century-Crofts.

CLARK, J. G. (1982). Counseling in a pediatric audiologic practice. *Asha, 24*, 521–526.

CLARK, J. G. (1983). Beyond diagnosis: The professional's role in education consultation. *Hearing Journal, 36*, 20–25.

CLARK, J. G. (1984). Counseling tinnitus patients. In J. G. Clark & P. Yanick (Eds.), *Tinnitus and its management: A clinical text for audiologists* (pp. 95–106). Springfield, IL: Chas. C Thomas.

CLARK, J. G. (1985). Tinnitus: The counseling imperative. *Hearing Journal, 38*, 23–25.

CLARK, J. G. (1987). Obtaining case history information. *Hearsay, 120*, 122.

CLARK, J. G. (1989). Counseling the hearing impaired: Responding to patient concerns. *Hearing Instruments, 40*(9), 50–55.

CLARK, J. G. (1990a). The "Don't worry, be happy" professional response. *Hearing Journal, 43*, 20–24.

CLARK, J. G. (1990b). Emotional response transformations: Redirections and projections. *Asha, 32*(6), 67–68.

COHEN, O. P. (1978). The deaf adolescent: Who am I? In A. I. Neyhus & G. F. Austin (Eds.), *Deafness and adolescence* (pp. 265–274). Washington: Volta Review.

GOODWIN, P. E. (1984). The tinnitus evaluation. In J. G. Clark & P. Yanick (Eds.), *Tinnitus and its management: A clinical text for audiologists* (pp. 72–94). Springfield, Il: Chas. C Thomas.

HAWKINS, D. B. (1986). Selection of SSPL 90. ASHA Clinical Workshop: Audiology. Speech presented at American Speech-Language-Hearing Convention, Detroit.

KILLION, M. (1988). The "hollow voice" occlusion effect. In J. H. Jensen (Ed.), *Hearing aid fitting: Theoretical and practical views* (pp. 231–234). Copenhagen: Stoutgaard Jensen.

LUTERMAN, D. (1979). *Counseling parents of hearing impaired children*. Boston: Little, Brown.

MITCHELL, C. J. (1988). Counseling for the parent. In R. J. Roeser & M. P. Downs (Eds.), *Auditory disorders in children* (2nd ed.). New York: Thieme Medical.

ROSS, A. O. (1964). *The exceptional child in the family*. New York: Grune & Stratton.

SANDERS, D. A. (1980). Hearing aid orientation and counseling. In M. C. Pollack (Ed.), *Amplification for the hearing-impaired* (2nd ed., pp. 343–391). New York: Grune & Stratton.

STONE, J. R., & OLSWANG, L. B. (1989). The hidden challenge in counseling. *Asha, 31*, 27–31.

STREAM, R. W., & STREAM, K. S. (1978). Counseling the parents of the hearing-impaired child. In F. N. Martin (Ed.), *Pediatric audiology* (pp. 311–355). Englewood Cliffs, NJ: Prentice Hall.

WEBSTER, E. J. (1977). *Counseling with parents of handicapped children*. New York: Grune & Stratton.

WILSON LEARNING CORPORATION (1978). *Managing interpersonal relationships*. Eden Prairie, MN: Wilson Learning Corporation.

chapter three

Conveying Diagnostic Information

Frederick N. Martin

It is not enough simply to provide accurate information. The manner in which that information is conveyed will have a direct bearing on both patient and family comprehension of results, as well as on their active acceptance of the recommendations given. In this chapter, Dr. Martin looks at the way audiologists present diagnostic and rehabilitative implications of audiological testing. In an effort to provide empathetic care, audiologists must learn to view themselves through the eyes of patients and families and to hear their own words as they sound to those most affected.

> Life is difficult.
> M. Scott Peck, M.D.
> *The Road Less Traveled*

INTRODUCTION

In what might seem like an absurdly simple statement, Dr. Peck sums up what we all know and often forget. Indeed, life can be very difficult even under the most normal circumstances. People demonstrate a wide range of abilities in coping with even the ordinary challenges of life, such as relationships with work associates, family, and friends; the rearing of children; or the management of money. For some people, at some times, just surviving is painful. However, all of the mundane problems of life may suddenly fade into insignificance when people receive news from health professionals that alters and further complicates their lives. The skill with which "bad news" is initially delivered may have a profound effect on acceptance of the disorder and all the efforts toward rehabilitation that become necessary.

Concerns have been expressed that modern medical technology may have caused interpersonal clinical skills to atrophy, which not only underserves patients, but takes away some of the joy that clinicians have, in the past, enjoyed with their patients (Rogers, 1989). After many years of teaching university students and surveying and observing the practices of my colleagues, I have come to have far less concern over the technical expertise that audiologists must have to administer and interpret their tests than I have about their abilities to share information with the very people they serve—their patients and the families of hearing-impaired individuals. Audiometric results are a routine matter to clinical audiologists, and after some time spent in dealing with patients the initial counseling experience all too often takes on the effect of a canned routine, in which the details of this or that test are explained so that the "average" person might understand them.

What audiologists often fail to integrate into their clinical activities is the concept that all people do not process new information with equal speed and accuracy. What the clinician views as the simple transfer of information may be a verbal blow to the recipients, and the clinical language may seem filled with strange and frightening words. Dealing with difficult information is sometimes impossible under the stress of the diagnostic situation and the revelation of a serious hearing difficulty. Audiologists must realize that the impact on patients of the diagnosis of hearing loss may be similar to the realization that they, or someone emotionally close to them, will be faced with a problem potentially threatening to a normal and healthy life. In order to deliver the best care to patients it is essential to understand their emotional reactions.

In Chapter 5, Dr. Van Hecke discusses the various stages of emotions, originally described by Kübler-Ross (1969) in her work *On Death and Dying*, and so they will not be iterated here. Luterman (1984) prefers the word *states* rather than *stages*. I agree with this for one does not simply move from one emotional stage to the next until the entire gamut has been run; that would be nice, but it is not so. Dr. Garstecki (Chapter 9) and Dr. Alpiner (Chapter 11) discuss the often-ignored fact that adult patients must also confront a variety of emotional states in adjusting to their hearing problems.

People who have been shocked, angered, or bereaved by bad news may temporarily discard these emotions only to reexperience them later. This may be true of all the emotional states, including those experienced by the parents of a child who has been diagnosed with an auditory disorder, or those emotions confronted by adults to whom the full nature of their hearing loss has finally been disclosed.

One might expect that learning of a handicap in a child would bring the parents closer together as they develop systems of mutual caring and support for each other. However, when tragedy strikes, parents often report increased marital difficulties. Not only do parents fail to understand the manner in which their partners experience grief, their different processes of coping interfere with each other, which causes discord, alienation, and often separation (Yalom, 1989, p. 142). After learning that a child has a hearing loss, mothers may feel a need to cease dwelling on their initial emotional reactions regarding their child, and often plunge into activities, including support groups, therapy, or learning all that can be learned about hearing loss, hearing aids, different processes of remediation, anatomy, pathology, and so on. Since men more often tend to suppress and evade their emotions, sharing often is more difficult for fathers. Both parents often feel guilty over their inabilities to cope and the hurt they bring on each other.

The guilt that both parents experience springs in large measure from the loss of control over what was perceived as a controllable situation: the rearing of a normal child. Parents feel that there must have been something they could have done to avert the hearing loss. Since many of us believe that our power is directly linked to our will, the comfort afforded by feelings of control over one's life is lost by what may be perceived as an irreversible experience, often called by philosophers a "boundary experience" (Yalom, 1989, p. 139). Some people never cease in their search for the reasons for the injustice that has befallen them, a pursuit that may obviate constructive action and create stress.

The stress that is added to the lives of individuals with hearing impairment, and those with whom they interact, can play a major role in acceptance of, and adjustment to, the handicap. Stress is an expected reaction to a communication disorder. Siegal (1986, p. 70) states that it is not stress itself that is damaging, but rather the ways in which people react to it. The stress comes less from the event itself than it does from the way it is interpreted (Siegel, 1986, p. 72), and stress can be extremely debilitating, both emotionally and physically.

Not all reactions to learning of a hearing loss are catastrophic, but relying on instinct, patient feedback, or cues from verbal and nonverbal behaviors to sense the emotions of others can be very misleading. It therefore behooves the audiologist, when delivering information about a hearing loss, to approach each case as if it were special, and the individuals potentially tormented by what the clinician may feel is just another run-of-the-mill hearing loss. Although most patients, or their care givers, will not appear to react with great emotion during an initial diagnostic interview, it must be remembered that clinicians need to develop an artful blend of emotional support along with content transfer. They must also know how to recognize situations that lie beyond their sphere of expertise.

Clinicians need to know when a referral is indicated for deeper professional counseling and how to go about this. Dr. Clark's discussions of the professional and nonprofessional counselor in Chapter 2 can be very helpful in this regard. Proper initial counseling may help us to recognize when we may be dealing with people in severe emotional trouble, and it may help to stave off deeper problems.

Finally, I want to stress the importance of kindness in dealing with patients. *Kindness* is an old-fashioned word, not often seen in the scientific literature. My son, a practicing anesthesiologist, has said that most of his colleagues believe that given a choice between a technically expert surgeon and one who is a good communicator, the former is preferable. It is my belief that the qualities of outstanding technical acumen can be combined with good listening and communicative skills if only we will believe it is important to do so. The proper approach to the diagnostic session that follows an initial hearing examination can contribute greatly to acceptance of a hearing disorder and the rehabilitative actions to follow.

PERCEPTIONS OF COUNSELING SKILLS

It is natural for people to hope for simple solutions to problems. If we are sick we want a prescription to alleviate the symptoms. Nobody enjoys surgery, but at least it is the surgeon who does the operation. We are accustomed to being passive recipients of the efforts of other people who cure our ills. As Luterman (1987) points out, audiologists are often eager and willing to step in and be "saviors" of their patients. The notion of "Do what I say and everything will be OK" sounds wonderful, but what the individuals on the receiving end of diagnostic information really need is time and help in learning to reach their own conclusions and make their own determinations about courses of action. This may require patients to progress at their own rates through various stages of adjustment.

Patient–clinician relationships often depend on the levels of control that are employed (Cassell, 1989). The clinician, usually being the individual with the higher level of control, often decides what is in the best interest of the patient, tells the patient what to do, and the patient is expected to comply. Interestingly, the Latin root for the word *client* is the same as for the verb "to obey." Less than complete compliance may be perceived as a lack of cooperation. An approach that exerts clinician control is believed by many clinicians to engender a form of paternalism, which offers comfort to the patient. Haug and Lavin (1983) found that older patients with lower levels of education were more accepting of this kind of relationship than younger, better-educated individuals who were more assertive and threatened clinicians with greater demands for information and explanation. Assertive patient behavior may be perceived as a reversal of the usual power relationship and may be threatening to the clinician.

Most people who have been critical of the counseling skills of professionals have based their criticism on personal experiences or on the anecdotal reports of others. In recent years, the professional literature has given scientific credence to much of the fear that audiologists and otolaryngologists have not been doing their counseling jobs as well as had been believed (Martin, George, O'Neal, & Daly, 1987; Martin, Abadie, & Descouzis, 1989). Studies of parental reactions to initial diagnostic counseling experiences show lingering resentment and anger over what is perceived as indifference and insensitivity on the part of clinicians. Often these emotions last for many years and are based on reactions to what they were told after the first diagnostic examination.

It should not surprise anyone that parents come to their child's initial diagnostic experience filled with hopes, no matter how unrealistic, that their worst fears will not be realized. That they may become shocked, upset, or disappointed is not surprising. One would not normally expect this to be the case with adults who have acquired a hearing loss. After all, most adults refer themselves for hearing evaluations, and it is expected that they would be aware of a hearing impairment and be more concerned with such matters as "What kind of loss do I have?" "How much loss is there?" "Will it get worse?" and "What should I do about it?" Recent research reveals that emotions run deeper in adult patients than had been supposed.

What studies now reveal is that, in many cases, the reactions on the part of adult patients may be as severe as those of the care givers of children with hearing impairments (Martin, Krall, & O'Neal, 1989). Although adults may verbalize their hearing difficulties with a seeming lack of emotion, they apparently also have fears and hopes regarding what they will be told. It is almost as though they were viewing the implications of their handicaps through a semitransparent screen, which is suddenly whisked away by the clinician, baring implications that are sometimes difficult to accept. Their reactions, like those of care givers, are often that they have been treated with insensitivity and even cruelty. A number of adults have stated that they were told curtly of an irreversible hearing loss and were rushed into making decisions, such as about the purchase of hearing aids, before they were adequately prepared to do so. Once again, resentment was expressed toward audiologist, physician, and hearing aid dispenser alike.

While there are some differences among patient reactions to the counseling skills of audiologists, otolaryngologists, and hearing aid dispensers, no one group emerges as clearly superior to the others. When investigation was made into audiologists', otologists', and otolaryngologists' views of their training and education as preparation for the interchange required at the time of delivering diagnostic information, it was clear that most are woefully underprepared for these experiences by virtue of course work and experience (Martin, Barr, & Bernstein, 1992). What separates those who are sensitive and empathetic from those who are cold and detached seems to depend more on the mentoring experiences clinicians had during their training, as well as their own individual personalities.

WHEN THE COUNSELING PROCESS BEGINS

Luterman (1987) could not have been more correct when he stated that the counseling process should begin at the time of the initial contact with the parents of children who are hearing impaired. There is every reason to believe that this is also the case for adults. With a little planning and forethought the time that passes from the making of the first appointment to the actual visit to the audiologist can be used advantageously in learning what will take place.

When an appointment for a hearing evaluation is requested, it is rare that patients can be seen immediately. Normally people are seen as soon as possible, but the realities of audiology practice do not always permit this. The person receiving telephone inquiries creates the first impression for all that is to follow. Clerks, receptionists, and secretaries are perceived as representing the attitudes of their employers, and it is the professional staff who are responsible for the behaviors of those who represent them. If the person on the telephone is cordial, friendly, and supportive, callers will have a more positive attitude about the services they will receive. Conversely, if that person is cold, indifferent, or unfriendly, a negative feeling may exist before the patient or family ever arrives.

After appointments are made, it is useful to contact the family by mail. Although this may add to the clerical duties and expenses involved, the use of word processors and simple computer programs can streamline this procedure. Families should be sent confirmation of their appointment dates and times, a map or general instructions for finding the facility, a copy of the case-history form that will be used, a release-of-information form, and a set of instructions for taking a hearing examination along with a brief explanation of what the tests mean (see Appendix 3–1). This last document can be kept by the family, and personal experience shows that not only is it referred to many times, but it is also shared with others who have an interest in hearing examinations and their interpretations. The first experience inside a sound-treated room, wearing uncomfortable earphones, listening to unusual sounds, and giving complete concentration to uninteresting stimuli can be difficult, and knowing what to expect can mitigate apprehension considerably.

There are many advantages to having families fill out history forms at home prior to appointment time. Uncertainties about dates of illnesses, onsets of difficulties, and enumeration of complaints can all be ironed out in privacy. The completion of the history form prior to the appointment does not replace history taking by the audiologist; it facilitates and enhances it. Having allowed people to consider their problems in light of the information that is needed for diagnosis can be very helpful. In part, it allows for a more open-ended approach to history taking so that what the individual tells the clinician is not limited to a closed set of responses. The patient history is often viewed as constituting as much as 50% of the diagnosis, and it should not be rushed.

Although history taking usually precedes the examination, if a young child shows fatigue or impatience it may be necessary to postpone the detailed history. A brief glance at what the parents have written at home will often allow the audiologist to make a game plan in terms of diagnostic approaches. Any good pediatric audiologist is fully prepared to begin a hearing evaluation immediately upon arrival of the child.

Although it is best for both parents to accompany their child to the clinic, this is often not the case. It is usually the mother who escorts the child to the examination. The person receiving the diagnostic information is then burdened with the responsibility of conveying that information to others who are critically involved. Aside from the emotions that can frustrate information transfer, it appears that there is often much confusion about what people are told about hearing loss, even when the recipients of the information are intelligent and well educated (Martin, Krueger, & Bernstein, 1990). Similar conclusions were drawn when mothers were interviewed after having received instructions from the children's pediatricians. Diagnostic terms may fail to convey meaning due to "doctors' and patients' failures to communicate in the same language" (West, 1984, pp. 97–98).

While it is often advantageous to have a significant other person accompany adult patients to the examination, this does not appear to happen often. However, the likelihood of a significant other attending the hearing evaluation is enhanced if the receptionist stresses the value of this when the appointment is made. Like care givers, adult patients can be helped by receiving printed materials prior to their appearance at the audiology clinic (see Appendix 3–2).

Although separation between the audiologist and family by a desk or table may be convenient for laying out forms and test results for description, it often creates a psychological barrier. Coming out from behind a desk may be perceived as a loss of power for clinicians and may create discomfort for them. At the same time, it can make for greater warmth among the parties. Except in dealing with very young children, the person addressed should be the patient. Teens and the elderly resent being discussed in the third person as if they were not present. The parent or adult child may be the target of counseling, but it is the patient who should be addressed. When the degree of hearing loss interferes with communication, the use of an assistive amplification device can be invaluable.

An all-too-common happening is that the care givers of children, or the significant others of adults, remain in the waiting room during the examination, or leave to return later. This is often their preference, even if they are given an opportunity to observe or participate in the examination. In my opinion, this choice should not be offered, but rather those accompanying the patient should simply be taken to the sound suite along with the patient. In the case of adults or older children, space should be made for these observers in the control room so that they can see and hear the test stimuli as well as the responses. In most cases, a running tutorial can be given by the audiologist so that a greater understanding of the test can take place. So often, in using this procedure, one hears comments such as, "I had no idea he had so much trouble understanding words. Why is that if the words are loud enough for him to hear?" A major opening for dialogue to follow has thus been created.

In the case of small children one parent can accompany the child into the test room, having been instructed to remain quiet and to maintain eye contact with the child in a supportive way. The parent should not be expected to cajole the child in terms of cooperation. The one weapon children have against their parents is refusal to comply. If sound field audiometry is to be done the parent should be fitted with hearing protectors and allowed to listen to the stimuli to which the child responds, or fails to respond. This has the effect of both illustrating to parents the kinds of difficulties their children may experience and integrating them into the examination process itself.

The diagnostic examination is completed when all tests that should or can be performed have been carried out. Often it is the young child, and not the audiologist, who determines when the examination is over. Experience teaches us to sense when we have pushed our patients' concentration and cooperation as far as is reasonable. The examination should be terminated before the child's frustration is the determining factor. In some cases more information is needed than has been acquired, which necessitates a return visit.

THE INITIAL PEDIATRIC DIAGNOSTIC COUNSELING PROCESS

The site for the counseling session that follows the audiometric examination should be carefully chosen. It should be comfortable and free of external distractions. Parents cannot give full attention to a conversation if they are distracted by a child who, by the time the examination is completed, may be restless and unhappy. An assistant is needed at this juncture to distract and entertain the child, preferably in another room. All interested parties should be present and made to feel at ease before counseling begins. Unfortunately, what is all too common is that we begin to speak before the patient/care giver is prepared to listen.

Beginning the first counseling session is often the most important feature of all that is to follow. Frequently what is called "counseling" is, in reality, the offering of details of testing, augmented by graphs (which just as often confuse as elucidate), followed by suggestions for remediation. There are better ways.

Patients/care givers may simply be asked what they know about the hearing loss, what they have learned from the testing, and what they wish to know. When we use this approach we may be surprised at how often people do not want to be told more than the "bottom line," which may be "Is my baby going to talk?" or "Are hearing aids necessary?" Studies indicate that while parents often claim that they want more information than they get, many clinicians believe they cannot initially handle more than a specific amount (Martin et al., 1987). This may create a major dilemma and challenges the notions of many audiologists that they know what is best for the family. Parents may be asked what they understand and do not understand about the extent of their child's communicative difficulty. Attempts should be made to learn the impact of the hearing loss on the child and on the family. It is far better to evoke questions than to produce a monologue.

SAMPLE DIALOGUE FOLLOWING A PEDIATRIC EVALUATION

Initial diagnostic session with a 3-year-old child who was brought to the clinic by his mother.

USUAL SCENARIO—Step 1

The mother has been sitting in the waiting room while two audiologists test her son. After testing is completed, the mother is taken to a conference room while the child is distracted with play, preferably in another room.

AUDIOLOGIST: "Our test results show that Colin has a profound hearing loss."
MOTHER: "Are you sure?" (This can't be true. Not my baby.)
AUDIOLOGIST: "He was pretty consistent in his responses and we believe we are

correct. Let me show you his audiogram and explain what these symbols stand for."

MOTHER: "Okay." (I don't know what all this means. I wish I could get out of here.)

AUDIOLOGIST: "Do you understand what the audiogram tells us?"

MOTHER: "I think so." (My husband will be furious. I won't remember any of this. Why did this happen to me?)

RECOMMENDED SCENARIO—Step 1

If sound field audiometry is done, the mother is provided with hearing protection and seated in the test room with the child and assisting audiologist. She is encouraged to observe her child's reactions and participate in the test in specified ways. Later, during the conference:

AUDIOLOGIST: "What did you think about Colin's responses to the sounds?"

Allow the mother to assist in verbalizing the diagnosis.

MOTHER: "I'm not sure. He seemed to respond mostly to the low-pitched sounds, and then only when they were very loud. I could hardly stand to listen to some of those loud tones."

AUDIOLOGIST: "That is the way it seemed to us too. What do you think this means?"

MOTHER: "I guess he *does* have trouble hearing."

Some acceptance is taking place.

AUDIOLOGIST: "I agree with you."

The audiologist dignifies and confirms the mother's impressions.

or

MOTHER: "Well, I think I saw a number of responses. I know him better than you do. He seems to respond to softer sounds at home than he did here. Also, he missed his nap today."

The mother is in denial.

AUDIOLOGIST: "You may be right. It is possible to be misled by young children and we don't want that to happen."

Attempting to convince the mother at this juncture that she is incorrect may result in alienation and delayed treatment for Colin. He may be taken to a different clinician or no further progress may be made for some time.

"Let's schedule him now for a retest."

Test results are not shown to the mother unless she asks to see them.

USUAL SCENARIO—Step 2

AUDIOLOGIST: "It is important that we not lose any more time."

There is an implication here that the parents have already wasted some time. This may add guilt and anger to the existing emotions.

"Here are some phone numbers of parents of deaf children."

The word "deaf" may conflict with any reference the audiologist makes to residual hearing because "deafness" to many people means no hearing at all (Ross and Calvert, 1967).

"I'd like you to call one of them right away. That can he helpful in your understanding and adjustment to Colin's hearing problems."

Talking to other parents often has the effect of comforting parents of the newly diagnosed child and relieves that feeling of being "in this fix alone."

RECOMMENDED SCENARIO—Step 2

AUDIOLOGIST: "Would you like me to give you the phone numbers of some parents of children with hearing problems like Colin's? They will be glad to share some of their experiences and that might be helpful to you."

The mother is given the option and is not told to do something she may not be ready to do.

MOTHER: "Okay." (This is a good idea. Maybe it will make me feel better and I'll learn something. I'll do it right away).

or

MOTHER: "Okay." (I'll need to think about this and talk it over with my husband. It may be embarrassing. I won't know how to go about it.)

or

MOTHER: "Not just now. I have to think about this for a while."

The mother may or may not intend to follow through on this suggestion.

AUDIOLOGIST: "That's fine."

The clinician is supportive of the parent's decision and does not attempt to rush her.

USUAL SCENARIO—Step 3

AUDIOLOGIST: "Now we need to talk about getting hearing aids on Colin right away and talk about getting him into therapy."

MOTHER: "Okay."

Mother sits politely but does not process what she hears. Her reports to her husband that night are incomplete and inaccurate and may cause disagreement between them.

RECOMMENDED SCENARIO—Step 3

AUDIOLOGIST: "Would you like to talk now about the options that are open to you to help Colin, or would you prefer to come back and discuss this at another time? Perhaps you can bring your husband with you when you return and we can run some additional tests on Colin to be certain we have consistent results."

MOTHER: "I'd like to discuss it now."

AUDIOLOGIST: "Fine."

The discussion is kept as nontechnical as possible. The mother is given some printed material to take home and an appointment is made for a revisit.

or

MOTHER: "I think I'm overwhelmed by all of this. I'd like to come back and talk when my husband is with me. Will that be all right?"

AUDIOLOGIST: "Certainly. I know that a lot of this is new to you. I think you're making a wise decision. Let's set up a time right now."

There are naturally many variations on the scene just described. No one is comfortable using the suggested words of others and we must each determine the approaches that make us most comfortable. Additionally, patient or care-giver reactions may evoke alterations in style and substance. In describing parallel difficulties in patient–physician communication, West (1984, p. 98) says, "In real life situations doctors and patients have no way of assessing one another's reactions to words that they use *as they use them* other than by observing the other's responses to them at that time." The main point is to allow individuals to make decisions as they go and not to rush them or bombard them with information that they cannot use at the time.

It is frequently of value to ask patients, or their companions, what their impressions were of the hearing examination after it is completed. Was a hearing deficit demonstrated? Does their observation square with previous conceptions?

Often it is advantageous to ask the patients/care givers for their impressions of the extent of the communicative difficulties that are experienced. For adults, self-assessment questionnaires have been very successful in some cases, as discussed in detail by Dr. Garstecki in Chapter 9. The extent to which the hearing loss impacts on patients and their significant others is often not directly related to the extent of the loss itself. Getting patients involved in discussion is often not easy to do.

We need to use verbal activity that encourages patient expression of ideas. These facilitating behaviors include questions, statements, or reflections and are discussed in more detail in Chapter 2. Patients are entitled to some form of verbal acknowledgment that the clinician has heard what they have said (Levenstein et al., 1989). Failure to receive this acknowledgment often results in mistrust and failure of patient compliance.

Stiles and Putnam (1989) point out that not all communication between clinicians and patients is verbal. Included in nonverbal activities are "tone of voice, gaze, posture, hesitations, laughter, facial expressions, touch," as well as many others (p. 215). Although clinicians may choose their words carefully, there is evidence that emotional states may be conveyed more clearly by nonverbal activities than by verbal communication. Each and every activity may affect the clinician–patient interaction.

THE INITIAL ADULT DIAGNOSTIC COUNSELING PROCESS

Although there are many exceptions, the majority of cases where initial audiological counseling is important involves children or adults with irreversible sensorineural hearing losses, whose causes are not threatening to the health or life of the individual. Such cases often become so routine to clinicians that they fail to recognize the importance of their words to their patients.

SAMPLE DIALOGUE FOLLOWING AN ADULT EVALUATION

Initial diagnostic session with a 45-year-old male who was accompanied to the clinic by his spouse.

USUAL SCENARIO—Step 1

The wife has been seated quietly with the clinician during the examination and has observed what has taken place. They are now seated comfortably in an office or conference room.

AUDIOLOGIST: "Let me show you the audiogram we drew based on the test you took when you listened for those soft tones. The red circles represent the intensity at which you could barely hear each frequency at threshold, and the blue X's represent your left ear. Intensity refers to the loudness of the tones, and frequency is a term for the different pitches you heard. Threshold is the intensity at which each tone was barely heard. The further to the right on the graph we go the higher the frequency, or pitch. The lower on the graph the louder, or more intense, each sound had to be before you could just barely hear it. The red and blue arrows represent your ability to hear by bone conduction."

Although the audiologist believes that defining new terms along the way means that the patient and his spouse follow their meaning, this is often not the case. Further, it is likely that even if the description just illustrated does convey meaning, it is unlikely that much of the information will be retained. Of course, there is a greater chance for accurate understanding and retention with the spouse present than if she were absent, partly because two heads are often, in fact, better than one, and also because the patient's hearing loss may interfere with the discrimination of critical words. The audiologist may feel comfortable using technical terms and may feel that educating the patient is important at this time, but a great deal of jargon has been used.

AUDIOLOGIST: "Do you understand the audiogram?"
PATIENT: "I think so."

There may be specific questions at this point, but it is likely that the patient may give the clinician the false sense of security that the information has been processed, simply because it is embarrassing to admit that it has not. Some individuals claim to have no questions because they have not understood enough of what has transpired to ask a question.

RECOMMENDED SCENARIO—Step 1

AUDIOLOGIST: "I know that took a long time. It can get very uncomfortable under those earphones in that tiny room. Do you have any impressions of the test or do you have any questions?"

The family can give cues about the depth of information they possess or wish to hear.

AUDIOLOGIST: "Would you like for me to give you my overall feeling of what we found or would you like to know the details of the test results?"

Again, the family is allowed to lead the way in determining how much depth is required.

SPOUSE: "Just tell us how much hearing loss my husband has and what can be done about it."

If the patient agrees this suggests that what is most desirable at this time is to cut right to the "bottom line." Like many others, these people want a professional interpretation of the test results and are no more interested in details at this point than they would be in the precise meanings of numbers on medical blood tests.

or

PATIENT: "Why were some of the tones softer than others and why was it so hard to hear those two-syllable words? When you gave me the one-syllable words I could make out some words clearer than others. Why was that?"

Some detail is required here.

AUDIOLOGIST: "You did a very good job of taking those tests. I deliberately made those sounds very soft so that you could just barely hear them—which allows us to compare your hearing for each of the sounds in each ear with how loud or soft they need to be for a person with normal hearing to barely hear them. The same is true of the two-syllable words; we wanted to know how your hearing compares to people with no hearing loss at all. The louder, one-syllable words were designed to find out how well you recognize the different speech sounds, to try to estimate the kinds of difficulties you have in speech communication. Do you want me to show you how these tests turned out and how we graph the results?"

A common error is to tell patients their speech recognition scores in percentages, which can create a variety of misperceptions; patients often confuse their speech recognition scores with percentage of hearing loss, a concept that is often ill advised in counseling patients. The use of single number designations like "You understood 80% in your right ear and 76% in your left ear" may be very far from accurate, since how much an individual discriminates is determined by a number of factors, not the least of which is the acoustic environment.

USUAL SCENARIO—Step 2

AUDIOLOGIST: "We find that you have what we call a sensorineural hearing loss. There is usually no medical treatment for this kind of problem."

The audiologist must realize that the patient may have been hoping for a reversal of the hearing problem. Hopes can be dashed at this point and further attention not forthcoming.

or

AUDIOLOGIST: "You appear to have what is called a sensorineural hearing loss. There is a great deal that may be done to improve the kinds of difficulty you are having in communication. Would you like to discuss some of these?"

This is a more accurate description of the hearing loss and creates a more optimistic outlook.

Frequently tests are performed that go beyond the routine measurement of hearing. Audiologists have a wide variety of site-of-lesion tests at their disposal. Usually these are called into use when there is suspicion of a neurological disorder. Detailed discussion of what these tests were designed to measure and their outcomes is often not fruitful, because they are unusual and unanticipated. In their zeal to provide complete coverage of the tests they have performed, audiologists may heap mountains of detail on patients, who listen politely in anticipation of learning new facts that are specific to their hearing problems. This deluge of technical information may be worse than a waste of time because the important messages may be lost in the garble of jargon that may accompany discussion of advanced tests. Clinicians might do well to reflect on their days as students and on the initial difficulty they might have had in grasping the full meaning of hearing tests in order to comprehend why it is not fruitful to overburden patients with extraneous information. Having said this, it is always essential to dignify any inquiries patients or their families have regarding specific tests with an appropriate explanation. Few things are more irritating to patients than a "you would not understand if I explained it" attitude on the part of any clinician.

When a number of tests have been performed, the audiologist may once again ask the patient (or family) whether he or she wants specific information and the nature of that information. Questions should be answered as completely and honestly as possible, avoiding technical language. Patients dislike the feeling of being rushed in the office of a professional person.

People often think of things they should have asked or comments they wish they had made after a situation has passed. If the relationship between patient and clinician is warm and cordial, the patient may be invited to telephone with further questions. Patients often leave the clinic believing they have understood what they have been told and later become confused or bewildered. Recognizing this 3 decades ago, Bailey and Martin (1961) recommended the use of a letter to be sent to patients several days after the diagnostic interview, repeating the findings and recommendations. The opportunity to read these letters in the privacy of one's home, away from the often-threatening environs of an audiological or medical setting, can be most useful. Perhaps more than informational, such letters send a message that the clinician cares for the patient personally and wishes to be of further assistance.

SPECIFIC DIAGNOSTIC INFORMATION

Tests of the auditory system can be divided into those of function and those of structure. The audiologist may be an expert in the former, but the latter must be carried out using imaging and other medical diagnostic procedures. Audiologists are frequently tentative about what they say to patients lest they step over the boundary that separates their specialty from the practice of medicine. I believe that the purview of the audiologist stops short of specifying etiology, but type and degree of loss, and even site of lesion, are part of the audiological province. Some specific diagnostic entities will now be discussed that involve the audiologist in direct information transfer regarding hearing test results.

Conductive Hearing Loss

One common finding is conductive hearing loss. With just the basic battery of tests it is often relatively easy to identify otitis media or serous effusion as the probable etiological factor. Although these problems are usually reversible, and are considered to be less serious in terms of communication deficits than sensorineural hearing losses, there is no way of knowing whether a patient or parent may react emotionally to learning of a conductive hearing loss. Nevertheless, in such situations it is not to the patient's advantage to delay treatment by staging a series of discussion sessions. Medical consultation should take place as soon as possible to avoid the possibility of such sequelae of middle ear disease as tympanic membrane perforation.

Otosclerosis is often another obvious diagnostic finding to audiologists, who must restrain their enthusiasm for conveying this medical diagnosis to the patient. It should be explained that the loss is conductive in nature and that a medical opinion is necessary to determine whether the loss is reversible. Depending on the patient's interest in detail, models and diagrams of the ear may be used to indicate the possible locations of lesions that may be causing the loss.

No promises should be made when referring cases with conductive hearing losses; however, audiologists should explain that the best chance for hearing to be improved is when prompt action is taken, and an immediate referral should be made back to the referring physician or to an otolaryngologist if the patient was self-referred. Copies of audiograms and tympanograms may be sent along with the patient.

The fact that audiometric data will accompany the patient to the physician does not negate the responsibility of sending a letter. Enclosed with the letter should be duplicate copies of the audiometric, tympanometric, and other findings, and an explanation of the reason for referral, along with a request to learn of the medical management and outcome. After medical treatment has been completed, follow-up hearing evaluations should be encouraged, since even in the case of prompt and adequate medical treatment a hearing loss may persist that requires audiological care.

Otoneurological Disorders

The motivated diagnostic audiologist is constantly on the alert for serious otoneurological symptoms. "All unilateral sensorineural hearing losses are acoustic neuromas until proved otherwise" is good advice by which to practice. The communicative skills of audiologists are challenged when their enthusiasm for an immediate medical consultation is frustrated by their inability to tell the patient precisely why this is necessary. We never know whether we have frightened people, even with seemingly benign statements like "I would like you to see a physician to determine whether there are any serious medical implications of your hearing loss." Sometimes it is helpful to explain that what is desired is the elimination of a diagnostic entity rather than its confirmation.

Sudden Hearing Loss

Sudden onset of hearing loss often constitutes a medical emergency. Prompt medical treatment may result in reversal of what seems like a profound, or even total, unilateral sensorineural hearing loss. In such cases, the audiologist should be firm in the recommendation for prompt otological appraisal. Without panicking the patient it should be explained that there are cases in which improvement in hearing may be forthcoming if treatment is administered in a timely fashion. The audiologist may even offer to make an appointment for the patient and, if this is agreeable, may make the telephone call while the patient is in attendance. If the audiologist enjoys a good reputation with the medical office being called, it is often possible for the patient to be "worked in" on the day of the call.

Tinnitus

It is rare to see hearing-impaired patients who do not make at least some complaint of tinnitus. In developing a case history the clinician should learn as much as possible about the tinnitus. In some cases it is important to make a medical referral if it is suspected that the tinnitus is a symptom of a medical condition. If this has been ruled out it becomes important to speak of ways to relieve the symptoms. If the recommended therapy involves medication or surgery, it is the physician who supervises the case; if the approach is the use of amplification, tinnitus maskers (the use of which has declined in recent years), biofeedback, or coping strategies, then it is the audiologist who is often the central figure.

The success or failure of a tinnitus management program, regardless of the procedure used, often turns on the relationship with the patient. Empathy and supportive counseling can be a valuable adjunct to therapeutic intervention. The interpersonal connection that is fostered in such situations may be the factor that determines the efficacy of the program.

Unilateral Hearing Loss

It has not been very long since we have begun to appreciate the extent of the handicap imposed by a unilateral hearing loss. Often patients have been addressed with such comments as "It is better to have no hearing in one ear and a normal ear on the other side than to have a mild hearing loss in both ears." These are words that are often not well received by patients who have great difficulty in sound localization and in hearing in noisy or acoustically competitive environments. Since their problem is so often misunderstood by others, when audiologists demonstrate that they do grasp the extent of the difficulties encountered by persons with unilateral hearing loss, this can be comforting to the patient.

Pseudohypacusis

The index of suspicion for pseudohypacusis goes up when clinicians learn that there is litigation involved with a hearing loss, that there may be a financial incentive, or that the diagnosis of hearing loss may lead to some exemption that is beneficial to the patient. Sometimes pseudohypacusis comes from unexpected places. For example, I have encountered university students who have feigned a hearing loss in order to receive a letter that will excuse them from their foreign language requirement. Suspicion is not evidence, and audiologists must not prejudge their patients' motives or morality.

In finding nonorganic hearing behavior in adults the audiologist is often freed from deciding what to say to the patient by the circumstances of the referral. In pension examinations, or when a hearing examination is paid for by an attorney opposing the patient's claim in a legal dispute, it is often inappropriate to discuss the test findings with the patient, and that should be explained. However, when patients are self-referred and are expected to pay for the examination themselves, the situation becomes much more delicate because statements that impune a patient's honesty are naturally met with resentment. In the present litigious environment it might be wise to imagine the patient's attorney present in the room with notepad and pencil in hand.

Since clinicians cannot know for certain what motivates pseudohypacusic behavior, the word *malingering* should never be used. Likewise, audiologists are not trained as psychiatrists or psychologists and should avoid discussions of psychogenic disorders. In most cases all that can be done is to explain to the patient that test results were too inconsistent to make a determination of the type and degree of hearing loss, and to offer to carry out further tests. The patient should understand that this position will be stated in any written reports that might be requested. Specific test results should not be discussed, especially those findings that give rise to the suspicion of pseudohypacusis. The last thing audiologists want to do is to function as tutors to help patients "beat" the next set of hearing tests they take.

It is expected that pseudohypacusic patients will be less than satisfied when their requests for corroboration of a claim have seemingly been denied. Further, if the clinician believes that a psychological consultation would be in the interest of the patient this must be pursued delicately. Such a recommendation, no matter how well intended, may meet with hostility, and the clinician must be prepared for remarks such as "Do you think I'm crazy?" The audiologist must maintain an air of diplomacy and calm professionalism. This is true in dealing with children as well as with adults.

The resolution of pseudohypacusis in children ranges from quite easy to very difficult. If the child is fabricating a hearing loss, discovering that the clinician knows that hearing is normal often causes the child to abandon this pursuit. The clinician can and should act as the child's advocate, since the parents may be annoyed and feel they have wasted time and money because a child did not pay close attention on a school hearing screening, or some other condition that led to the test. It can simply be stated, in the child's presence, that tests show the hearing to be normal. If this is a one-time thing for the child the situation may end on that note.

Audiologists should remain alert for persistent symptoms of pseudohypacusis, which may represent a child's unspoken call for help during times of emotional stress. If there is persistent demonstration of nonorganic symptoms, the child should be excused from the conference and the parents helped to decide what it may be that is causing the pseudohypacusic behavior. Is the child calling out for attention? Is there something going on in the home that is threatening to the child's security, such as an impending divorce, new baby in the family, move to a new home, recent death, or some kind of abuse? Is there a problem in school that may be excused if the child is somehow handicapped? The parents should be helped to decide whether a referral is indicated for in-depth counseling.

Noise-Induced Hearing Loss

Although it is rare that audiometric findings alone allow for assuredness in assessing etiology, the combination of case history and audiometric configuration often allows the audiologist to conclude that an individual hearing loss has probably been caused by exposure to intense noise. In such cases it is often appropriate for audiologists to express their concerns over the dangers of further noise exposure, an effort that is often met with frustration.

There are numbers of times when patients are seen (these are usually males, although not exclusively) whose progressive hearing loss can potentially be traced to shotguns or rifles used in sports shooting. When caution against continued use of guns without hearing protection is met with refusal to comply, or denial of the relationship between gunfire and hearing loss, there is little the clinician can do. Even more upsetting than adult refusal to avoid noise exposure is the knowledge that parents will allow their children to be exposed to dangerous sound levels such as firecrackers, firearms, or loud music.

Experienced audiologists know that "scare" techniques are no more successful in preventing gun lovers from using their guns than are physicians' attempts at frightening their diabetic patients into dieting. Concerns over future damage to hearing may be expressed, disposable hearing protection devices can and should be dispensed as part of the day's "package," along with demonstration in their use, and the patient should be encouraged to return for periodic hearing examinations to check for progression. Care should be taken that patients do not sense disapproval on the part of the clinician; otherwise rapport may be destroyed and follow-up not obtained.

Presbycusis

Aging is expected to be accompanied by serious afflictions. Unlike stroke, heart attack, or osteoporosis, hearing loss is considered by some professionals to be more of an annoyance than a serious medical condition. Elderly patients do not appreciate an attitude that says, "Of course you have a hearing loss; you are fortunate to have lived long enough to earn one." While this sentiment may not be verbalized, it is often inferred by patients from the behavior of their clinicians. The older person's withdrawal from social gatherings, the theater, or attendance at religious observances is often the result of the hearing loss.

The kinds of difficulties that patients have experienced should be discussed in as much detail as the patient's state of mind will allow. The family may even learn much from statements made by patients in the clinic. This is far more important than conveyance of specific diagnostic information. The patient should be treated with the utmost respect, and all comments should be made directly to them rather than to accompanying family members. Demonstration of the use of room lighting, the ideal geographic arrangement of talkers, the paraphrasing of misunderstood statements, and similar suggestions can be very helpful to all the persons involved. Dr. Trychin's discussion of coping strategies in Chapter 10 provides more detail on this subject.

In recent years a familiarity in communication has developed and is often tacitly deplored and occasionally verbally objected to by elderly persons. Addressing patients by their first names has become routine in many business and professional situations, probably in the belief that informality breaks down unnecessary barriers. It is not possible to treat individuals with too much respect, and the appropriateness of titles like Ms., Mrs., or Mr. is never in doubt. Elderly persons often feel they have already lost some of their dignity, and the audiologist should not contribute to this belief.

Central Auditory Processing Disorders

Often, in routine hearing testing, the type or degree of hearing loss does not square with the patient's complaints about difficulty in hearing and understanding speech. It is appropriate to carry out a battery of tests for central auditory processing disorders whenever such a problem is suspected. Whether or not the results on these tests are positive, the audiologist must use experience and intuition in deciding on referral for further testing and examination.

Learning of a child's central auditory disorder may impact on parents in ways similar to learning of a hearing loss. They have been told that there is "something wrong" with their child, and that he or she is less than perfect. After the test results have been explained, it is again useful to try to evoke statements from the parents that will assist them in accepting a referral. Terms like *brain damage* should be scrupulously avoided.

It is helpful for audiologists to explain the nature of central auditory disorders and offer coping strategies. After the diagnostic findings have been explained, provision of printed materials and an appointment for further discussion should be provided. A discussion of the kinds of difficulties the patient is experiencing is much more helpful than diagnostic labeling and shows that the clinician is concerned and insightful. Since many areas of the United States, including many school districts, do not have ready availability of support services for children with central auditory processing disorders, the audiologist should assist in finding the proper assistance for the child.

Some patients request diagnostic testing with a complaint of hearing difficulty, especially in untoward listening situations, although results suggest normal hearing sensitivity and there is no evidence of a central disorder. This is a phenomenon that has only recently been reported in the literature, although experienced clinicians have observed it for some time. Some of these individuals successfully use personal amplification devices. Research is needed to understand this phenomenon, but until our understanding is increased such complaints should not be dismissed or treated as trivial.

REMEDIATION

Diagnostic hearing tests are not a goal in themselves. Along with the patient's history, they are designed to aid the clinician in helping the patient. Often the audiologist is the person who guides patients in improving their abilities at communication and adjustment to the problems that accompany hearing impairments. Aural habilitation and rehabilitation inspired the genesis of the profession of audiology, and they remain central to its practice. Most approaches to aural habilitation or rehabilitation begin with some consideration given to personal amplification devices.

For a wide variety of reasons the number of people who are advised to wear hearing aids has increased steadily over the years. Modern technology has improved the instruments themselves, the often-important aspect of cosmetic appeal, and the means of appropriate fitting. Addressing hearing aid acceptance for children is discussed in detail in Chapter 7 and for adults in Chapter 9. The words spoken about amplification at the time initial diagnostic findings are reported sets the scene for patient willingness to pursue the use of amplification. Often, being told that hearing aids are needed has a depressing effect on people. Adults may feel suddenly old, and parents may be concerned that their children will look odd or pitiful. If the disappointment at being told that a hearing loss is irreversible is followed immediately by recommendations for amplification, with its attendant expense and difficulties, the patient may be overwhelmed and incapable of following through. Clinicians must decide on the advisability of when to make recommendations for amplification. It is common to find ear molds in audiology clinics that have been made for patients who have not returned to pick them up, or to receive the hearing aid evaluations they agreed to participate in just a week earlier.

Further, most audiologists would probably agree that simply fitting a hearing aid to a patient often does not guarantee successful use. Many clinics "bundle" the price of the hearing instrument with a program of aural rehabilitation. How this is handled is determined by the philosophy of the individual clinic, but some care after fitting is required in all cases, even those that appear easy to fit. Individual attention is required in the prescription of other amplification devices as well as hearing aids.

Introducing assistive listening devices and systems to people is discussed in detail by Dr. Garstecki in Chapter 9. These instruments have proved so useful to so many patients that they should be described or demonstrated to patients and their relative merits outlined. Provision of printed or videotaped materials regarding these devices, to be discussed at a second meeting, may be an appropriate means of handling this important and often-overlooked means of improving patient communication. This is equally important for adults and for children.

When a significant and irreversible hearing loss is found in a small child, the clinician has so much to discuss with the care givers that one hardly knows how and when to begin. The parents cannot be rushed into these discussions, and yet they cannot be postponed until the family thinks of its own questions to ask. Audiologists are naturally anxious for parents to learn about support groups, amplification systems, contact with other parents or care givers, aural habilitation teams, and methods of rehabilitation. However, time must be provided for discussion, educational materials must be supplied, families should feel they have the privilege of changing their minds, and clinicians must show respect for decisions that they believe are incorrect. The clinician must educate the care givers so that they can make informed decisions about how their children are to be educated. Although each of us has a preferred system by which we believe most children with hearing impairment should be managed, that system will not work unless the family believes in it. For further discussion the reader is referred to Dr. Johnson's discussion of educational issues in Chapter 8.

While there may appear to be less drama in working with adults or adventitiously hearing-impaired teenagers, their needs are no less critical than the parents of small children with hearing impairments. Research has shown that these individuals desire enlightenment about their problems, and the audiologist is the ideal person to educate and inform them so that their rehabilitation takes on more depth than the historical approach using drills and repetitive activities.

CONCLUSION

Much of what is of value to patients and those concerned about them emerges from the initial diagnostic counseling session. If people have respect for and feel respect from their clinicians, the relationship to follow has gotten off to a good start. The shock of learning of a disorder may be present even if the diagnosis is anticipated. At the time clinicians attempt to share their knowledge and opinions, technical expertise must become secondary to kindness, sensitivity, and common sense. In an average career each audiologist has an often-profound impact on literally thousands of lives, often at the time of the first diagnostic hearing evaluation. That is a tremendous responsibility, and its significance should never be underestimated.

REFERENCES

BAILEY, H. A. T., & MARTIN, F. N. (1961). Letter to the patient with a sensori-neural hearing loss. *Laryngoscope, 71*, 562–567.

CASSELL, E. J. (1989). Making the subjective objective. In M. Stewart. & D. Roter (Eds.), *Communicating with medical patients* (pp. 13–23). Newbury Park, CA: Sage.

HAUG, M., & LAVIN, B. (1983). *Consumerism in medicine: Challenging physician authority.* Beverly Hills, CA: Sage.

KÜBLER-ROSS, E. (1969). *On death and dying.* New York: Macmillan.

LEVENSTEIN, J. H., BROWN, J. B., WESTON, W. W., STEWART, M., MCCRACKEN, E. C., & MCWHINNEY, I. (1989). Patient-centered clinical interviewing. In M. Stewart & D. Roter (Eds.), *Communicating with medical patients* (pp. 107–120). Newbury Park, CA: Sage.

LUTERMAN, D. M. (1984). *Counseling parents of hearing-impaired children and their families.* Boston: Little, Brown.

LUTERMAN, D. M. (1987). Counseling parents of hearing-impaired children. In F. N. Martin (Ed.), *Hearing disorders in children* (pp. 303–319). Austin, TX: Pro-Ed.

MARTIN, F. N., ABADIE, K. T., & DESCOUZIS, D. (1989). Counseling families of hearing-impaired children: Comparisons of the attitudes of Australian and U.S. parents and audiologists. *Australian Journal of Audiology, 11*, 41–54.

MARTIN, F. N., BARR, M., & BERNSTEIN, M. (1992). Professional attitudes regarding counseling of hearing-impaired adults. *American Journal of Otology. 13*, 279–287.

MARTIN, F. N., GEORGE, K., O'NEAL, J., & DALY, J. (1987). Audiologists' and parents' attitudes regarding counseling of families of hearing-impaired children. *Asha, 29*, 27–33.

MARTIN, F. N., KRALL, L., & O'NEAL, J. (1989). The diagnosis of acquired hearing loss: Patient reactions. *Asha, 31*, 47–50.

MARTIN, F. N., KRUEGER, J. S., & BERNSTEIN, M. (1990). Diagnostic information transfer to hearing-impaired adults. *Tejas, 16*, 29–32.

ROGERS, D. E. (1989). Out of touch: Is technology widening the emotional moat between doctors and their patients? *Wall Street Journal*, pp. R38–R39.

ROSS, M., & CALVERT, D. R. (1967). The semantics of deafness. *Volta Review, 69*, 644–649.

SIEGEL, B. S. (1986). *Love, medicine & miracles.* New York: Harper & Row.

STILES, W. B., & PUTNAM, S. M. (1989). Analysis of verbal and nonverbal behavior in doctor–patient encounters. In M. Stewart & D. Roter (Eds.), *Communicating with medical patients* (pp. 211–222).

WEST, C. (1984). Medical misfires: Mishearings, misgiving, and misunderstandings. In *Routine Complications.* Bloomington: Indiana University Press.

YALOM, I. D. (1989). *Love's executioner, and other tales of psychotherapy.* New York: Harper Perennial.

APPENDIX 3–1

Forms to be sent to families prior to escorting a child to the clinic for a hearing evaluation:

1. Letter of confirmation of appointment
2. Instructions for what will take place during the pediatric examination
3. Authorization for release of information

LETTER OF CONFIRMATION OF APPOINTMENT

Thank you for calling The University of Texas Speech and Hearing Center to schedule an evaluation for _____ . The evaluation is scheduled for _____ . Please fill out the enclosed form(s) as completely as possible and bring these forms with you at the time of your appointment.

Please fill out the packet of forms enclosed as completely as possible prior to the evaluation. This will assist the audiologist in performing a thorough examination. The evaluation of hearing in children assesses hearing for speech, hearing for tones, and measurements of eardrum function. A description of each of these areas is provided in the following sheet entitled "Instructions for Pediatric Hearing Evaluations," to help you feel more comfortable with the examination.

We would like to suggest that when you come to the clinic to have your child's hearing evaluated that you invite another person, for example a spouse or close friend, to accompany you. This is not required, but we find that it is often helpful to have an interested party present when we review the test results.

Again, thank you for calling The University of Texas Speech and Hearing Center.

Sincerely,

Enclosures

INSTRUCTIONS FOR CHILDREN'S HEARING EVALUATIONS

On the day of your appointment you and your child will be met in the clinic lobby by the audiologist, who will receive the packet of information you have been sent. Some general observations of your child will be made before actual testing begins. Whether we review the history information you have brought before we begin testing or after completion depends on a number of factors, including how important we believe it is to start testing immediately.

You will be asked to accompany your child into a sound-treated room. We may ask you to hold her or him on your lap. One audiologist will be with you and your child, and the other audiologist will be in an adjoining room with your spouse, if he or she is present, operating the test equipment. The precise type and order of testing will depend on your child's age and ability to cooperate.

Sounds may be presented through earphones, if they will be tolerated, or through loudspeakers. Your child's responses will be carefully observed as he or she is trained to look for the sound, place a block in a box after hearing each sound, or by some other technique. Attempts will be made to assess your child's ability to hear tones of different pitches and to hear and discriminate different speech sounds. If the test is completed satisfactorily we will be able to draw and show you an *audiogram*, which is a graph that represents your child's ability to hear tones of different pitches.

Following (or in some cases preceding) the tests for tones and speech, the function of your child's eardrums will be assessed. He or she will first be examined with an ear light. Then a snugly fitting plastic piece will be inserted into one ear while a headphone will be placed over the other ear. The following sensations will be perceived: a humming sound, some slight pressure changes, and a series of loud tones. There is no danger to your child's ears or hearing from this procedure and no active cooperation is required, except that she or he sit or lie quietly. This test is called *acoustic immittance* and gives us a great deal of information about possible fluid behind the eardrums as well as the function of certain muscles in the ear that are related to how we hear. On completion of the test we will be able to show you a graph called a *tympanogram*, indicating how well your child's eardrum moves in response to sound and changes in pressure.

After all tests are completed your clinicians will discuss their findings and explain what they mean. This is an ideal time for you to ask whatever questions you have so that we can agree on whether some course of action is needed and what that action should be. We will, of course, review all these instructions with you when you arrive at the clinic, and we hope you will feel free to ask questions at any time.

AUTHORIZATION FOR RELEASE OF INFORMATION

Re: _____ , _____ _____
last name   *first name*   *middle initial*

       I, the undersigned, authorize The University of Texas Speech and Hearing Center to acquire and/or release professional information from and to my child's physician and/or other professional personnel involved in the evaluation and management of requested services.

Signed: _____

_____
relationship to child

_____
date

       I, the undersigned, authorize The University of Texas Speech and Hearing Center to use information, photographs, sound recordings, video recordings, and other records or materials that have to do with my child's testing or therapy at this Center, for educational, scientific, or professional purposes.

Signed: _____

_____
relationship to child

_____
date

APPENDIX 3–2

Forms to be sent to adults prior to appearance in the clinic for their hearing evaluation:

1. Letter of confirmation of appointment
2. Instructions for what will take place during the examination
3. Authorization for release of information

LETTER OF CONFIRMATION OF APPOINTMENT

Thank you for calling The University of Texas Speech and Hearing Center to schedule an evaluation for _____ . The evaluation is scheduled for _____ . Please fill out the enclosed form(s) as completely as possible and bring them with you at the time of your appointment.

Enclosed you will also find a set of instructions for taking the hearing examination, along with some samples of the words that will be used during one of the tests. Please read these materials over before the evaluation, for they explain the meaning of some of the tests performed. Instructions will be repeated prior to each hearing test.

We would like to suggest that when you come to the clinic to have your hearing evaluated that you invite another person, for example a spouse or close friend, to accompany you. This is not required, but we find that it is often helpful to have an interested party present when we review the test results.

Again, thank you for calling The University of Texas Speech and Hearing Center.

Sincerely,

Enclosures

INSTRUCTIONS FOR TAKING THE HEARING EXAMINATION

As a part of your examination you will receive several different hearing tests. The results of these tests will help us determine the type and degree of hearing impairment you have so that we may best advise you regarding your hearing difficulties.

The tests are divided into three parts: (1) hearing for speech, (2) hearing for tones, and (3) measurements of eardrum function. Here are a few simple instructions to make these tests go more quickly and easily for you and to ensure the accuracy of the test results.

You will be seated in a sound-treated room. A pair of earphones will be placed over your ears or a button will be held to your forehead or behind your ear by a metal or plastic strap. This equipment will fit snugly but should not be uncomfortable.

For your first speech test you will hear some two-syllable words like *sunset* or *airplane*. Please repeat each word you hear, even if you have to guess. Some of these words will be too faint to hear but try to repeat as many as you can. Do not be concerned over missing some of the words, since it is expected that this will happen. Please do not watch the examiner's face because this may interfere with the accuracy of the test. From this examination we can determine your *speech reception threshold*, which tells us how loud speech must be before you can barely understand it. On page 2 you will find an alphabetical list of the words that will be used. Please familiarize yourself with this list.

For the next tests you will be asked to listen closely and respond to some very soft tones in one ear. The test will be repeated in your other ear. As soon as you barely hear each tone please signal the clinician. You may be asked to press a button, raise your hand, or give a verbal response. There will be a series of such tones of different pitches, first in one ear and then in the other. Each time you are aware of a tone, even faintly, please signal. On the basis of this test we can determine your hearing levels for *air conduction* and *bone conduction*, so that we can draw your pure tone *audiogram*. The audiogram gives us information about how well your ears hear sounds across a wide range of pitches.

You will then be given a list of 50 one-syllable words, which you will be able to hear at a comfortable loudness level. Each word will be preceded by the phrase "Say the word . . . " You are asked merely to say the last word of the phrase. For example, if the examiner says "Say the word *boy*," you simply repeat *boy*. If you are not certain of the word please try to guess and repeat the word that it most sounds like. This test may be repeated at a louder level. This will give us your *speech discrimination* or word understanding score for each ear.

It may be necessary to introduce a continuous windlike noise into one ear while your other ear is being tested. This noise, while loud, is harmless, and will help to ensure that the ear not being tested does not take part in the test. Simply try to ignore the noise and concentrate on the test signal.

Another routine test will measure the movement of your eardrum. Your ear will first be examined with a special light called an otoscope. Then a tightly fitting plastic piece will be inserted into one ear. An earphone will be placed over your other ear. You will note the following sensations: a humming sound, a sensation of slight pressure, and a series of loud tones. There is no danger to your ears or to your hearing from this procedure. Although this test takes only a few minutes, it provides us with a great deal of information about your eardrum, your middle ear, and the nerves that go from the ear to the brain and back. This procedure is called *acoustic immittance* and requires only that you sit quietly. No response on your part is necessary.

The examining audiologist will be glad to answer any questions you might have regarding these instructions or the test results. These instructions will be explained in greater detail during the testing session.

Please feel free to ask questions at any time.

Thank you,

The words used to test your *speech reception threshold* will be taken from the following list. You do not need to memorize these words but please look over the list.

airplane	armchair
birthday	doormat
eardrum	farewell
iceberg	mousetrap
mushroom	northwest
playground	railroad
sidewalk	stairway
sunset	

AUTHORIZATION FOR RELEASE OF INFORMATION

Re: _____ , _____ , _____

          last name   *first name,*   *middle initial*

      I, the undersigned, authorize The University of Texas Speech and Hearing Center to acquire and/or release professional information from and to my physician and/or other professional personnel involved in the evaluation and management of requested services.

Signed: _____

_____

                                           date

      I, the undersigned, authorize The University of Texas Speech and Hearing Center to use information, photographs, sound recordings, video recordings, and other records or materials that have to do with my testing or therapy at this Center, for educational, scientific, or professional purposes.

Signed: _____

_____

                                         date

chapter four

Genetic Counseling

Shelley D. Smith

Research on a variety of genetic disorders continues to bring a broader understanding of the interrelationship between genetics and the auditory system. While genetic counseling is clearly an area involving information transfer, the information will be most readily received and understood when couched within the type of emotional support counseling advocated throughout this text. Toward this end, Dr. Smith stresses the need for audiologists to gain a greater understanding of genetic principles and genetic counseling as an adjunct to comprehensive patient care and referral.

> The deeper we get into reality, the more numerous will be the questions we cannot answer.
>
> *Spiritual Counsels and Letters*
> *of Baron Friedrick Von Hugel*
> (Douglas V. Steere ed.)

INTRODUCTION

Genetic evaluation and counseling involve the accurate diagnosis of the cause of hearing loss and the sharing of information on the genetic and medical aspects of the condition with the family. In order for this to occur, there should be close cooperation between the geneticist and clinicians in the hearing sciences. In addition, the audiologist in particular can serve as an important liaison between the patient and the geneticist, both preparatory to the genetic evaluation and to reinforce the counseling afterward. The purpose of this chapter is to review the basic principles behind the evaluation and counseling.

GENETIC FACTORS IN HEARING LOSS

Clearly, there are many different causes of hearing loss. It has been estimated by numerous researchers that about half of the cases of profound sensorineural hearing loss in children are due to genetic factors (Fraser, 1976; Morton, 1991). The genetic contribution to milder types of hearing loss or to late onset hearing loss is less studied, but is undoubtedly significant. For example, at least 70% of cases of otosclerosis have a clear genetic cause (Morrison & Bundey, 1970). Within genetic hearing loss, there are many different forms with different characteristics and modes of inheritance (Figure 4–1). In some of these, the hearing loss is part of a *syndrome* with associated physical or medical findings. Often these other characteristics are more serious than the hearing loss, and recognition of the syndrome can be important for treatment. Other cases are *nonsyndromic*, in that the responsible genes cause only hearing loss.

To briefly review, *genes* are the codes in the DNA (dioxyribonucleic acid) and serve as blueprints for growth, development, and function. DNA has a double helical structure; that is, it looks like a twisted ladder. The rungs of the DNA

FIGURE 4–1 Causes of Profound Congenital Deafness. The relative proportions reflect several different studies. See Morton (1991) for a review.

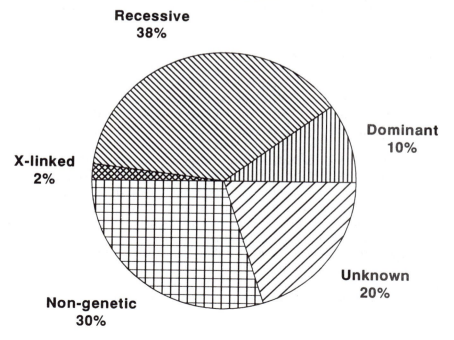

ladder are made of one of four bases, and the order of the bases down the ladder constitute the genetic code for proteins made by the cell. The genes are arranged linearly along the DNA molecule, and the molecules are packaged into separate *chromosomes*. There are 23 pairs of chromosomes in all, 22 pairs of *autosomes*, and one pair of *sex chromosomes*. One chromosome from each pair is inherited from the mother and the other from the father. Thus, all of the genes come in pairs. One chromosome from each pair is selected at random for inclusion into the egg or the sperm, so that, for each child, there is a 50-50 chance that a given chromosome will be passed on. Genetic disorders can be caused by errors at the gene level or at the chromosomal level.

For most genes there are different possible codes, called *alleles*. For example, a gene influencing eye color could have several possible alleles, each producing a different color. The term *genotype* refers to the alleles in a given pair, and *phenotype* refers to the physical outcome. If both of the alleles in the genotype are the same, the person is said to be *homozygous*; if they are different, the genotype is *heterozygous*. For the eye color example, the genotype for a person inheriting a blue color gene from each parent would be blue/blue (homozygous), and the phenotype, the resulting eye color, would be blue eyes. The genotype for a person inheriting a brown color gene from one parent and a blue color gene from the other would be blue/brown (heterozygous), and the phenotype may be hazel. If the phenotype in a heterozygote reflects only one of the two alleles, that allele is said to be *dominant*, and the other would be *recessive*. That is, if a person with a blue/brown genotype has brown eyes, the brown allele would be dominant, and the recessive blue allele would be expressed only in people with the homozygous blue/blue genotype. Since an individual with blue eyes would have inherited one blue allele from each parent, each parent must carry at least one blue allele.

Autosomal Recessive Inheritance

Many of the genetic syndromes with deafness are inherited in an autosomal recessive manner. About 80% of the cases of genetic congenital profound deafness are recessively inherited, with about half of these being syndromes with additional physical findings. Syndromes can be diagnosed either by specific laboratory tests or by recognition of a pattern of physical findings, but genetic nonsyndromic types of deafness can be very difficult to diagnose.

Generally, a child with a recessive hearing loss has two hearing parents, both heterozygous *carriers* of the recessive allele. With each pregnancy, there is a 25% chance that both parents will pass on the recessive allele and the child will be homozygous and have the hearing loss. Each hearing child would have two out of three chances of being a carrier. For the next generation, the chance that either the person with the hearing loss or the sibling that is a carrier would have a child with the same hearing loss would depend upon whether the spouse also carried the same gene, since the child would have to inherit the gene from each parent. Individually, these genes are rare in the general population, so as long as they do not marry a relative, the chance of hearing loss in the next generation would be small. The exception to this would be that often deaf people choose to marry other deaf people. If two deaf people with exactly the same genes for recessive hearing loss have a child, all of their children would be deaf. If they have different forms of deafness, even if they are recessively inherited, all of their children would be hearing. Since there are many different forms of recessive nonsyndromic deafness, and at this time they are indistinguishable, it cannot be determined whether two parents have the same type until after they have had a child.

If the hearing loss is nonsyndromic, or the physical features of a syndrome do not appear until later in life, the only way to determine that the cause is genetic may be through the family history; either another sibling or very close relative with the same condition, or relatedness (*consanguinity*) between the parents. However, when families are small, it is quite likely that they will not have a second deaf child, since the chance would only be 25% for each pregnancy. Thus, even when recessive inheritance is the cause of the hearing loss, the family history is usually negative, so many nonsyndromic recessive cases go undiagnosed even after an extensive evaluation. In that case, it is impossible to determine whether a hearing couple with one child with deafness of unknown etiology has a 25% chance of recurrence in future children.

Autosomal Dominant Inheritance

With dominant inheritance, only one gene in the pair needs to code for a condition in order for the person to show the condition phenotypically. In nearly all cases, people with a dominant form of hearing loss are heterozygous; that is, they have one allele for hearing loss and one allele for hearing. This is partially because the genes are rare in the population and it is unlikely that both parents would have the same dominant condition and both pass the allele to a child. Also, although theoretically a person who is homozygous for a dominant condition should be no different from one who is heterozygous, for many conditions this is not the case. The homozygous person may be much more severely affected, or the condition may be lethal, producing a miscarriage.

In a fully dominant hearing loss, the hearing loss usually can be seen going from generation to generation. One parent will have the condition, and each child would have a 50-50 chance of inheriting it. However, there can be exceptions to this pattern. Some dominant genes are not fully *penetrant;* that is, they do not always show up phenotypically in the heterozygous person. When this happens, the gene may appear to "skip" generations. The gene does not actually skip, since it has been transmitted faithfully, but the phenotype may not be present, due to the influence of other genetic or environmental factors. This can complicate genetic counseling. For example, it may be thought that a hearing person who has a parent with a dominant form of deafness did not inherit the deafness gene and would have no chance of passing it on to his or her own child; but if the gene is actually present but not penetrant, there would actually be a 50% chance that the child could inherit it. Yet there would still be a chance that it would be non-penetrant in that child, so that while the chance of transmission would be 50%, the actual chance of deafness would be less.

Another complication of some dominantly inherited syndromes is variable *expression*. This means that there can be different phenotypic manifestations of the gene, and an individual with the gene may show one or more of the signs. Waardenburg syndrome is a classic example of a condition with variable expression, since a person with the gene may have one or more of the four major signs: deafness, white forelock, heterochromia (different-colored eyes), or dystopia canthorum (placement of the inner corners of the eyes closer to the pupils). The geneticist has to be aware of all of the possible manifestations in order to recognize the presence of the gene in the family.

It is also possible for a person to have a dominant disorder when neither parent has the gene, through the process of new *mutation*. Mutations occur at a low but consistent rate in everyone, but often the changes are in insignificant parts of the genetic material and are not noticed, or they may be recessive. In some cases, though, a random mutation can change a "normal" gene into one producing a dominant syndromic or nonsyndromic hearing loss. In this case, the chance that the parents would have another child with hearing loss would be quite low, but the child would have a 50% chance of passing the gene on to his or her children. In a deaf child with hearing parents, differentiating the situation of new mutation from nonpenetrance (or even nonpaternity) can be difficult, and again the correct diagnosis may go undetected.

X-Linked Inheritance

As mentioned above, one pair of chromosomes is termed the sex chromosomes. Females have two *X chromosomes*, while males have one X and one smaller *Y chromosome*. The X chromosome carries many genes with a variety of functions, while the Y primarily carries the code for producing a male. Genes on the X chromosome are termed *X-linked*, and among them are several recessive alleles that cause hearing loss. If a female has one of these alleles on one X, the normal dominant allele on the other X can counteract it. However, if that allele occurs on the X in a male, his Y chromosome does not have a corresponding gene, and the recessive gene can show up. If a woman is heterozygous for an X-linked form of hearing loss, she will have normal hearing and is a carrier. Each of her sons would have a 50% chance of inheriting the hearing loss, and each daughter would have a 50% chance of being a carrier. When a male with X-linked hearing loss has children, his sons would not have the hearing loss (since they would have had to inherit his Y to be a male) and all of his daughters would be carriers. This produces a very characteristic pattern of inheritance in a family, where only males have hearing loss, they are related through hearing females (e.g., two male cousins whose mothers are sisters), and there is no male-to-male transmission.

As with the other modes of inheritance, there can be difficulties in recognizing X-linked recessive conditions. By chance, a boy may not have any affected male relatives, so the family history would be negative even though the gene has been present in several women. It is also possible for a male to have an X-linked recessive condition as the result of a new mutation.

Chromosomal Syndromes

In some cases a genetic condition can result from an error at the chromosomal level, where there is extra or missing chromosomal material. These are generally detected by doing a *karyotype*, in which cells (usually from blood) are cultured and the chromosomes are studied under a microscope. As a rule when the autosomes are involved, the larger the chromosome material involved, the more serious the syndrome. For example, Down syndrome is caused by extra material from chromosome 21, either an entire chromosome or certain critical parts of it. The term *trisomy* refers to an entire extra (third copy) of a chromosome. Trisomies for other, larger chromosomes are more severe, and most are not compatible with life, resulting in early miscarriage. Babies with trisomy 13 and trisomy 18 may live to birth and a few may live a number of years, but are more severely involved physically and cognitively than children with Down syndrome. Abnormalities of the sex chromosomes are less severe and may even be unnoticed, as in boys with an extra Y chromosome. At least one X chromosome must be present, however.

Parts of chromosomes may be *deleted* or *duplicated*, with the physical findings depending upon exactly what part of a chromosome is involved. Individually these abnormalities are usually quite rare. If a baby is found to have a chromosomal abnormality, a literature search will probably be necessary to see if any other children have been described with the same or similar abnormality in order to determine what types of problems may be expected in the future. In some cases where there is extra chromosome material it may be difficult to determine which chromosome it came from, or in some cases the deleted or added material may be so small that it is difficult to see with microscopic studies. Newer molecular methods will be able to help resolve these diagnostic difficulties.

In cases where there is an entire extra chromosome, the parents' chromosomes are generally normal and the recurrence risk is 1% or less, unless the mother is over age 40. For some reason, the chance of a conception with an abnormal number of chromosomes increases in any woman as she gets older. Where there are duplications or deletions, both parents need to have chromosome testing, since one could carry a "balanced" rearrangement, in which all of the chromosomal material is present, but part of a chromosome has been moved (translocated) to another chromosome. In this case, there is a chance that another baby could be born with only one of the rearranged chromosomes (unbalanced).

It is very important that the family understands the type of chromosomal abnormality in the child, and that difficulty in identifying the abnormality or in finding reports of children with similar problems can make it very difficult for us to make predictions.

After their baby girl was born, the family's pediatrician was concerned that the facial features were unusual, and a karyotype was requested. This showed that there was a small piece of extra material on chromosome 18, but the microscopic study could not identify which chromosome this extra piece came from. Thus, she was "partially trisomic" for an unknown segment of chromosome. We saw the family in clinic when the baby was 3 months old. She was growing well and did not have significant health problems, although development was slightly delayed. We explained that, since the extra piece of chromosome could not be identified, we could not make exact predictions on how she would do in the future, but that most children with extra chromosome material have at least some physical and cognitive delays. We encouraged them to enroll her for the school-sponsored infant stimulation services to help maximize her potential. Several weeks later, I received a telephone call from the mother, who was quite distraught at some information she had received from a school librarian who had offered to do a computerized search for her. Unfortunately, the librarian had searched under "Trisomy 18," and those reports predicted a very bleak outcome. I was able to reassure the mother that the information was not appropriate for her child, and that we had no reason to believe that she would be as seriously affected. The girl has continued to be somewhat delayed, but does not appear to be severely retarded.

This example illustrates two problems. First of all, we were not able to tell the family exactly what to expect in the future, since we could not compare their daughter's chromosomal abnormality with any in the literature. This was naturally frustrating to the family, and they accepted the librarian's offer of help. However, the terminology used in chromosomal abnormalities can be confusing, and an error in interpretation led to very misleading information.

Multifactorial Inheritance

Some genetic conditions appear to be caused by a combination of several genes and nongenetic factors that determine susceptibility. The classic example has been cleft lip and palate, which was thought to be due to the additive effect of many genes. More recent studies suggest that only a few genes are involved, and it may be that most "multifactorial" conditions are actually due to single genes with reduced penetrance. However, since the factors that influence penetrance may include other genes, the distinction between the two models blurs. In practice, the chances of recurrence of a multifactorial condition are determined empirically, and are generally low, on the order of 5% if the family history is negative.

GENETIC EVALUATION

Families may come to a geneticist for a number of reasons. They may want to know the cause of the hearing loss, whether it is likely to progress, whether there are any associated physical or medical problems currently present or that may develop in the future, and what the chance is that the hearing loss or syndrome will occur again in the family. The purpose of the genetic evaluation is to try to identify the cause of the hearing loss. Without the correct diagnosis, it is very difficult to give an accurate answer to the family's questions about cause, prognosis, and recurrence.

A genetic evaluation is usually done by a team. Generally there is a clinical geneticist with an M.D. and a genetic counselor with a master's degree or a nurse with training in genetics, plus any other consultants specializing in the condition the client has. Previous medical records are reviewed, and the genetic counselor takes a detailed medical and family history. This history generally covers at least three generations, including medical and physical information on grandparents, aunts, uncles, and cousins, as well as parents and siblings. The extent of the family history will depend upon the suspected diagnosis. Because of the possibility of variable expression of a genetic syndrome, the person taking the family history has to be familiar with the various manifestations of the syndromes and must be sure to ask the appropriate questions. A family who has a deaf child may think it very strange when the geneticist asks them if they have any relatives with one blue eye and one brown eye, but this question is necessary if Waardenburg syndrome is suspected! Records may be requested on other family members as well, or they may be asked to come to the clinic for examination.

The clinical geneticist does a thorough physical evaluation looking for signs of a genetic syndrome. These signs may be quite distinctive, leading to the immediate diagnosis of a syndrome, or they may be very subtle, and the geneticist must recognize what physical features are important and which ones are part of normal variation. Often a given physical feature occurs at a low frequency in the general population, but attains significance if found in combination with other specific features.

A 5-year-old boy was referred to the genetics clinic for a moderate hearing loss of unknown etiology, which had just been diagnosed. He came in with his mother and 4-year-old sister. The mother told me that she suspected that her husband also had a hearing loss, but he refused to have his hearing tested. As I started to take the family history, the mother interrupted me with a question. "You know, my son has a little pit in front of his ear, and so does his father. The doctors have told me that it doesn't mean anything, that lots of people have them, but I think it must be related." She was quite pleased when we agreed with her. We explained that isolated ear pits can occur in the general population, but that when they occur with hearing loss, it can be a sign of autosomal dominant inheritance, and can be part of the branchio oto renal syndrome. This syndrome is quite variable, but can include ear or cervical pits, hearing loss, and kidney problems. We recommended that both children have renal ultrasounds, and that her daughter also have her hearing tested, even though she did not have the pits. We made the same recommendations for their father and his siblings. The renal ultrasounds on both children were normal, but it was found that the daughter had a hearing loss very similar to her brother's. The father still declined testing, but the paternal grandmother had her hearing tested and hearing loss was confirmed.

Depending upon the findings in the history and examination, specific medical or laboratory tests may be done to reach a diagnosis. For example, in the case of a single child with a profound hearing loss and vestibular dysfunction, an ophthalmological examination (including an electroretinogram if the child is old enough to cooperate) should be done to rule out Usher syndrome Type I, in which retinitis pigmentosa develops in adolescence. A CAT (computerized axial tomography) scan of the inner ear may be done to rule out a cochlear malformation, or renal studies may be done, since there are a number of syndromes that involve hearing loss and kidney problems. It will often be recommended that both parents and any other siblings should have hearing tests.

GENETIC COUNSELING

When all of the information has been gathered, the interpretation is given to the parents. If a diagnosis has been made, the condition and its medical and genetic implications are reviewed. As has been discussed above, however, situations such as singleton nonsyndromic recessive hearing loss, new dominant mutation, or a previously undescribed collection of physical findings can complicate the ability to give an accurate diagnosis or chance of recurrence. Unfortunately, lack of diagnosis is not uncommon in clinical genetics. Regarding the subspecialty of dysmorphology (the study of birth defects) a prominent dysmorphologist, Gorlin (1991), has stated:

> There is probably no other area of endeavor in which failure to diagnose is accepted as the norm. Could one practice surgery or civil engineering or law and fail so often, yet be considered an expert? Under no circumstances! Nevertheless, it has been demonstrated repeatedly that the best of us has no greater than a 20% overall rate of success. Surely it must be the only field in which one can perform so dismally yet be considered competent (p. vii).

In cases when the cause of the hearing loss cannot be identified, the reasons for the lack of diagnosis should be explained to the family. Often, the geneticist will want to follow up in a year or so to see if there are any medical changes that may reveal a syndrome, or if there are any new medical or genetic discoveries in the literature that might give a diagnosis. The audiologist can be an important adjunct in the process by referring the family back to the geneticist if any medical or audiological changes are noted. Even in situations where the diagnosis is unknown, it may be possible to give estimates of the chance of recurrence based on previous population studies.

A number of studies of nonsyndromic deafness have been done to determine the proportion of genetic cases and the chance of recurrence (Smith, 1991), and the resulting figures have been fairly consistent among studies. When both parents are hearing, the family history is negative, and their first child is profoundly deaf, the chance of recurrence in a second child is about 10%. This would reflect an average between the probability that the cause is autosomal recessive, with an actual chance of recurrence of 25%, and the probability that the cause was not genetic or was due to a new mutation, with a very low chance of recurrence. The fact that the figure is an estimate must be explained to the family, and it would need to be revised after the next child is born. If the next or any subsequent child is born deaf, it would be presumed that the actual cause is autosomal recessive inheritance (assuming that a separate cause of deafness is not identified) with a chance of recurrence of 25%. If the second child is hearing, the estimate for deafness in a third child would decrease to about 7%, reflecting the somewhat greater probability that the actual cause has a low chance of recurrence (Bieber & Nance, 1979).

When one parent has nonsyndromic deafness and the other is hearing, the chance that their first child would be deaf is about 7%; but once a deaf child has been born to the couple, the most likely explanation is that the deaf parent has a dominant form of deafness, and the estimated chance of recurrence in a subsequent child goes up to 40% (Bieber & Nance, 1979). The chance of deafness is not fully 50%, since the gene could have reduced penetrance.

If both parents are deaf, and the cause is unknown for each of them, the chance that their first child will be deaf is about 10%. If the child is hearing, the chance of deafness in the next child is even lower; if the child is deaf, the chance increases to about 60%, since it is possible that both parents have the same form of recessive deafness and the actual chance of deafness is 100%. If there is at least one deaf child and one hearing child, the most likely explanation is that one parent has a dominant gene, and this is reflected in the estimated chance of recurrence of about 33% (Bieber & Nance, 1979).

The purpose of genetic counseling is not just to give medical and genetic information, but also to support the family as they deal with the information. The standard for geneticists is to be nondirective as much as possible (Ad Hoc Committee on Genetic Counseling, 1975); that is, to empower the family to make decisions that are in accord with their own situation and beliefs. In practice, it is recognized that it is impossible for a counselor to be completely impartial, and that subconsciously the counselor's own biases may influence the way the information is presented to the family. This can be especially dangerous if the counselor is not familiar with the deaf community and culture, and assumes that a couple is concerned about the "risk" of deafness, when in actuality they may just be curious about the chances of deafness in their offspring, or may prefer to have a deaf child. For that reason, the geneticist, and audiologist as well, should be careful not to use potentially pejorative terms such as *recurrence risk, disorder, handicap*, or *abnormal gene.*

Not only are there ethical reasons for giving the family accurate and complete genetic information, but there are also legal risks if the information is not provided. In one malpractice suit, professionals were sued when deafness was not diagnosed in a child before their second child was also born deaf (Pelias, 1986). Presumably, if they had known that the first child was deaf, they could have been made aware that there was a chance that the second child could also be deaf. In the same way, failure to accurately diagnose a syndrome that has potential medical complications or for which prenatal diagnosis would be available could also put a clinician in legal jeopardy. Documentation of the evaluation must be placed in the medical chart, and the family's consent is often sought to release the information to their local physician as well. To ensure that the family understands and remembers the counseling, a copy of the report or a letter written in lay language is also sent to them. An example of such a letter to hearing parents of a deaf child is included in Appendix 4–1; however, each letter will have to be tailored to the family's specific questions and to their level of understanding of genetic principles.

ISSUES IN GENETIC COUNSELING

The types of questions and problems that arise in genetic counseling in hearing-impaired individuals and their families will depend on the consultand (the person seeking counseling) and the type of hearing loss. Whether the consultand is hearing or deaf may have a great influence on his or her view of hearing loss and decision to seek genetic counseling. Factors such as age of onset, degree of loss, family history of hearing loss, and whether the condition is syndromic or non-syndromic also affect the perception of "burden" of the condition (including the possibility that it is not seen as a burden at all). Even in situations where the diagnosis, prognosis, and chance of recurrence are equal, individuals will differ in the questions they feel are important and their responses to the information. With that in mind, the following examples are given to illustrate the situations that can occur.

Hearing Parents with a Child with Congenital, Profound, Nonsyndromic Deafness

To begin with, it is often difficult for families and professionals to realize that the etiology of deafness in this situation can be genetic, and that a genetic evaluation is appropriate. If genetic principles are not understood, the absence of a positive family history can lead them to assume that the deafness is not inherited. Parents may examine every illness the child had before the deafness was detected, or any possible complication of pregnancy or delivery, in an effort to identify a cause. Along with this can come feelings of guilt and blame (depending upon the parent's perception of the deafness): if only the illness had been cured, if only the mother hadn't taken that medication, and so on. Although a genetic evaluation may not identify a precise cause (and the complications in determining the etiology in this situation have already been described), it may be possible to rule out other causes, and the possibility of a genetic cause can be raised. This has its own potential to create feelings of guilt, but we will often try to help the family see genes as random and impartial, and not something that could have been controlled. It may also be pointed out we all carry recessive genes that can cause serious medical problems in our children. The risk that the child will actually have one of these problems is solely a matter of chance, the chance that our spouse carries the same gene and the chance that both happen to pass it on to the child. Rather than taking responsibility for events they could not have controlled, the parents can be supported in exploring constructive ways to accept the deafness and help their child with any problems it may pose.

When it is not possible to establish a diagnosis, the family is left in an uncomfortable position. While it may be helpful to realize that a number of conditions with serious medical problems may have been ruled out by the evaluation, they are still left without answers to their questions. Instead, they have a wide range of complicated possibilities, each with a statistical probability: autosomal recessive inheritance, new dominant mutation, and, if the child is a boy, X-linked inheritance; along with an equal possibility that the cause is largely nongenetic. Estimates of the chance of recurrence can be given, but it must be clear that these are estimates and will change with changes in the family.

Finally, the family's perception of the risks will depend on how they see the "burden" of deafness.

A young hearing couple from an urban area suspected that their 1-year-old son had a hearing problem, and audiological studies confirmed that he was deaf. The pregnancy had gone well, the child had been healthy, and no one else in the family was deaf, so this was totally unexpected, and the parents were devastated. After an extensive medical and genetic evaluation, no cause could be identified. The family understood that there was a possibility that the cause could be recessive, with a 25% chance of recurrence. They became excellent advocates for their son and were active in the school system and with other parents of deaf children. He progressed well in school and in communication skills, and had a good self-image. Still, they waited 10 years before they felt they could try another pregnancy. The next child, a girl, had an ABR (Auditory Brainstem Response) while still in the newborn nursery, and this showed that she was also profoundly deaf. Again, the parents were devastated. However, they have continued to work with her and in the community, and both children have done well.

This family was a model for how one might want the parents to react; they were active and supportive of their son without being obsessively involved, and they had a close relationship with him. It would be easy to assume erroneously that the acceptance of their son and his deafness would mean that they would not be concerned if another child was born deaf.

A rural family had a 3-year-old deaf son. It has taken some effort, but they had obtained educational services for him, and he was progressing in his communication skills. When the family came to the genetics clinic, the mother was already pregnant with her second child. The genetic evaluation did not identify a diagnosis, and in the counseling session I told them that the chance could be 25% that the child she was carrying could also be deaf. Her response was, "Well, we've already learned sign language—it wouldn't be any problem to sign to this child, too." The second child was born hearing, and they named him "Tom," which they felt would be easy for their deaf son to say.

This illustrates the range of reactions people have, and that the counselor should not prejudge. I had been quite worried about telling this mother about the chance of recurrence in her unborn baby, since my previous experience had been that hearing couples often were upset by the possibility of recurrence. However, this could raise another question: Was this family's reaction a symptom of denial, or a sign of adjustment?

Acceptance of Deafness

The acceptance of the risk of having a second deaf child has sometimes been taken as an indication of whether the family has fully accepted the first child. Does a family's unwillingness to take that risk negate the value of the deaf child? Or is the first family described above especially honest with their own feelings and abilities to take on the challenges a second time? The second family may be showing better adjustment to the deafness, or they may not fully perceive the needs that their deaf child will have. The counselor (audiologist or geneticist) has to remember that the family's perception of the risk of deafness will depend upon the family's own background, expectations, and abilities, and we need to be sensitive to these differences and to be able to support the family without judgments as to whether their reaction reflects "acceptance" in our eyes.

The issue of acceptance can be taken even further, though, into an area where many geneticists are very uncomfortable. What if prenatal diagnosis becomes available for deafness? What would the use of such a test in a second pregnancy, and even the termination of the pregnancy, say about the value of the first child, or about deaf people in general? Certainly, deafness is not a life-threatening condition, and many deaf individuals would assert that it is not even life-limiting. However, in the course of studies to determine the genetic cause of deafness, the ability to diagnose prenatally will arise, even if it is not the purpose of the research. Should this test be denied to a family who asks for it? Legally, can it be denied?

Clarke (1991) and others have pointed out the serious dilemmas and contradictions facing geneticists when we try to decide who should have access to prenatal diagnosis, even though it seems that these decisions must be made. Most geneticists will decline to do prenatal diagnosis solely for selection of sex; yet in an era where a pregnancy can be legally terminated for no more reason than inconvenient timing, can information that would influence the decision for termination be withheld? Can counseling be truly nondirective if the counselor makes a conscious decision whether to inform a family of the possibility of prenatal diagnosis? In the current legal climate, doesn't the family have the right to complete information, and the autonomy to make a decision based on that information? On the other hand, it has been my impression that most geneticists, especially those who have worked with deafness, would find it very difficult to be "nondirective" in such a case, and are themselves very much opposed to termination of a pregnancy solely for the indication of deafness. These are pressing ethical problems, and no answers have been found. Analogous situations arise now, when comparatively minor sex chromosomal abnormalities are found in the course of prenatal diagnosis for more serious conditions. Generally the approach has been to describe the implications of the abnormality completely enough so that the family understands that the condition could be quite minor, but to still leave the decision of termination up to them. To withhold the information would leave the geneticist in legal jeopardy.

Adult with Congenital Profound Deafness

It has been recognized for many years that deaf people often do not receive genetic services (Nance, 1971). Part of this may be due to lack of information that the person's deafness may be genetic and that genetic evaluation is available, but it is also true that deaf people may avoid geneticists. Many people in the general public have the misconception that a genetic counselor is going to tell them whether they should have children, and deaf people in particular may share this, especially since there were individuals in the "eugenics" movement around the turn of the century who did discourage intermarriage among deaf people.

Another reason deaf people may not request genetic services was articulated in a recent workshop on genetics and hearing loss at the Eighth International Congress of Human Genetics in 1991. A deaf speaker expressed the opinion that deaf people who sought genetic counseling had not fully accepted their own deafness; if they had, they would not care whether their child was deaf or hearing. Still, when counseling has been offered by geneticists who are familiar with deafness and the deaf culture and can communicate with deaf people, deaf adults have sought counseling (Arnos, Israel, & Cunningham, 1991). As in any other population, the reasons for desiring genetic information are quite varied.

Two young people who were engaged to be married came in for counseling. The woman was deaf from birth and had a deaf brother, so it was assumed that the cause of her deafness was autosomal recessive. Her fiance was deaf following meningitis at age 2. They were quite concerned when they received the information that the chance was very small that their children would be deaf. How would the child learn to communicate with speech, when they both used sign? I reassured them that, while the child might use sign as a "native language," there would be ample opportunities through such things as television, preschool, and hearing friends and family for the child to learn to speak well.

A deaf couple from a rural area had two deaf children. They came to the clinic to learn the chance that their next child would be deaf, and if anything could be done to maximize the chance of a hearing child. The family history was compatible with autosomal recessive inheritance for both of them, so it was explained that the chance could be as high as 100% that their other children would also be deaf. In their area there were virtually no other deaf adults their age, and very few other deaf children, so they saw deafness as a limitation to their interaction with the surrounding community. We discussed the hope that attitudes were changing and that there were more opportunities in education and employment for their children. We also discussed the current limitations of genetic research to reverse deafness. As part of a multidisciplinary educational evaluation for their children, they were also able to talk with a psychologist about their feelings.

For some families, a one-time genetic counseling session cannot provide the support that they need, and it is important to find someone locally who can follow up with them. For this family, it would also be helpful to try to connect them with organizations for deaf adults, even if they were not located in their own community.

A young woman with Waardenburg syndrome came in to the genetics clinic to get information on the condition. Although she had known the name of the syndrome for many years, she did not know the genetic mechanism and was very interested in the explanation of genes and dominant inheritance. She was also very interested to learn which physical features were part of the syndrome. We discussed that the gene for one form of Waardenburg syndrome had been localized, and she was quite indignant that geneticists might want to use this information to "cure" her deafness, as she said. On the other hand, she had been told in the past that she should not marry a man with Waardenburg syndrome because there would be a chance that they would have a child with serious birth defects, and she did see this as a problem (the actual risk for this has not been established, but is theoretically possible that the homozygote could have serious physical defects).

This woman came from an extensive deaf family and was active in the deaf community in her area. She identified with her deafness and her culture rather than seeing it as a handicapping condition. Genetics for her was primarily of interest intellectually, except for the possibility that she might have a child who would have problems that she did see as handicapping.

These families saw deafness and recurrence in their children quite differently, as could be expected from any group of people coming from very different backgrounds. Their own experiences are going to influence how they accept their own deafness and whether they are concerned about the presence or absence of deafness in their children.

Adult Onset Deafness

In general, deaf or hard-of-hearing adults who were previously hearing see their deafness quite differently from congenitally deaf adults. They are not part of a deaf community, but see themselves as being excluded from the hearing community. They often come to a geneticist hoping that genetic research has found a way to cure or stop the progression of the hearing loss. Many forms of progressive nonsyndromic hearing loss are autosomal dominant, so their children are at 50% risk, but at this time a test does not exist to detect the gene presymptomatically except possibly in some large families. As a result, the parents may feel helpless in their inability to stop the hearing loss in their children.

A young father from a small town was referred to the genetics clinic because he had a moderate to severe progressive hearing loss and his son had just been identified with a mild hearing loss. The father's mother also had a hearing loss, but it had not been noted until she was in her late 40s. The father, who was in his 20s, had recently obtained hearing aids. He had felt very uncomfortable wearing his hearing aids in public in his hometown because he had never seen a young person with hearing aids, and had felt that his condition was very unusual. While in a fast-food restaurant in Omaha, he had been quite surprised to see another man his age also wearing hearing aids. He also felt very guilty that his son had apparently inherited the hearing loss from him. He was relieved when we told him that we had seen many adults with hearing loss, and that the type of dominant progressive hearing loss that appeared to be in his family was not uncommon. We were able to put him in touch with organizations for hard-of-hearing adults so that he could get their newsletters and make connections within the state. Further testing of his family showed that his brother was also developing a hearing loss, and he was referred to an audiologist for follow-up. Although he still felt bad that his son had a hearing loss, the genetic explanation helped the father feel less guilty about it, and he realized that his attitude could be a good model for his son to follow in accepting the hearing loss. The family also volunteered to participate in research to identify genes causing dominant progressive hearing loss.

A family with otosclerosis was asked about their attitudes toward the condition and how geneticists could be of help to them. The family members, a mother and her four adult children, all felt that otosclerosis was a significant problem in their lives. While they wanted to know the genetic basis and the chance that their children would also develop otosclerosis, they were much more desirous that genetic research would find a way to "eradicate" the gene from their family. I explained to them that, while genetic research may find ways to prevent the hearing loss through correction of a gene or a gene product within the ear itself, at this time geneticists are reluctant to change a gene in the germ line; that is, to alter a gene that is going to be passed on to future generations. We do not know the entire function of each gene, and it is possible that it is important in some other part of development, or could provide an important function in future generations that is not required in our current environment. The family was comfortable with this explanation, and we discussed the importance of early detection and potentials for prevention in the future.

Syndromic Deafness

In cases where deafness is part of a syndrome, the associated medical problems can compound the problems posed by the deafness, or they may be much more serious than the deafness itself. In fact, hearing loss may go unnoticed in children with multiple handicaps, and it is important that they be tested well to be sure that an untreated hearing loss is not adding to their difficulties.

The counseling problems presented by a genetic syndrome will vary according to the syndrome itself. Usher syndrome can be used as an example. Usher syndrome Type I involves congenital profound deafness and vestibular dysfunction, with subsequent development of progressive visual loss due to retinitis pigmentosa in adolescence. (Usher syndrome Type II is similar except that the hearing loss is less severe and vestibular function is normal.) Both types are inherited as autosomal recessive traits. Since the signs of retinitis pigmentosa do not appear until the child is older, the deafness initially appears to be non-syndromic. The family will not know that their child has a recessive form of deafness, let alone that the additional vision problem will develop. While they may be willing to accept a possible 25% chance of deafness, the combination of both deafness and vision loss is usually seen as a much greater burden, and a 25% risk of Usher syndrome may be seen as unacceptable. Unfortunately, the second child may be born before the first child is diagnosed as having Usher syndrome. It is important that the possibility of Usher syndrome is raised in any child with deafness of unknown etiology, and that the family is encouraged to follow up with an ophthalmologist. An electroretinogram (ERG) may be done, and certainly the family should be advised to look for signs of nightblindness, restricted peripheral vision, or sensitivity to light. Since there is currently no treatment for retinitis pigmentosa, the question has been raised as to when a screening for Usher syndrome should be done. Would an early diagnosis unnecessarily stigmatize a young child, when there would be no difference in treatment? Clearly, the ability to give an accurate genetic diagnosis is one argument for early detection. Also, the gradual development of nightblindness can be unnoticed by teenagers, and they may put themselves in danger by walking or driving at night. It has also been argued that early diagnosis can give the child the opportunity to accept and prepare for an adult life with decreasing vision. However, not all families may accept that view.

A routine ophthalmological evaluation of a 10-year-old girl with profound congenital deafness revealed the first signs of retinitis pigmentosa, and the diagnosis was confirmed by an ERG. She was not aware of any symptoms. The parents were told of the diagnosis of Usher syndrome and the disease was described in detail. They elected to tell two of the girl's teachers, but despite the concerns of the geneticist and the other professionals involved with the girl, the family decided not to tell their daughter or any other professionals in their home community. A few family members were told. The family was given information regarding Usher syndrome and was encouraged to contact other organizations such as the Retinitis Pigmentosa Foundation and Gallaudet College. They declined further genetic follow-up and did not inform their daughter of the diagnosis until she noted the symptoms herself. The family then attended a summer program on Usher syndrome at Gallaudet, and I understand that the girl is adjusting well, although I have not had further contact with the family.

This was a frustrating situation for the counselor involved, but she respected the parents' wishes and provided the information they requested. Fortunately, she could also ensure that other support systems were put in place.

The preceding examples have been given to illustrate the wide range of feelings and attitudes families have when they come to a geneticist, and the different reactions they may have to the information. It is impossible, then, to give definite recommendations on what should and should not be said to families, except that the counselor, whether audiologist or geneticist, needs to be sensitive to the possible differences. This idea was brought out very strongly at the 1991 March of Dimes/Birth Defects meeting where there was a symposium on Huntington's chorea, a dominant disorder of progressive neurological deterioration that starts in adulthood. Five young adults at risk for the disease were asked what a geneticist could say that would help a person in their situation. They all responded that, as they were all different people, no one thing would have meaning for all of them. It was more important that the counselor be available and willing to listen, and to try to help them with their own unique problems. The audiologist and geneticist also have to realize when the difficulties require more extensive help than they are able to give, and when they must explore other resources for referral.

COOPERATION BETWEEN GENETICISTS AND OTHER PROFESSIONALS

In the genetic evaluation of a hearing-impaired individual, it is vital that the geneticist work closely with audiologists and other professionals who deal directly with clients and their families. To begin with, it is usually the audiologist or otolaryngologist who makes the diagnosis of hearing loss and is in the best position to refer the family to the geneticist.

The indications for referral to geneticists are quite broad. Certainly it is more likely that a diagnosis will be reached when there are distinct physical features that suggest a genetic syndrome, but this should not be the only guideline, since many genetic forms are nonsyndromic. Similarly, positive family history cannot be taken as the sole criteria. Genetic hearing loss can be congenital or late onset, sensorineural or conductive, progressive or stable, bilateral or unilateral, so one cannot go by the characteristics of the hearing loss. Referral to a geneticist is justified in any person who has a hearing loss of unknown etiology. In fact, one should be careful to critically examine the presumed etiology unless it has been well documented.

A 6-year-old boy who was referred to the genetics clinic had a high frequency sensorineural hearing loss. He had been scheduled for genetics as part of a multidisciplinary evaluation, and the parents wondered if they really needed to be seen by a geneticist. They explained to me that the hearing loss was the result of trauma at birth, and it was noted in the medical record that the birth had indeed been traumatic, with shoulder dystocia that resulted in temporary paralysis of the arm. The father also had a high frequency hearing loss, but had been first noted when he was in ninth grade, and had been attributed to a blow to the ears shortly before the hearing loss was diagnosed. Audiological testing showed that the configuration of hearing loss was very similar between father and son, and the family history further showed that a maternal uncle of the father's also was reported to have had a hearing loss. On that basis, a CAT scan of the temporal bone was done on the son, and he was found to have a Mondini malformation of the cochlea. A CAT scan on the father revealed a similar malformation. His mother had normal hearing and a normal CAT scan, but an old audiogram from the decreased uncle showed the same configuration as those from father and son. Instead of being nongenetic, it appeared that the cause of the hearing loss in this family was an autosomal dominant gene with reduced penetrance. The family found this explanation to be fascinating, and the mother felt less guilty about the difficult delivery.

There are also times when genetic counseling is indicated even when the cause is known to be nongenetic. Usually the genetic information is given to the parents when the children are young, and it may not be conveyed to the children as they reach adulthood. This was pointed out to me quite clearly when a 15-year-old boy who was deaf following meningitis at age 2 asked me if there was a chance his children would be deaf. Although his parents knew that the cause of his deafness was not genetic, no one had talked with him about it. I explained that they would not inherit deafness from him, but that the chance of having deaf children would depend upon whether his future wife would be deaf and what the cause would be. In addition, a geneticist can also explain the nongenetic mechanism and implications of conditions such as congenital rubella (Arnos et al., 1991).

For the legal reasons cited above, it may be especially important that each appropriate family is informed that genetic evaluation is available, and that the referral be documented in the patient's chart. For example, the notation of the discussion with the patient can be made in an audiological report for the medical chart, in a letter to the referring physician or agency, or in the "recommendations" section of the audiogram itself, depending upon the practices in the audiology clinic.

In discussing the genetic referral with the family, it is very helpful if the audiologist can explain the purpose of the evaluation, the type of information that will probably be requested, and the possible outcome, along with the information that counseling is nondirective. The genetics clinic may be able to provide brochures or handouts that explain the evaluation.

Geneticists also need to rely on the expertise of the audiologist and physician in determining the significance of various findings. For example, if the parent of a child with profound hearing loss is found to have a high-frequency hearing loss, the geneticist needs to consult the hearing professionals to determine if the parent's loss could be due to noise or some other factor, or if it could be a clue to a genetic factor. In trying to compare serial audiograms or audiograms between relatives, the geneticist needs the audiologist's expertise in determining if differences are due to acceptable error or if they are significant.

Although geneticists try to make themselves available to families after the evaluation is completed, this may be difficult if the family lives some distance from the clinic. The audiologist is likely to be in more direct contact with the family, and may be in a position to help reinforce the basic principles of the genetic counseling if the family has questions or is confused, and can help to identify a problem that would require follow-up by the geneticist.

CONCLUSION

Genetic factors cause a significant proportion of cases of hearing loss. The types of hearing loss run the gamut from congenital to adult onset, mild to profound, progressive or stable, sloping or flat, syndromic or nonsyndromic, and all of the major genetic modes of transmission are represented. Determining the cause of the hearing loss in an individual case can be quite difficult. When a diagnosis is made, the family can be given information on the genetic basis, the prognosis, and the chance that it could occur in other family members. Even when cause remains unknown, useful information can be conveyed to the family through genetic counseling.

Audiologists can be an important part of the genetic evaluation process. They are often in a very good position to refer the family to a geneticist and to explain the purpose of the referral to them. They can provide valuable information on the nature of the hearing loss to the geneticist and can help interpret the results of various audiological tests. They can also help after the evaluation, noting when reevaluation or further counseling may be necessary.

The principles of counseling are very similar for audiologists and geneticists, although the issues they face can be quite different. In either profession it is important to be open and understanding, and to present the information in a manner that is sensitive to individual differences.

In the future, geneticists hope to be able to delineate the different types of syndromic and nonsymdromic hearing loss and identify the genes that cause them. This information would be vital in giving accurate information to the families and in treatment of the hearing loss when this is desired. However, this research will be impossible without collaboration with experts in hearing loss who can help diagnose causes, characterize types of hearing loss, and identify significant variations that may differentiate the effects of individual genes.

ACKNOWLEDGMENT

I would like to acknowledge the many helpful and stimulating discussions on these topics with Susan Tinley, M.S., R.N.

REFERENCES

AD HOC COMMITTEE ON GENETIC COUNSELING, AMERICAN SOCIETY OF HUMAN GENETICS. (1975). *American Journal of Human Genetics, 27*, 240–242.

ARNOS, K. S., ISRAEL, J., & CUNNINGHAM, M. (1991). Genetic counseling of the deaf: Medical and cultural considerations. In R. J. Ruben, T. R. Van De Water, & K. P. Steel (Eds.), *Genetics of hearing impairment* (Vol. 630, 212–222). Annals of the New York Academy of Sciences.

BIEBER, F. R, & NANCE, W. E. (1979). Hereditary hearing loss. In L. Jackson & N. Schimke (Eds.), *Clinical genetics: A source book for physicians* (pp. 443–461). New York: Wiley.

CLARKE, A. (1991). Is non-directive genetic counseling possible? *Lancet, 388*, 998–1001.

FRASER, G. R. (1976). *The causes of profound deafness in childhood.* Baltimore: Johns Hopkins University Press.

GORLIN, R. J. (1991). Forward. In J. M. Aase, *Diagnostic dysmorphology* (p. vii). New York: Plenum Medical Book Company.

MORRISON, A. W., & BUNDEY, S. E. (1970). The inheritance of otosclerosis. *Journal of Laryngology and Otology, 84*, 921–932.

MORTON, N. E. (1991). Genetic epidemiology of hearing impairment. In R. J. Ruben, T. R. Van De Water, & K. P. Steel (Eds.), *Genetics of hearing impairment* (Vol. 630, pp. 16–31). Annals of the New York Academy of Sciences.

NANCE, W. E. (1971). Genetic counseling for the hearing impaired. *Audiology, 10*, 221.

PELIAS, M. Z. (1986). Torts of wrongful birth and wrongful life: A review. *American Journal of Human Genetics, 25*, 71–80.

SMITH, S. D. (1991). Recurrence risks. In R. J. Ruben, T. R. Van De Water, & K. P. Steel (Eds.), *Genetics of hearing impairment* (Vol. 630, pp. 203–211). Annals of the New York Academy of Sciences.

APPENDIX 4–1
SAMPLE COUNSELING LETTER

August 27, 1991

Mrs. Anna Day
444 S. 44th St.
Omaha, NE 68131

Re: Johnny Day
     bd 7/3/85

Dear Mrs. Day,

It was a pleasure to meet you and your son, Johnny, and his sister, Leigh, at the Genetics Clinic on August 16, 1991. This letter is to briefly review your discussion with Dr. Alan and me.

As we discussed, the fact that Johnny has a sensorineural hearing loss, the ear pits, and small pits in his neck means that he has a condition called the Branchio-oto-renal (BOR) syndrome. The term *branchio* refers to the area around the ear and neck, "oto" refers to the ear, and "renal" refers to kidney problems. Since you have found that Leigh also has a similar hearing loss, it is very likely that she also has BOR. Not everyone who has this condition has all of the findings, so the children may not have the renal problems that can go along with this. However, it is important for them to get renal ultrasounds to be sure that they do not have a kidney malformation that could lead to problems later, and I understand this has been scheduled by your doctor.

The Branchio-oto-renal syndrome is a genetic condition caused by a single gene. Genes are the small bits of information that we inherit from our parents. All genes come in pairs, with one inherited from our mother and the other from our father. One of these genes, which is usually inherited from one of the parents, can cause Branchio-oto-renal syndrome. However, individuals who have this gene may only have a few of the characteristics of BOR. That is, they may have any combination of the primary characteristics; hearing loss, ear pits, pits or cysts in the neck, or kidney malformations. The hearing can range from normal to hard of hearing to a significant hearing loss such as Johnny has, and it is sometimes a nerve loss, sometimes conductive, or it may be both. It may also be progressive, so it will be important to keep testing Johnny's and Leigh's hearing. Since Johnny's father also has ear pits and a hearing loss, he also has the gene for BOR. You have told us that Mr. Day's mother also has a hearing loss, so he may have inherited it from her.

Anyone who has BOR has a 50-50 chance of passing that gene on to a child. Since the genes come in pairs, a child could either inherit the BOR gene or the normal gene in the pair. We would not be able to predict the types of hearing problems they may have, however. Similarly, the kidneys may be normal, or they may have a slight malformation which does not cause any real problems, or there may be severe problems including missing kidneys. This could be important for any future children you and your husband might have. You have told us that you are not planning any more children, but if you happen to get pregnant again, you may want to have an ultrasound of the baby's kidneys during the pregnancy. This could be important information in planning the rest of the pregnancy and delivery. For example, if a kidney malformation was found that would require immediate surgery after birth, you would want to be sure the baby was born in a hospital that could provide that kind of care. Even if the prenatal ultrasound appears normal, it should also be repeated after the baby is born. We would be happy to go over this in more detail with you if you become pregnant. Johnny and Leigh, and anyone else in the family who is found to have BOR, may also wish to see a geneticist when they are planning to have a family so they can get the most up-to-date information. Specifically, it would be important for Mr. Day's brother, Douglas, to be seen to determine whether he has any of the signs of BOR, since he and his wife are planning a family. We could see them, or any of your other relatives who are interested, in the clinic here or we could refer them to a geneticist in their area. I am enclosing an article on BOR from the *Hereditary Deafness Newsletter of America* that goes over this condition in more detail, and you may want to share the information with your relatives.

　　I hope this information is helpful to you. As we discussed on the telephone, I will plan to see you again in the clinic in September when your husband can also be present. In the meantime, if you have any questions, please feel free to contact me at (402) 498-6622 or write to me at Boys Town National Research Hospital, 555 N. 30th St., Omaha, NE 68131.

Sincerely,

Shelley D. Smith, Ph.D.
Medical Geneticist

cc:　W. Kimberling, M.D.
　　　211 W. 33rd St.
　　　Omaha, NE 68104

chapter five

Emotional Responses to Hearing Loss

Madeleine L. Van Hecke

Adult patients, as well as parents and family members of children with impaired hearing, may be profoundly affected by the diagnosis of permanent hearing loss. In this chapter, Dr. Van Hecke presents some of the emotional responses that may occur when the fact of hearing loss is actually confronted. Within her discussion, Dr. Van Hecke considers some of the major illusions of life and how these are necessarily altered for families and patients as they confront hearing impairment during various life stages.

The cataclysm has happened, we are among the ruins, we start to build up new little habitats, to have new little hopes. It is rather hard work: there is now no smooth road into the future: but we go round, or scramble over the obstacles. We've got to live, no matter how many skies have fallen.

D. H. Lawrence
Lady Chatterly's Lover

INTRODUCTION

Audiologists, like others who enter the health professions, often have altruistic reasons for doing so: We want to make a significant difference in people's lives. With such hopes, we are understandably disappointed when our clients apparently resist our efforts to assist them. For example, in one study only about half of the elderly individuals who had serious hearing impairments used their hearing aids "more than occasionally," even though they said they found the aids beneficial (Christian, Dluhy, & O'Neill, 1989). Today's sophisticated technology will be of limited use unless audiologists can also address the psychological factors that affect hearing-impaired individuals.

The gap between our desires as clinicians to enhance our clients' lives and the extent to which we address their emotional needs remains marked, as Dr. Martin illustrates in Chapter 3. Over two-thirds of the adults responding to the survey conducted by Martin and his colleagues felt that the evaluator showed no concern for their feelings (Martin, Krall, & O'Neal, 1989). Clients report feeling angry, depressed, anxious, self-conscious, embarrassed, inferior, and isolated. They may have a sense of imposing on others or of being patronized or exploited by others. As one 65-year-old woman urged audiologists:[1]

> Try to understand that the client is going through a very traumatic experience. Clients are faced with a loss that in all probability will only get worse with age, a loss that affects every part of their life: home, office, social affairs. Trying to cope with such a loss is devastating and overwhelming, and they need help from everyone they come in contact with.

Similar pleas to "give emotional support" and "validate the client's feelings" were expressed by many others who answered a questionnaire from Martin and his colleagues.

THE THERAPEUTIC ALLIANCE

How can clinicians respond to appeals for more sensitivity to clients' emotional reactions? Some audiologists may be concerned that addressing the psychological needs of clients involves counseling that goes beyond our training and prescribed role. But as Dr. Clark's examples in Chapter 1 illustrate, the clinician's role is often one of educating, supporting, and acting as a sounding board to help clients make decisions. These are all aspects of "supportive counseling," a kind of counseling that can occur naturally within the relationship that the audiologist has with clients.

The following words of one 53-year-old man[1] emphasize that clients expect professionals to be competent and to communicate treatment options honestly and clearly: "Keep abreast of recent developments in assistive listening devices. Give the patient advice on protecting what hearing he or she has left. Be able to give the patient an honest appraisal of his prospects for surgically correcting or improving the hearing." But in expecting professionals to keep abreast of the field, this client may also be pleading: "Give me hope that whatever can be done, will be done—assure me that I won't miss an opportunity because you are ignorant." In asking for an honest appraisal of the situation, the client may also be saying: "Don't let me remain anxious and uncertain if you do know some things for sure."

Clinicians recognize that their first obligation is to be competent practitioners in their field, and they are usually well trained to respond to requests for information. What is more difficult is to also react to the underlying concerns that the client's words and tone imply.

Sensitive clinicians who pick up on a client's underlying concerns can then respond to these worries. Comments like "You don't want to be left in the dark. You want to know whatever I think about what is happening" allow the client and clinician to explore concerns and to lay the foundation for how they will work together. In so doing, they establish a "therapeutic alliance," the mutual understanding that they are working together toward a common goal.

Establishing an alliance with clients is perhaps most crucial when working with parents of hearing-impaired children. Professionals are often tempted to dominate conversations with their advice. Asking first what parents have already been told or have already tried conveys that the audiologist wants to work with them to address their children's problems.

In addition to encouraging a genuine dialogue with clients, clinicians who want to establish partnerships with their clients must see them as people. The following words of one 43-year-old woman[1] remind us of this.

> First remember that you are dealing with another human being. I have found that audiologists tend to retreat behind their technology and testing machinery. The majority of them have made me feel like a walking audiogram. Ten percent of an audiological exam is taken up with making contact with the client and ninety percent with testing and billing. I think these proportions should be reversed, or at least made equitable.

One psychologist observing optometry students noted that they tended to bury themselves in the technological aspects of the exam and missed data available from the clients themselves. Problems occur when practitioners "orient themselves to the patient's chart instead of the person in the chair . . . " (Cole & McConnaha, 1986, p. 922). Students and less experienced practitioners may relate to clients in a mechanical style because they are more confident when they follow a practiced routine. More experienced professionals may deliver news in a routine fashion because the process has become so familiar to them. In both cases, clients sense that their reactions and concerns are secondary to the standard script the practitioner is delivering.

Professionals need to encourage clients to ask questions and to express their doubts. This allows us to respond to clients emotionally at the same time as we clarify misconceptions or supply reassuring information. As one 50-year-old woman commented:[1] "Don't get impatient and brush off the patient's questions as not accepting 'minor difficulties.' [Don't] take questions about [hearing] aids personally; patients who ask questions aren't necessarily saying you did not fit them with the right aid." Asking clients "How is it going?" invites their reactions and shows that we see their dissatisfaction as a problem for us to consider together, rather than a nuisance that we want to avoid.

In addition to searching for objective expertise, clients seek a genuine, human response from the professionals whom they consult. Whether we are addressing parents or hearing-impaired adults, our attitude can show that we see the client as a person first and appreciate his or her individuality. We can ask parents: "What are some of the ways in which Jimmy is special to you?" or "Tell me a little about what kind of baby Sarah is?" We can show an interest in the lives of our adult clients beyond the sphere of their hearing conditions.

Prior to audiological testing, the clinician looks over the information forms that the client has filled out, and comments: "I notice that you work in an automotive plant. What's that like for you?"

CLIENT (SMILING): "Boring. But I'm hoping that they'll train me for a different section which I'd like better. It's more technical, it would be a promotion. But now I don't know. . . . "

CLINICIAN: "Are you afraid the hearing problems you've been having might keep that from happening?"

CLIENT: "Yeh, well, I don't know. But I know sometimes I'm not following my boss's directions and he gets mad. I guess I'm not always hearing him right. It's hard, the plant is so noisy. But I don't think he understands . . . so I don't know what he'll do about recommending me for the other job."

Asking questions about an individual's job or favorite recreational activities and then learning how the hearing loss might be affecting these areas show that we see clients as people and not as diagnostic puzzles to be solved. Other questions (Zamerowski, 1982, p. 49) that might be helpful include: "What's going through your mind? What does this mean to you? How will this change your life?"

The practitioner needs to at least glimpse "what it's like to be you" in order to understand what sort of assistance would be most helpful to an individual client. The answer to this question depends, to some extent, on the person's stage of life.

THE IMPACT OF HEARING LOSS DURING DIFFERENT LIFE STAGES

When clinicians are more aware of the issues all of us face at different life stages, they can be more sensitive to the potential influence of a hearing condition. Although a detailed analysis of human development is beyond the scope of this chapter, the ways in which clients' life stages might affect the impact of their hearing loss can be illustrated.

Infancy

Infants need care givers who respond sensitively to their needs: adults who will feed them when they are hungry, warm them when they are cold, move them into the center of a noisy family gathering when they are bored, and move them back into the quiet darkness of a back bedroom when they are overstimulated and need sleep. They also need adults with whom they interact playfully, providing an experience that both parties enjoy. This kind of responsive care giving and mutuality creates a bond between infants and care givers. The result is that infants develop the conviction that they are lovable and loved, which Erikson (1950) referred to as a "basic sense of trust."

As Schlesinger (1978) has so sensitively conveyed in her work, communication limitations can interfere with this process. Hearing-impaired infants may respond less to their care givers and fail to enter into the playful verbal games common between hearing infants and adults. Parents who are unaware of their child's hearing problems may feel frustrated in their attempts to engage their baby. Parents often feel a sense of personal rejection when they are unable to soothe or entertain their infants, especially when they do not understand what is causing their child's diminished responsiveness. On the other hand, when parents do realize that their child is hearing impaired, they may be devastated by the news. It is difficult for them to be emotionally available to their baby because of their own grief and anxiety about their child's condition. The audiologist can support parents in their distress and at the same time help them recognize the nonverbal ways in which their babies are trying to communicate.

Preschool

During the early preschool years, children must gradually resist their natural inclination to be the center of the universe. They must learn to share, to control their angry outbursts and demands, to wait their turns, and to cooperate with the authority of adults. At the same time, they need to develop a sense of "autonomy" and pride in their new-found independence as they insist upon zipping up their own jacket or mixing their own chocolate milk, rather than feeling consumed with "shame and doubt" (Erikson, 1950). Preschoolers are more able to cooperate with authority while sustaining their dignity if they are given reasons for the rules they are asked to observe and are allowed an appropriate degree of independence. Parents of hearing-impaired children must determine how much independence to grant their children who are less able to hear warning signals or to comprehend directions. Moreover, when their children's ability to understand verbal communication is limited, it is very difficult for parents to try to explain: "Not here . . . not now . . . not under these circumstances because . . . " rather than simply exclaiming "No!"

During the later preschool years, children are faced with the challenge of developing a sense of "initiative versus guilt," practicing adult roles as they scold their dolls, pretend to drive a car, or imagine themselves to be doctors, nurses, firefighters, and grocery clerks. To sustain a sense of positive initiative, hearing-impaired children need models of hearing-impaired adults in positive roles and meaningful answers to their repeated question: "Why?" They also need to express the exhuberance of this stage in their imaginary play, and not be stymied by too many hours of passive speech training.

Finally, preschoolers need reassurance that they are not to blame for the communication difficulties they are having. As Piaget (1932) discovered, preschool children are so egocentric in their outlook that hearing-impaired pre-schoolers are likely to assume they are "bad" for causing whatever problems are associated with their condition. Sensitive audiologists can encourage parents to notice signs of their children's fear or guilt and provide reassurance. Even when children are too young, or too limited in their communication ability to under-stand complicated explanations, they can be reassured through caring touch. Parents can "hug their children and be close to them when words fail. Reaching out physically is the clearest communication of reassurance and comfort" (Bristor, 1984, p. 31).

School-Age Children

School-age children need to develop a sense of competency, a sense of "industry versus inferiority." They are trying to master a host of learning tasks: how to read, draw a house, catch a ball, get a pillow into a pillowcase, make a friend. Like all children, the positive self-esteem of hearing-impaired children is at risk when they are overhelped, underchallenged by easy tasks, or defeated by overly difficult tasks. Clinicians can help parents determine reasonable but challenging goals and discover areas in which their child's talents can be expressed and acknowledged. Audiologists can show the kind of faith in the child's abilities that the parents themselves must sustain.

Hearing-impaired children in school also need to find peers who affirm them. As the child grows older, the family's acceptance is no longer sufficient: The child yearns to be included in a group of friends, sought after as a member of the team, invited to the party. While all children struggle with achieving acceptance outside of the family, this task may be more difficult for hearing-impaired chil-dren depending upon their school and social situations. By this time in their lives, children with hearing problems are more able to have a direct relationship with their audiologist. Some school-age children may confide their concerns and disap-pointments more freely to a caring professional than to their parents whom they hope to protect from worry.

Adolescence

The major psychological tasks facing adolescents are establishing a sense of identity (Erikson, 1950) and becoming more independent, able to make decisions about their lives and take responsibility for those decisions. Adolescents with an acquired hearing loss need to formulate a sense of identity that comes to grips with having a handicap. Their sense of identity includes an increasing awareness of their likes and dislikes, strengths and weaknesses, beliefs and ethics and hopes. A hearing impairment raises questions: "Will I be able to succeed in college?" "Will I be accepted in a profession even if I gain the necessary educational credentials?"

Most fundamentally, an impairment raises the question of how hearing-impaired adolescents see themselves in relation to others with a similar condition. The process of defining themselves involves identifying with groups and other individuals. Like all adolescents, hearing-impaired teenagers need to develop bonds with friends as they move toward adult independence. They need friendships that provide an island of safety as they explore both the wide world beyond their families and the inner world of their own dreams, hopes, and fears. If adolescents reject others who are like themselves, they are deprived of the peers who could best understand their struggles and provide support. For these reasons, the most valuable contribution that clinicians make to adolescents might well be in helping them connect with adolescent members of the deaf community.

Susan, a teenager who has recently experienced a sudden shift in her hearing, says: "I can't help it. I think of deaf as stupid. I watch some of the kids using sign language and I think: That's not me. I don't belong with them. But then when I see my old friends, they act so strange. Sometimes I think they just include me out of pity." A sensitive clinician might respond: "You don't feel like you belong with other teenagers who have hearing problems but you also don't feel like you belong with your hearing friends the way you once did. It must be very hard to feel like there's nowhere you completely 'fit in.'"

The sense of not belonging is a difficult experience at any age, but it is particularly troubling during the teenage years when friends are crucial and adolescents are trying to understand "who they are." This clinician's response might help Susan explore a positive identity that included her hearing limitations.

Young Adulthood

The two major tasks facing young adults is to develop intimate relationships with others (Erikson, 1950) and to begin to carve out a life that might fulfill a dream they have formed (Levinson, 1978). This dream involves images of how they would like to live, including whether or not to marry or have children and what sort of success to pursue. It might involve romantic images of living on a cliff overlooking the ocean or picturing themselves heading a Fortune 500 company.

It is easy to imagine how a hearing loss might threaten both intimacy and the nature of these dreams. Young adults in their twenties are already wondering: "Will I find someone to love who also loves me? If I find someone, will we be able to sustain intimacy?" A hearing loss raises new doubts about the ability to be in a love relationship. Similarly, if a dream requires activities that are difficult or impossible to pursue with a hearing condition, young adults have lost not only some hearing ability but their vision of what their lives would be like.

Thirty-Something

Among the men whom Levinson (1978) studied, there seemed to be a transition time at around age 30 when many of them questioned their life structures. Was this really the sort of work they wanted to do? Was this marriage all they had hoped it might be? A reassessment of their earlier decisions occurred, often followed by changes designed to bring these men closer to the fulfillment of their dreams. They created modified life structures that they then spent their 30s developing and strengthening by investing themselves deeply in their work, families, friendships, and communities. Similar statements may be true for women in this age group as well.

It is difficult for adults to continue investing energy in these areas when they experience hearing loss. Hearing-impaired adults need understanding to work through the problems they encounter, to protect what they have built so far, and to plan for their futures. This understanding is hard to find when family members act as though hearing difficulties are a "result of distraction, lack of concentration, and unwillingness to communicate rather than the consequence of a hearing problem" (Hetu, Lalonde, & Getty, 1987, p. 142).

Mrs. Jacobs, who experienced a moderate hearing loss in her mid-30s, confides: "At dinner time, I can't keep track of the conversation. Sometimes I still ask people to repeat what they've said, but it gets so tiring. Half the time I just stay quiet and pretend I've understood."

It is hard for hearing professionals to imagine how frustrating it is to continue trying to communicate, especially in group settings, and how tempting it is to simply withdraw.

Workers who experienced occupational hearing loss reported that they often used strategies like Mrs. Jacobs's (Hetu et al., 1987). These included pretending to understand while keeping silent (67%), trying to guess what was said (40%), and simply accepting that they would lose the stream of conversation (36%). Helping clients learn more positive coping strategies would enrich their relationships with both friends and families. In Chapter 10, Dr. Trychin presents a number of approaches to improve communication and relationships.

Hearing loss may also affect occupational success. A recent study of hard-of-hearing and deaf clients showed that the income of both groups was lower than that of the general population (Mowry, 1988). Though it varied from one occupation to another, hard-of-hearing individuals earned an average of 8.5% less than their counterparts in similar jobs, while deaf individuals earned 19% less.

The Midlife Crisis and Middle Adulthood

Though researchers disagree over whether the turmoil of midlife is great enough to warrant the title "crisis," most of them believe that people often experience a period of serious questioning around ages 40 to 45. Many people have experiences at this time that remind them of their own mortality, such as the illness and death of their parents and the appearance of the first clear signs of their own physical aging. A hearing loss at this time is likely to trigger or intensify this crisis. When we begin to measure our lives in terms of "time left to live" rather than "time since birth," we feel a time crunch. The coming years constitute our "last chance" to analyze what we want from life and to pursue it.

The difficulties that hearing-impaired adults encounter during this life stage may cause them to question their ability to achieve their dreams. One researcher found that 41% of those interviewed reported significant problems at work because of their acquired hearing loss, while another 23% stated it had led to changes in their jobs or prospects (Beattie, 1984). As one woman commented:[1] "I have managed to be successful in my job but I have paid in stress and exhaustion. I learned to stay one step ahead and do better work than my co-workers and I learned to anticipate. I have always felt inferior to hearing people." Though there are individual differences, it is clear that the ramifications of a hearing loss during adulthood can be profound.

The Mellow 50s

In their early 50s, many adults experience another "settling down" period that is a more mellow and satisfying time than earlier life stages. Children may be launched on their own; grandchildren may be appearing. Financial security is often greater than at any previous time. Many people at this time become satisfied with the level of their career success and no longer devote evenings and weekends in an attempt to "get to the top." They are then able to pursue activities and relationships that they ignored during their younger adult years when they were preoccupied with family life and with developing their careers. They may also emphasize "generative" activities, such as involvement in community affairs or in ecology, as they try to positively influence the world that will continue beyond their lives.

Experiencing a hearing loss at this time may seem especially cruel, particularly when it diminishes some of the hearing-impaired adults' recently discovered enjoyment. They may have realized that their family relationships were more important to them than climbing up another notch on the ladder of success, only to find themselves having difficulty understanding the higher-pitched voices of their grandchildren or struggling even to understand their children's words. If they are experiencing difficulties at work due to their hearing loss, they may find themselves pressured to consider early retirement with its concomitant drop in financial resources. At a time when they are most able to give of their expertise and time to future generations, they may be least able to communicate their ideas or to work actively with groups. Moreover, a physical disability at this time intensifies fears of aging. As one woman commented:[1] "I have an enormous fear of becoming a lonely old deaf lady."

Late Adulthood and Old Age

The aging process represents a psychological challenge to older adults. Western society values youth, beauty, health, physical strength, speed, and success. Older people are often declining in these areas, as well as experiencing the loss of friends and family through death, illness, or relocation after retirement. A hearing loss represents yet another in this series of losses, all signs that they are aging and coming into the last stage of life.

According to Erikson (1950), this is when adults review their lives and seek to find meaning in them. This stage of life is often reflected in two contradictory images. The positive image is that of older people whose wisdom and experience allow them to continue enriching the lives of others, to come to terms with their own mortality, and yet to live life fully for as much time as they have left. In Erikson's terms, these individuals have attained a sense of "integrity," based on the belief that their lives were worth living. The negative image is that of a self-absorbed, complaining, embittered older person who feels cheated by what life has had to offer.

In Chapter 11, Dr. Alpiner provides a discussion of the challenges involved in counseling geriatric patients and their families. Only two points will be emphasized here. First, a hearing loss is likely to exacerbate other problems related to aging. For example, many older people feel isolated even when their hearing is intact; this isolation may increase with their decline in hearing. Second, other losses they have experienced will come to mind in response to this newest setback. This means that the grief many people experience in response to hearing loss is likely to be intensified for older clients. On the positive side, working through their reactions may engage older people in the life review process in a way that leads them to integrity.

TELLING OUR STORIES

Having a sense of the ways in which a hearing problem might influence individuals during different life stages can be helpful, but can never convey the unique situation of each client we see. As Perry (1970) often says, every person is far more complex than any theory. In order for us to have an appreciation of the particular people in our care, we need to hear them "tell their stories."

Psychological research demonstrates that our perception of events, and the meaning they hold for us, is far more important in determining the impact of those circumstances than are the actual events themselves. For instance, researchers attempting to measure "quality of life" have learned that individuals' *perceptions* of factors such as health, social support, and financial adequacy influence their quality of life far more than objective measures of these same determinants (Magilvy, 1985). The significance of this understanding for audiologists can be seen clearly in a study of elderly persons with hearing problems (Calvani, 1985). Their answers to a questionnaire indicated the extent to which their hearing impairment disrupted their social functioning and caused them emotional distress. The scores for those individuals who, in terms of objective measures, had a mild hearing loss were especially revealing. Their "hearing handicap" scores ranged from "mild" to "severe." This finding emphasizes that the effects of a hearing loss are determined by what that loss does to our lives as much as by the extent of sound attenuation.

Bicknell (1984) suggests that in speaking with handicapped individuals, professionals should ask themselves the following questions:

What does it mean?
To this person?
To have this handicap?
At this time in his life?
With these caretakers?
In this environment?
And in this peer group? (p. 357)

Asking questions like "What is your major concern about your hearing problem?" gives people a chance to "tell their stories."

One psychologist experienced a serious hearing decline while he had a private therapy practice. He became unable to hear what his clients were saying when the level of their voices dropped as they became sad or distressed. At these crucial moments when they most needed to be understood, he was least able to hear them. Unless hearing aids or other treatment could improve the intelligibility of their words for him, the psychologist felt he would have to end his profession.

An audiologist who understands what a hearing loss means to this man is not likely to congratulate him on having the rest of his senses intact or on being young enough to retrain. Instead, the clinician can work with him on strategies to improve his communication with clients.

"Telling their stories" to empathic listeners can be emotionally healing to clients, but they need to hear us respond to them in return. One 34-year-old woman urged clinicians to search for ways to communicate:[1] " . . . don't give up on talking—come closer; write; find something that works. Have an amplifier available both to help communicate and as an introduction to the existence of assistive devices." Clients expect professionals in the field to understand their communication difficulties and try to address these. When we fail to do so, they are angry and skeptical about the genuineness of our concern. As one 65-year-old woman pointedly asked:[1] "Why is it that otologists and audiologists do not know any sign language? Why do they wear beards and mustaches that make lip reading impossible?" Such comments underscore our clients' belief that we are failing to see the world through their eyes—or, rather, that we are failing to imagine what it would be like to hear through their ears.

EMPATHY

Empathy is the capacity to so clearly understand how other people experience the world that their reactions make sense to us and we begin to share their emotional response. We "feel with" them. It describes a deceptively simple task that can be extraordinarily difficult to achieve. Noddings (1984) gives an instructive example:

Suppose that I am a teacher who loves mathematics. I encounter a student who is doing poorly, and I decide to have a talk with him. He tells me that he hates mathematics. *Aha*, I think. *Here is the problem, I must help this poor boy to love mathematics, and then he will do better at it.* What am I doing if I proceed in this way? I am not trying to grasp the reality of the other as a possibility for myself. I have not even asked: *How would it feel to hate mathematics? . . . What reasons could I find for learning it?* (p. 15)

There are many parallel situations in which clinicians are likely to feel frustrated rather than empathic. Clients may state that they have not used their hearing aids because they make them irritable and jumpy. They may announce that asking others to repeat "just isn't worth the trouble" so they have withdrawn from social interaction.

Mrs. Eliot, who was recently widowed, returned to her audiologist thinking that her 3-year-old hearing aids simply needed some adjusting. Instead, she needed new aids. Returning after her first week with her new aids, Mrs. Eliot says: "I might as well have just stayed with my old aids. Or just forget it all together. These new ones aren't making things any better. I could have flown to visit my daughter for what these cost!"

It is difficult to resist the urge to defend against Mrs. Eliot's protestations and explain the ways in which her condition has changed that make it impossible for technology to help her as much as it did in the past. It is hard to ask ourselves first: How would it feel to have adjusted to hearing aids only to realize that you will have to do this all over again, with probably less satisfaction than the first time? How would it feel to be recently widowed and to have forfeited a visit to your daughter in order to pay for your hearing aids?

The most direct and painful means of seeing the other's reality as our own is to experience it ourselves. Lustbader (1991) describes how Dr. Oliver Sacks's practice of neurology was transformed after he himself experienced hospitalization and nursing home care:

> I came to realize, as did my patients, that there is an absolute and categorical difference between a doctor who *knows* and one who does not, and that this knowing can only be obtained by a personal experience of the organic, by descending to the very depths of disease and dissolution. (Sacks, 1987, pp. 202–203)

This idea of being transformed by personal illness is also the theme of the 1990 film *The Doctor*, publicized as "A story about a surgeon who became an ordinary patient and then became an extraordinary doctor." Statements made by the doctor in the film, like Sacks's comments, imply that only by experiencing a hearing impairment ourselves can clinicians "really" know what it is like and thus develop the kind of empathy that will transform our work.

Perhaps this is why some hearing-impaired people urge professionals to engage in "simulation" exercises to create a temporary experience of what it is like to have a disability. One 60-year-old client[1] recommended that not only clinicians, but the families of hearing-impaired individuals, should "put in soft ear plugs for a day—then try to converse. It's an embarrassing, painful situation, and most enlightening."

We can also try to find the common ground we share with our clients by connecting their dilemmas with parallel ones of our own. We may not have experienced a hearing loss, but we have felt the same emotions in other circumstances. As one example, the pain of exclusion is a familiar one for many of us. From our youth, we remember the overwhelming need for acceptance and the humiliation of standing on the outside, not getting the joke, or not being chosen for the team. Recalling these times may help us understand the pain of social isolation experienced by many hearing-impaired individuals.

It may be true that hearing people cannot "really know" what it feels like to have a hearing loss. There will always be limits to the extent we can identify with another person's experiences. But in listening to our own clients, attending support groups, engaging in simulation exercises, and recalling our personal times of loss and pain, we can be more sensitive to the distress of those for whom we care. As we become more empathic, we will find our clients expressing their concerns and feelings more freely and with more intensity. This creates another dilemma: How do we respond to their pain?

Just Listening

What can we do when our clients express their troubled feelings to us? One of the most difficult things for us to do is to "just listen." "Just listening" runs counter to what we have been taught. We have learned that when people are depressed, we should try to cheer them up. When they are angry, we urge them to calm down. When people blame themselves, we tell them they shouldn't feel guilty. If they tell us how anxious they are, we tell them not to worry so much.

Another factor that makes it difficult for us to allow clients to simply tell us how badly they are feeling is that most of us are very uncomfortable with silence. In social interactions, there is an almost audible sigh of relief when someone opens up a new conversational line that will not only fill the current gap but sustain talking through the next few minutes. When a client is not speaking—struggling to control his or her emotions, searching for words to express his or her thoughts, or dissolving into tears—we are strongly tempted to fill the silence with our own words. Doing so may prove to be counterproductive.

"Troubles Talk" and Problem Solving

A final factor which affects many of us is our inclination to respond to distress with problem solving. Tannen (1990) describes problem-solvers who see little point in listening to repeated descriptions of difficulties from people who are unable or unwilling to work on solutions. But when people engage in what Tannen calls "troubles talk," they are seeking reassurance that they are not alone, that others understand and empathize with their reactions. They become frustrated when listeners respond with strategies for solving their difficulties; their listeners, in turn, are annoyed when the troubled person rejects advice or help. As one baffled man demanded: "Why *wouldn't* I want to help people solve their problems if I care about them?"

Tannen believes that men are more likely than women to respond to the distress of those whom they love by trying to "fix" things, either directly or through helpful advice. But whatever our gender, those of us in the helping professions need both capabilities. We need to collaborate with our clients in actively searching for solutions to their dilemmas when they are ready to do this. We also need to be able to "just listen," to validate that they are not crazy and that we understand that they are in great pain: the pain of grieving.

It is particularly crucial to receive our clients' grief and "just listen" when we cannot truly "fix" their hearing loss. On the other hand, we know that this business of "accepting" and "receiving" feelings is not quite so simple. How do we accept someone's feelings of depression without appearing to concur that the situation is hopeless? How do we accept their feelings of guilt without joining in their self-blame? We need to take a closer look at the nature of mourning and the "fine line" that the sensitive clinician walks.

GRIEF

Many of the emotions experienced by hearing-impaired individuals parallel the feelings of grief described by Kübler-Ross (1969) in her work with terminally ill patients. One 42-year-old man urged clinicians:[1] "Recognize that a hearing loss is one of the most depressing things a person will ever have to endure. It is like a 'death.'" The grief model assumes that persons with acquired hearing loss mourn the diminishment of the quality of their lives. The assumption is that hearing-impaired people, like others who grieve, can eventually arrive at some sense of peace and acceptance after struggling through the feelings of guilt, depression, and anger, which are part of the mourning process.

How might this happen? In the midst of their grief, people yearn for some way to make sense of their pain, to search for meaning in this experience. As Moses and Van Hecke-Wulatin (1981) suggested, fundamental philosophical issues may underlie the emotions of grief. Through mourning, individuals come to grips with those issues and often experience a spiritual change in their attitudes and values as they resolve them (e.g., Schneider, 1983).

DENIAL

Denial refers to the sense of disbelief and unreality people sometimes experience when they hear shocking news. They may feel oddly detached, reporting later, "I heard the words, I knew what the words meant, but somehow they weren't real to me." They may find themselves focusing on some trivial detail, mentioning that a plant needs watering or that the button on the clinician's jacket is coming loose. Parents often experience intense shock and disbelief when first informed of their child's disability. One mother described her sense of unreality: "I was stunned. . . . I felt like a spectator in a dream. I just knew I would wake up and everything would be all right" (Bristor, 1984, p. 29).

Researchers suggest that denial may be the reason some individuals fail to perceive their hearing difficulties. In one study of elderly patients in a physician's general practice, for example, the percentage whose audiometric results indicated a hearing impairment was much greater than the number who reported experiencing hearing problems. Moreover, 27% refused to believe the test results when given them (Gilhome-Herbst & Humphrey, 1980). Some of this discrepancy may occur because the hearing decline has been a slow process to which individuals have unconsciously adapted. However, it seems likely that their need to protect themselves from bad news also causes them to ignore difficulties they are having. As one 36-year-old female said:[1] "I was shocked and tended to deny the situation. The audiologist failed to give me support and as a result I still have trouble accepting it. Audiologists tend to lose sight of the fact that those test results involve *people!*"

Mrs. Haldeman is listening to the third audiologist she has consulted. Once again, she insists that the audiologist's diagnosis must be wrong, since her 3-year-old daughter can hear her name whispered behind her back. "Show me!" demands the audiologist. Mrs. H. turns her child around and whispers "Mary!"—stamping her foot on the wooden floor at the same time. The child turns to the vibration and smiles. Her mother then looks victoriously at the audiologist. Instead of arguing with Mrs. Haldeman, the sensitive audiologist might say: "The idea of Mary being deaf seems almost impossible for you to accept. Can you tell me a little bit about what it would mean to you if somehow my assessment were correct?" (Moses & Van Hecke-Wulatin, 1981, p. 254)

The professional's natural reaction to denial is to try to counter it with irrefutable evidence. But it is difficult, if not impossible, to break denial down through logical argument.

If Mrs. Haldeman were able to confide her fears about Mary's future, the audiologist would be able to empathize with her dread. A thoughtful response might be: "If you really believe that things will be that bad for Mary, I can certainly understand how terrible it would be for you to accept that my diagnosis might be even a little bit accurate." With these words, the audiologist is able to walk a fine line: showing empathy for the parent without inadvertently supporting her denial.

In the case of adults with an acquired hearing loss, the clinician can ask clients to describe the reasons they initially sought an evaluation and the ideas they had about what the problem might be. The professional can empathize with the shock that must occur when individuals who hoped to dismiss the concerns of their spouses as overreactions, or who thought they merely needed some wax removed from their ears, are given a much more serious diagnosis. Most importantly, the audiologist can listen sensitively to what impact it would have on the person's life "if it were true" that total recovery is not possible or that continuing deterioration is likely. In learning of their clients' fears, clinicians can offer reassurance and hope that they will be supported as they seek the information, treatment, and coping strategies that will help them sustain the quality of their lives as much as possible.

DEPRESSION

At the simplest level, individuals with a hearing impairment experience sadness for what has been lost. They miss what once gave them pleasure: hearing the shouts and laughter of children on their way home from school, listening to music or attending films and lectures, being comforted by the sound of waves crashing on the shore. Hearing loss also diminishes the quality of their intimate conversations. The day-to-day "schmoozing" and quick-witted joking that was once part of their companionship with others may have turned into a source of frustration as they ask for repetition or misunderstand one another. They yearn for past times when communication and the closeness it engendered were a joy rather than a struggle to achieve.

The sense of loss may be pervasive:

> "It affects me in every conceivable fashion. It limits social activities, limits cultural activities, limits communication. It affects your well-being, insofar as you're isolated. Depending on the situation, and people, you even feel ignored and stupid, and consequently very exasperated." (Magilvy, 1985, p. 142)

As this quotation suggests, the reactions of others may make us feel stupid or embarrassed, threatening our self-esteem and increasing our depression.

Depression and Self-Esteem

Everyone needs acknowledgment that they are valued and valuable people, capable of intelligent thought and of contributing to those around them. This sense of personal value can be threatened when individuals must struggle to take a simple telephone message or when others react to them with annoyance or impatience.

Still worse is to be ignored entirely. Imagine the people whose hearing limitations exclude them from participating in family conversation at Thanksgiving dinner. They feel unacknowledged in a way that quiet members of the group do not. They are visible and present, as are the dishes on the table. But they have become like the cups and saucers we reach over for cream and sugar. The conversation and laughter move back and forth over them, insensible to their presence. It is as if they have ceased to exist for the rest of the family. The terms *social isolation* and *loneliness* used frequently by authors describing the experiences of hearing-impaired individuals (e.g., Christian et al., 1989) seem woefully inadequate to capture the sense of exclusion in this situation. Certainly audiologists do not want to contribute to their clients' sense of being excluded by addressing their hearing companions while ignoring the hearing-impaired person.

Depression and Dependency

Depression may also be a reaction to the "dilemmas of dependency" that hearing-impaired persons may experience. It is difficult to rely on the patience of others to repeat what they have said, to ask others to coordinate a meeting or make telephone calls, or to request that others take our needs into account as they plan a recreational event. Lustbader (1991) describes the uneasy connection between dependency and resentment:

> Giving help eventually embitters us, unless we are compensated at least by appreciation; accepting help degrades us, unless we are convinced that our helpers are getting something in return. (p. 18)

Thus, one 43-year-old woman whose illness forced her to depend on others described "a relentless pressure to please—to prove myself worth the burdens I impose" (Lustbader, 1991, p. 18). Sometimes the desire to reciprocate makes people feel they must comply with all the wishes and whims of those who help them. They may respond to this dilemma by becoming chronically angry, demanding, and cantankerous. Many, however, find it difficult to express their frustration and anger to those on whose kindness they depend. Instead, they try to be the good patient, the good spouse, or the good grandpa—cooperative and smiling and undemanding. When their tolerance reaches its end, they find themselves lashing out at the receptionist who can't tell them how much longer they will have to wait, or the grandchildren whose chatter makes it impossible for them to follow a favorite television program. When the dust settles, they are left with an uneasy mixture of guilt and resentment.

Depression and the Illusion of Power

At a philosophical level, depression may be a reaction to the loss of an illusion. Gould (1978) argues that adults try to procure a sense of safety by continuing to believe unquestioningly in a set of childhood illusions. One of these illusions is that adults can be all-powerful, that they can "fix" whatever goes wrong. Accustomed to temporary physical problems, people expect to recover and return to their lives as they were before the illness or disability. A permanent hearing loss forces them to come to grips with the limits of their power.

Professionals who encourage those who are depressed to talk about their feelings offer them a rare opportunity to feel less alone with their fears, their sense of helplessness, and their frustration with their inadequacies.

A 70-year-old resident of a retirement home explains why he no longer tries to connect with others:

"I used to go down to the lobby for coffee hour, but it was too hard for me to hear what people were saying. If more than one talks at once, forget it—I can't hear a thing. They all laugh, and I don't know what's so funny. You feel like an idiot, nodding and smiling when you don't know what the heck is going on. I can't keep asking people to repeat things for me. As it is, I can tell I'm a burden to have around. I can picture them saying under their breaths when they see me 'Oh, no, look who's coming.' So I don't go any more. It's not worth it" (Lustbader, 1991, p. 139).

The "fine line" that the sensitive audiologist walks with the depressed person is the line between empathizing with their feelings without concurring with their darkest views of what life holds for them. We might comment, "Right now, it feels as if you have no choice except to withdraw . . . that must be a terrible feeling." This kind of remark can communicate empathy while at the same time implying through our tone that there might be other options.

Through their depression, hearing-impaired individuals mourn their inability to restore their own functioning to its previous level or to attenuate all the negative repercussions that their hearing condition imposes. As they sit with someone who listens to their frustration and depression, they begin to explore what it means to be satisfied with only partial control of their lives. But as one 34-year-old man notes, this process takes time:[1] "I was severely affected by the diagnosis of my hearing loss. I am only now climbing out of the pit of fear and depression in which I've been trapped. . . . "

ANGER

It is easy to imagine how all of the experiences that are capable of provoking depression might also trigger anger. Realizing the ways in which their lives have been diminished, hearing-impaired individuals feel angry at what they have lost and ask: "Why me?" Ignored by others, they may sit alone with a sense of retaliation. Seeing others exasperated by their difficulty in hearing them or being accused of only listening "when they want to," they may counterattack with accusations that others are mumbling. Persons with hearing problems may be astounded at the intensity of their resentment toward those who continue to listen and communicate so easily, enjoying what they have lost without apparently appreciating its worth.

Sometimes the anger experienced by hearing-impaired individuals is a natural response to the reactions of others. A 52-year-old female, offering advice to others with a hearing loss, warned:[1] "Be prepared to have people treat you like a moron at times." How could anyone not be angry in response to such treatment? However, people with hearing problems also experience anger that is less in response to specific situations and more like a pervasive undercurrent in their lives. They may recognize times when they feel chronically angry, or when their anger strikes them as being unwarranted or out of proportion to the situation triggering it.

Anger and the Illusion of a Just World

Indiscriminate anger may be a reaction to the shattering of a second illusion that once provided a cushion of safety: the illusion that the world is a just place in which good things happen to good people and bad things happen to bad people. Thus, the anger a hearing-impaired person experiences may include an intense sense of being betrayed: This was not the way life was "supposed to be." When the hearing loss occurs at the same time as other stresses, their sense of justice may be especially outraged. They think: "It isn't fair that after I've already suffered so much, this should be happening to me too." The loss of the illusion that life is fair raises the philosophical issue of how to live in a world that is often unjust, a world in which evil actions frequently appear to result in prosperity, while honesty and integrity apparently lead to deprivation.

People often try to talk themselves out of this underlying anger. They say: "It doesn't really make sense to be angry; there's no one really to be angry *at*." Yet to work through their feelings of anger, clients need to ventilate their frustration with someone who affirms that these emotions are natural reactions. As one 33-year-old woman urged clinicians:[1] "Don't be afraid of the anger and the pain of grief." People with hearing limitations need professionals who are able to help them experience and explore their anger. This, in turn, eventually allows them to restructure their inner sense of justice and discover meaningful ways to live with the "unfairness" that a handicap represents to themselves and other family members.

GUILT

Beyond seeking information about the nature and extent of their hearing loss, individuals most commonly press for an answer to the question "What caused this?" Behind this question is the human need to make sense out of life's experiences. But when people must live with a limitation, they ask this question with more than curiosity: They ask it with a concern that something they have done or failed to do might have contributed to the problem. They think about the past and wonder if the days of their trapshooting, the band they played in, or the noisy plant they worked in may have caused their present condition.

People with hearing problems seem to be searching for an answer to the question "Who is responsible for this happening?" When their answer is someone other than themselves, their nagging sense of guilt is transformed into anger. If God seems responsible, they blame God. If they were genetically vulnerable to developing hearing problems, they may blame their parents. If they believe their workplace should have instituted more stringent noise abatement rules, they blame their company.

In contrast, when individuals feel they are responsible for contributing to their condition because they "should have known better," they feel guilty. This is especially true if they believe their disability is placing a burden on others. If the hearing loss has reduced their income because of job limitations or the expense of their care, they may feel guilty each time other family members deny themselves a dinner out or a new coat. Even if the hearing loss was totally outside their control, they may feel guilty about its repercussions on others. If their spouse's social life has become more limited because of their difficulty in participating, they may add the burden of guilt to the other difficulties they face.

Guilt and the Illusion of Control

Parents of children with hearing problems may be especially vulnerable to feelings of intense guilt. Gardner (1968) argues that the guilt reaction that parents of severely ill children experience represents their attempt to maintain a sense of control over life-threatening events. The belief that "If I had only done X or not done Y my child would be fine today" leads to devastating feelings of guilt—but it also implies that people have the power to prevent terrible things from happening. Letting go of the illusion that adults can always protect those whom they love would release them from guilt, but it carries with it an enormous price. Without this tacit belief, people experience the anxiety that comes from acknowledging "the fragility and transitoriness of life" (Shapiro, 1983, p. 917) and their relative helplessness in altering its course.

One young mother, who had continued teaching during her pregnancy despite her husband's objections, contracted rubella and blamed herself when their child was born deaf and brain damaged. "It's not your fault!" her doctor responded. "You might have caught the measles from one of the kids on your block even if you hadn't still been teaching." The mother shakes her head, fighting tears. Responding more sensitively, the clinician might tell the mother: "If you truly believe that you caused your child's impairment, no wonder you feel so badly. Tell me more about it" (Moses & Van Hecke-Wulatin, 1981, p. 256).

Parents who are struggling with guilt need an empathic listener who walks a fine line, confirming that the parents' feelings are legitimate without concurring in the parents' self-blame.

As parents and clients experience and explore their feelings of guilt, they reevaluate the degree of control they have over life events, and therefore the degree to which they are accountable for what occurs. They find a way "to avoid the absurdity of assuming full responsibility for all life events, and the equally absurd position of disclaiming any responsibility" (Moses & Van Hecke-Wulatin,

1981, p. 255). The professional working with guilt-ridden parents can help them explore these issues by listening to them "tell their stories," and by suggesting that self-forgiveness is possible in those areas where they judge themselves to be truly liable.

ANXIETY

An acquired hearing loss, particularly one in which the individual's condition is likely to worsen over time, raises great anxiety about the future. How bad is the condition likely to become? Will the individual become totally deaf? What will be the impact on employment, personal life, dreams? To what extent will assistive devices and coping strategies effectively diminish the problems encountered? The fact that these questions cannot be answered unequivocally heightens the hearing-impaired person's anxiety.

In response to the audiologist's question about how things are going, Mr. O'Malley says: "Well, not so good. I mean since you told me last week—I don't know—I can't concentrate at work, I'm not sleeping well. To be honest, sometimes I feel like I'm going crazy. The other day I couldn't hear the person on the phone and I thought I might start screaming or something." (Mr. O'Malley begins laughing in an embarrassed way.) "I don't know—maybe I need a mental ward as much as a hearing aid!"

The emotional roller coaster that people find themselves on when they grieve can make them fear that they are going crazy. Clinicians can reassure clients that their reactions are normal by stating: "Most people have a lot of reactions to a hearing loss. Sometimes they feel like they are going crazy because they can't predict how they are going to feel from one moment to the next."

Losing the illusions of a controllable and just world that once provided a sense of safety also contributes to the anxiety of people who experience a hearing loss. Their lives may be permeated with a terrible sense of vulnerability. The diminishing of this anxiety is one significant benefit of working through the philosophical issues connected with grief. Sometime during this process, many individuals begin to experience "acceptance."

Acceptance

Bristor (1984) defines acceptance as "transcending loss," feeling "serenity without passivity" (p. 29). The following words capture this feeling:

Sometimes I'm not sure what my disability is. Is it being paralyzed, or does that add a laughably small increment to the primordial handicap of being human? . . . We are not perfect; we are never what we would wish to be—however beautiful, good, gifted, serene, or strong we appear. These imperfections must be accepted without rancor before we can get on with the real and simple business of psychological development—doing the best we can with whatever we've got. (Vash, 1981, p. 130)

Like the other emotions associated with grieving, acceptance takes time. People move in and out of acceptance in various forms before achieving a more permanent resolution. With a hearing problem, the "invisible" handicap, it may be more difficult for individuals to bring themselves to this acceptance. Professionals have a fine line to walk here as well. Recognizing that many individuals with hearing problems feel embarrassed about wearing hearing aids, the audiologist may promise them that they will be fitted with the most inconspicuous model available. At the same time, we may try to assure clients that a hearing impairment is nothing to be ashamed of. As one 56-year-old woman noted:[1]

> We call it an invisible handicap and then try to keep it as invisible as possible, preventing people from helping us. The hearing aid industry would serve us better by selling their aids in decorator colors to draw attention to them rather than hiding them, thus alerting the people to whom we talk that we have a problem.

THE CHALLENGE TO PROFESSIONALS

Grieving is a slow process. During mourning, individuals move back and forth from one emotion to another. Often it is hard for them to know themselves exactly how they wish others to respond. Sensitive clinicians may sometimes feel caught between a rock and hard place. "Don't mislead us by giving us false hope and acting like a hearing aid will solve all our problems," protests one client, while others remonstrate: "Give people hope!" Similarly, most people wish they had more emotional support:

> I feel I should be told the truth right out but with concern for my feelings. That's what everybody seemed to try and overlook. I cried a lot and they saw it but nobody seemed to know how or didn't want to deal with my fear or feelings (30-year-old female).[1]

However, some prefer a more impersonal approach:

> I like the way I was dealt with. They gave me all the facts. There was no B.S. about it. They told me what the chances of getting better were (slim and none). They told me about hearing aids but they would use them as a last resort. Then I was left on my own, which was what I wanted (29-year-old male).[1]

Experienced audiologists know that the treatment that individuals want varies not only from person to person but even from moment to moment with the same client. Within a single discussion, clients might move from simply ventilating feelings to engaging in more active problem solving to exploring a philosophical dilemma. The sensitive professional moves with them, trying to provide what they most need at each point: comfort, practical suggestions, information, silent acceptance, reassurance.

Dedicated professionals might easily feel overwhelmed by the enormity of this task, which implies that we become proficient in counseling psychology as well as maintaining state-of-the-art expertise in our own fields. We might feel anxious or depressed at what this demands, asking: "How can I do all of this?" We might protest that "it isn't fair" when we are stereotyped as part of a "cold, uncaring, and money-mad" medical world despite our efforts. We may feel guilty when we fail to help someone, wondering, "Did I do enough?" "Should I have done something differently?" Our dream, in which we imagined ourselves making a difference in the lives of appreciative clients, is threatened by the indictments conveyed by many of the comments in this chapter.

Ironically, these experiences may provide a foundation for the empathy professionals need. These emotions remind us that our work confronts us with the same philosophical dilemmas our clients face. We, too, must sustain a realistic sense of competency while recognizing that there are limits to our ability to help. We must maintain a reasonable sense of responsibility for the outcomes of our efforts while recognizing the limits of our control. We must find a sense of purpose in a sometimes unjust world. And like our clients, we too mourn a dream: the dream of what we thought our professional lives would be like. Striving to resolve these issues in our own lives creates a kinship with grieving clients—which can be the bedrock of our partnership with them.

CONCLUSION

Audiologists enter their profession hoping to improve their clients' quality of life. To be effective, audiologists need to empathize with their clients' emotional reactions to developing a hearing disorder. This chapter describes how clinicians can respond more sensitively if they consider their client's life stage, listen actively to individual clients' "stories," and learn how to respond to the emotions of grief that many clients experience.

REFERENCES

BEATTIE, J. A. (1984). Social aspects of acquired hearing loss in adults. *International Journal of Rehabilitation Research, 7*, 215–216.

BICKNELL, J. (1984). The psychopathology of handicap. *Annual Progress in Child Psychiatry and Development*, pp. 346–363.

BRISTOR, M. W. (1984). The birth of a handicapped child—A wholistic model for grieving. *Family Relations, 33*, 25–32.

CALVANI, D. (1985). How well do your clients cope with hearing loss? *Journal of Gerontological Nursing, 11*, 16–20.

CHRISTIAN, E., DLUHY, N., & O'NEILL, R. (1989). Sounds of silence: Coping with hearing loss and loneliness. *Journal of Gerontological Nursing, 15*, 4–9.

COLE, K. D., & McCONNAHA, D. L. (1986). Understanding and interacting with older patients. *Journal of the American Optometric Association, 57*, 920–925.

ERIKSON, E. H. (1950). *Childhood and society.* New York: Norton.

GARDNER, R. A. (1968). Psychogenic problems of brain-injured children and their parents. *Journal of the American Academy of Child Psychiatry, 7*, 471–491.

GILHOME-HERBST, K., & HUMPHREY, C. (1980). Hearing impairment and mental state in the elderly living at home. *British Medical Journal, 281*, 903–905.

GOULD, R. (1978). *Transformations: Growth and change in adult life.* New York: Simon & Schuster.

HETU, R., LALONDE, M., & GETTY, L. (1987). Psychosocial disadvantages associated with occupational hearing loss as experienced in the family. *Audiology, 26*, 141–152.

KÜBLER-ROSS, E. (1969). *On death and dying.* New York: Macmillan.

LEVINSON, D. J. (1978). *The seasons of a man's life.* New York: Knopf.

LUSTBADER, W. (1991). *Counting on kindness: The dilemmas of dependency.* New York: Free Press.

MAGILVY, J. K. (1985). Quality of life of hearing-impaired older women. *Nursing Research, 34*, 140–146.

MARTIN, F. N., KRALL, L., & O'NEAL, J. (1989). The diagnosis of acquired hearing loss. *Asha, 31*, 47–50.

MOSES, K., & VAN HECKE-WULATIN, M. (1981). A counseling model re: The socio-emotional impact of infant deafness. In G. T. Mencher & S. E. Gerber (Eds.), *Early management of hearing loss* (pp. 243–278). New York: Grune & Stratton.

MOWRY, R. L. (1988). Quality of life indicators for deaf and hard of hearing former VR clients. *Journal of Rehabilitation of the Deaf, 21*, 1–7.

NODDINGS, N. (1984). *Caring.* Berkeley: University of California Press.

PERRY, W. (1970). *Forms of intellectual and ethical development in the college years: A scheme.* New York: Holt, Rinehart, & Winston.

PIAGET, J. (1932). *The moral judgment of the child.* New York: Macmillan.

SACKS, O. (1987). *A leg to stand on.* New York: Harper & Row.

SCHLESINGER, H. S. (1978). The effects of deafness on childhood development: An Eriksonian perspective. In L. S. Liben (Ed.), *Deaf children: Developmental perspectives* (pp. 157–167). New York: Academic Press.

SCHNEIDER, J. (1983). *The nature of loss, the nature of grief: A comprehensive model for facilitation and understanding.* Baltimore: University Park Press.

SHAPIRO, J. (1983). Family reactions and coping strategies in response to the physically ill or handicapped child: A review. *Social Science and Medicine, 17*, 913–931.

TANNEN, D. (1990). *You just don't understand.* New York: Morrow.

VASH, C. L. (1981). *The psychology of disability.* New York: Springer.

ZAMEROWSKI, S. (1982, July). Helping families cope with handicapped children. *Topics in Clinical Nursing,* pp. 41–56.

NOTE

1. These unpublished comments were written in response to a questionnaire distributed as part of the research reported by Martin et al. (1989).

chapter six

Counseling Children with Hearing Loss and Their Families

Dale V. Atkins

In this chapter, Dr. Atkins stresses the audiologist's need to bring a child's entire family into the rehabilitation process. This process becomes more effective if the audiologist can open avenues for family members to grow and develop through interaction with others who have traversed the same path. As discussed by Dr. Atkins, the audiologist has much to learn from the family, and that learning is considerably enhanced through the audiologist's own artful use of listening skills.

Her words rinse through my thoughts, clear as water, disconnected as rain.

Michael Dorris
A Yellow Raft in Blue Water

INTRODUCTION

Families with children who are hearing impaired, like all families, interact among themselves. The common need of a family's members are met through mutually beneficial interactions. Whenever one person in the family has a problem, the impact is felt by each other member. How a problem is dealt with by every member of the family will resonate in everyone, particularly the parents, sisters, brothers, and grandparents. Striving for a "new normalcy," one that meets the needs of each individual, is the biggest challenge facing any family with a child who has a hearing loss.

There is no clearly defined set of personality attributes, coping strategies, attitudes, or feelings that characterize a healthy and productive family with a child who is hearing impaired. Each family is unique. However, we can learn from those families who have loving, productive, satisfying, and joyful lives.

In my work with families, I have identified the following characteristics that help families function successfully:

- An attitude of acceptance
- An environment where people are encouraged to feel good about themselves
- A mutual respect
- An ability to listen to one another
- A sense of humor not used at the expense of others
- A willingness to adapt to change
- A flexibility of roles
- A drive for excellence with realistic expectations
- An ability to experiment with different problem-solving techniques
- An acknowledgment of feelings and other points of view
- An appreciation of difference

People in successfully functioning families can discover strengths they never knew they had, thus allowing relationships to reach new depths. Previously held beliefs about one another are often disproved, and aspects of their individual natures emerge in ways they did not think possible.

Rearing a child with a hearing impairment is a challenge to a person's will, spirit, and belief system. Everything that was previously taken for granted is suddenly questioned. Parents reevaluate themselves, their friendships, family relationships, and the society in which they live because of the roles they must now assume.

I'd like to think that I remember all of the parents, siblings, and grandparents I have ever met. Certainly, I have learned from all of them, and each has been unique and has touched my heart and my life profoundly. I am and will always be deeply grateful to all of the families who afforded me the privilege of being a part of their lives while they experienced many dramatic and difficult changes.

Parents benefit by sharing experiences. I consider my role to be that of a messenger. In this chapter I will explore the concerns of audiologists, parents, siblings, and grandparents in the context of our multicultural world. If I can articulate what parents and professionals have shared with me so that others can hear their words, feel their pain, experience their resolution, and gain strength from their hope, I will have achieved my goal.

FAMILIES IN NEED

Frequently families experience a restructuring process while they are adapting to life with a child who has a hearing impairment. Relying on the help of others can be difficult, but for some it can afford a family an opportunity to tap resources that were previously undiscovered.

Jonathan and Mary discovered their son Chad (now 7 years old) had a hearing impairment when he was 2 years old. At that time Mary was pregnant with their second child. This pregnancy confined Mary to bed while Chad's hearing impairment required that he be seen by audiologists and tutors several times a week. Jonathan traveled for business and was not a reliable child-care provider. Mary's sister became the support person taking Chad to his appointments, working with him and sharing with Mary and Jonathan what she had learned. The financial pressures increased when Mary later became unemployed. But the support of her sister and the knowledge that Chad was receiving the help he needed considerably alleviated their emotional stress.

Mary and Jonathan faced their child's hearing impairment when least expected. The diagnosis is unfair, unpleasant, and unwanted, and since it cannot be undone, it must be dealt with. Some of us are better able than others to deal with acute and ongoing crises.

When the suspicion of hearing loss is confirmed, there is often much sadness, guilt, anger, and remorse. Suddenly, the parents do not feel they know what to do, they question everything they know about their child, and they wonder how they will ever relate to this child, who is different from the one they expected. Feelings of growing competency with their own parenting skills are called into question while they worry about what will happen to their children, their relationship, their family. These feelings are complex and confusing. Unanswerable questions are asked and heighten frustration and feelings of isolation.

Factors Influencing Family Adaptation

The emotional, practical, and social aspects of life are dramatically altered when a child who is hearing impaired is in the family. Parents abandon parts of themselves as they refocus or redefine their priorities. Good friends are asked to accommodate to their pressing demands. New friendships are formed because old ones may no longer meet the parents' needs. Choices are made in favor of one member of the family at the expense of another.

The following factors are among those that influence family adaptation when a child with a hearing impairment is in the family.

Marital harmony or dissonance. The presence of a child with a hearing impairment in a family can emphasize strong and weak points in a relationship. Aspects of the marriage that may not have seemed significant become prominent while each parent attempts to integrate what it means to have a child with a hearing impairment.

Single-parent families. The demands on single-parent families are keenly accentuated when a child has special needs. Significantly more resources (emotional, time, and money) are needed, thus requiring much more of the single parent. These families must have access to support services, other parents, and audiologists with whom they can discuss alternative child-rearing approaches, educational options, and other pertinent matters related to their children.

Step-parenthood. Whether or not step-parents understand and can adapt to the impact of hearing impairment in their lives may not be apparent until they have assumed some of the parental responsibilities. Among the issues that are relevant to all step-parents are how much and what type of commitment and obligations they have in the child's life.

Family size. Large families can significantly affect the quality of the parent–child and sibling bonds. Families with "unwanted" children often experience the strains of parental ambivalence, causing difficulties not only between generations but between siblings. Children in large families have usually learned to wait their turn, share, and appreciate one another as members of a group. The opportunities for socialization and a sharing of responsibilities increase when there are many brothers and sisters. Families who have children with hearing losses are expected to participate in their children's school and therapy programs. This can be taxing on any size family.

Birth order. In families of all sizes, birth order may have an impact on parent–child and sibling interactions. Oldest children tend to be given more responsibility for their younger charges, and appear to be task oriented, serious, and high achieving. Parental behavior is usually different toward each child. Frequently expectations and demands are higher on the firstborn. When the firstborn child has a hearing impairment, those expectations may be altered with later-born children needing to fulfill the parents' dreams for the firstborn.

Sex and age spacing of the children. Some families prefer boys to girls or girls to boys. If a family holds one or the other sex in higher esteem, this can seriously affect the child's self-image and the relationships within the family. If a boy was desired and one was born, then he surely has luck. If a girl was born to a family that wanted a boy, she may internalize their disappointment. Siblings who are close in age can have tremendous benefit for the child who is hearing impaired. The hearing sibling serves as an important language and socialization model. However, the strain on the parent to attend to the needs of a few children close in age may be overwhelming.

Economic status and its constancy. In instances when a hearing impairment is diagnosed, aside from the stress accompanying this event, there are often tremendous financial restraints on the family. Most often, choices are made in favor of the child with the greatest need.

Parental employment. A two-income family may shift to a single-income family if one of the parents becomes more fully involved in a child's education or therapy program. This may be done willingly or resentfully. In some instances, one or both parents may restructure employment to earn more income or to be available for family-centered programs. Additional jobs and longer hours may be required to pay for the additional services.

Coping strategies. Understanding the depth and range of feelings that will be present is an important first step in developing coping strategies. Attempting to discover and understand the attitudes that each of us has about hearing impairment, children with disabilities, parents of children with disabilities, and people who work with them is an important component of coping effectively. Good time management for ourselves and the children helps to facilitate the coping process.

Expectations of self and others. All of us have an image of ourselves and our children, those who work with them, and those who are in professions we have held in either high or low esteem. The challenge is to keep our expectations "realistically high" so that we are always challenged and have the opportunity to appreciate our successes when they have been achieved.

Temperamental match between parent and child. A child's hearing impairment may or may not contribute to temperament. Some children are slower to warm up to than others, and their parents may have difficulty relating to the child. Generally, personalities that are evident early on do not have to do with hearing impairment.

Styles, values, and beliefs about rearing children. We may or may not have a philosophical approach that works for all of our children. Attempting to be true to ourselves *and* recognizing the needs of our children as individuals can be a good mix for learning the healthiest way to rear children.

Style of communication. Our style of communication, whether appeasing, combative, assertive, aggressive, cooperative, or empathetic, will be tested while we are facing ourselves, school personnel, other parents, audiologists, and hearing aid dispensers. In order to achieve goals more effectively, it is helpful for parents and audiologists to examine and adjust communication styles.

Approaches to problem solving. Since there are many approaches, most of us resort to familiar patterns we observed or developed in childhood. Some of us avoid or ignore problems; some of us hope another person will "rescue" us. Others of us are combative, not giving up without a fight. Since parents and professionals need to work as a team, it is useful to employ creativity while collaborating to solve problems.

Types of acute and chronic stress. Meeting the needs of a child with a hearing impairment can stress emotional and financial resources. Other stressors that may exist have to do with health and illness of other family members, employment and job satisfaction, and other conditions that demand attention.

Adaptability to change. Some of us take to change more comfortably than others. When facing hearing impairment, the most fundamental change that occurs is the view we have of ourselves and our children. Some of us fear that we will not be able to adapt; we can resent the need to change and resist adjusting in ways that are unfamiliar despite the fact that they may be helpful.

What "difference" means to the family. Our view of ourselves and our family is questioned when we discover that our child has a hearing impairment. How this is treated by others can contribute to our feeling a part of or apart from our family and larger community. The difference in our family can make us feel diminished, enhanced, unusual, or a host of other feelings.

Support system within the family. How we manage with the help we have or do not have can determine how well we adapt to life with a child who has a hearing impairment. Calling upon those who are close to us for help is often difficult due to the nature of preexisting relationships, availability, and logistics.

Previous exposure to hearing impairment or disability. Our attitudes are often a reflection of our previous experience or lack thereof. For many of us, exposure to hearing-impaired people may have been limited to a person distributing cards displaying the finger spelling alphabet, an aged family member who uses a hearing aid, or some preconceived notion of "deaf and dumb." It is sometimes difficult to challenge old attitudes to allow for the inclusion of new thoughts.

Joanne, a young, single mother, discovered that her 2-year-old son was hearing impaired after he recovered from spinal meningitis. "I have no idea what is in store for me. I feel I have to fasten a seat belt for a very scary roller-coaster ride. Sure, I'm glad he's alive, but I'm devastated that he's deaf."

Having survived the fear that her son might die, she was faced with another unknown, the world of hearing impairment. She had to overcome feeling helpless and isolated. What helped her the most was tracking her own progress and that of her son by keeping a diary. When Joanne compared herself to her friends or compared her son's progress to the hearing children at the playground, she felt even more depressed and hopeless. Whenever she met new people, she tried to develop friendships with those who seemed interested in her, who encouraged and supported her and her effort. She reevaluated the quality of her existing friendships and how she spent her time. Frequently she felt as if nobody was in as bad a situation as she. These moments passed if she let herself experience them. She understood that they had more to do with dashed hopes, unrealized expectations, and her disappointment with the unpredictability of life. Sometimes, her tension manifested itself in severe headaches, and she often lost her temper over insignificant things.

Over time, Joanne rediscovered things she used to do for herself but had stopped doing. She took walks, spent time with good friends, and went bowling. She enjoyed these brief "escapes" and trained herself not to feel guilty about participating. This helped to restore her faith in herself and in her life.

CHALLENGES FACING THE AUDIOLOGIST

The audiologist's role is complex and multifaceted. To be most effective with families of children who are hearing impaired the audiologist must posses a working knowledge of hearing impairment and the various medical and educational approaches to its remediation as well as a sensitivity to families and an appreciation of their struggle in adapting to hearing impairment. Audiologists are keenly aware of the potential perceptual, speech, communication, cognitive, social, emotional, educational, intellectual, vocational, parental, or societal problems that can arise if a child possesses a congenital hearing impairment that is severe enough to prevent the child from hearing speech prior to being fitted with a hearing aid (Boothroyd, 1982). Their purpose is to help the child and parents overcome the disability of hearing impairment to the greatest extent possible. Since the task is tremendous and implementing audiological habilitation programs early in a child's life is a crucial factor of success, an audiologist can feel pressure to "succeed" with a child.

In Chapter 3, Dr. Martin discusses important considerations for audiologists to consider when participating in initial diagnostic counseling. To enhance their effectiveness, audiologists need to have an ongoing support system and a strong sense of self.

Everyone who works with families of hearing-impaired children, like the families themselves, needs a support system that consists of open, compassionate, understanding people who are good listeners. It can be draining to work with parents who are in crisis. To manage their own stress, audiologists need to create a network of both work-related supports and personal support resources.

The task of helping families to create or maintain adaptive resources at this difficult time can be tremendously stressful for the audiologist. These stresses are similar to and reflective of the families' difficulties. It is not uncommon for audiologists to be reminded of their own personal losses when working with these families. Just as parents express feeling vulnerable, audiologists, too, can become acutely aware of their own susceptibility.

Audiologists enter a family's life when family members are grief-stricken, overwhelmed with personal pain, sadness, or confusion. A common grief response is withdrawal, and it is extremely difficult to reach people who are removed. While experiencing enormous anguish, parents are forced to enter a world that threatens the family's stability. The audiologist is always coping with the stress of others and feeling their pain while trying to help them to cope. In order to help the families, the audiologist must be secure, approachable, and accepting, with an excellent and realistic sense of timing for giving information.

Parents, regardless of their culture, have various explanations about the cause of their children's hearing impairments. They may believe it to be the result of real problems such as the result of a medical condition, genetic incompatibility, ototoxic drugs, noise, or even imagined sources such as punishment by God or ancestors' curses for actions or thoughts of the parents or their relatives. Frequently, behavior and receptivity to the intervention or support of other parents or professionals are dictated by a person's belief system. Audiologists need to be aware and accept that these are forces that should be addressed.

Parents initially meet with the audiologist at a time of acute crisis when they are highly anxious about whether their child can hear. Since a common parental reaction to the news that a child is hearing impaired is denial, frequently parents believe that the diagnosis is wrong. Anger directed toward an audiologist can be present for months or years, possibly affecting the relationship between the audiologist and parents.

Mismatched Expectations

Generally, there is much information to be shared, and the audiologist may feel a sense of urgency for the parents to respond to the challenge and follow up on suggestions that will benefit their child. Parents are not always able to appreciate the audiologist's perspective, and consequently, it may leave the audiologist with intense feelings of frustration and loss of enthusiasm.

Parents who appear to make progress are the ones who follow up on suggestions and perform in a certain way. The parents who need the most encouragement are generally those who are unable to assimilate the information at a rate the professional feels is appropriate. The audiologist must attempt to maintain a balance for the family, not overwhelming them with too much information at one time, so that the family can continue to move ahead.

There are significant personal challenges to audiologists who interact with families of hearing-impaired children. They must continuously cope with their own expectations and those of their clients. Expecting families to follow a progression of stages (e.g., shock, recognition, denial, anger, resolution) that leads to a final state of acceptance unfairly imposes a rigid standard on what is a highly personal process that is neither predictable nor linear. Audiologists who are interested in counseling families must approach them and the process without attempting to control their experience and without imposing goals or success criteria. There is no "correct way" to adapt to life with a hearing-impaired child.

Audiologists can experience significantly high levels of stress when they operate under an unyielding set of standards or ideas that relate to the manner in which parents "should" adapt. They must allow the parents to lead. When parents are allowed to address their concerns in a supportive, nonjudgmental environment, their level of anxiety usually diminishes. All too often, audiologists see families in a busy clinical or office setting where appointments are tightly scheduled. Time is frequently the situational stressor that provokes a common experience among audiologists, that of never being away from the office.

Exploring Viable Options

It is the responsibility of audiologists to help parents to have access to information so that they can make informed decisions that are best for them and their family. Often these decisions need to be made quickly and without adequate information, although there may be several sources of input (Pearlman & Scott, 1981). Too frequently, parents and audiologists feel that one approach is superior and then become closed to learning about other methods, sometimes feeling threatened by their mere mention. Because an audiologist is affiliated with an Auditory–Verbal, Oral–Aural, Cued Speech, Total Communication, or Sign Language program is not reason enough to withhold information from parents about other approaches.

Learning about other philosophies or methods opens the door for discussion and inquiry. Parents obviously need to learn about hearing impairment, and they deserve to have the various options presented to them as alternatives from which they can choose wisely. Initially confused, parents often put audiologists and other professionals in the uncomfortable position of feeling they are supposed to tell the parent what to do. Over time, parents become better prepared to make their own decisions, relying on the audiologist less for direction and more for guidance. Ideally, parents emerge as "case managers" working within an interdisciplinary team (Marlowe, 1991).

Despite the fact that audiologists are knowledgeable about hearing impairment, there is a significant number who do not regularly visit classrooms or educational centers. Programs with differing philosophies and techniques need to be seen so that audiologists and parents of hearing-impaired children can be well informed of all alternatives, not just those they espouse. There is no reason that some audiologists are not current regarding various approaches and developments in the field. Parents need to be able to depend on audiologists as informed sources in order to make the best decisions for themselves and their families *without ever feeling that they have failed or disappointed the audiologist or others working with their children.* Sometimes being informed requires knowledge beyond the scope of our chosen profession. An example of this occurs when we attempt to better understand people of an ethnic origin differing from our own.

Multicultural Considerations

About 50 million (21%) of the 240 million citizens in the United States are African American, Hispanic, or Asian. By the year 2000, it is projected that one out of every three Americans will be nonwhite. "Hispanics are among the most rapidly growing and the youngest of minority groups in the United States as reflected in the increase in Hispanics among school-age deaf population" (Rodriguez & Santiviago, 1991, p. 89). We have an obligation to become familiar with cultures that are different from our own. Clearly, there is no *one* African American, Hispanic, or Asian cultural type, but we need to learn more than many of us already know to understand and serve all families in the best way possible.

In the 25 largest urban school systems, the majority of students are ethnic, racial, or linguistic minorities. The demographics continue to have a profound impact on programs for the hearing-impaired children as well as programs for parents. Making efforts to minimize the problems that may arise from cultural differences can be achieved only by developing awareness of the needs among the cultural groups. Sensitivity to these differences is a basis for developing trust and creating an open forum for sharing problems and examining possible solutions.

Developing an Awareness to Different Cultures

It is probable that audiologists and others working with families from different cultural backgrounds have little awareness of those people and their circumstances. This can create unnecessary boundaries to communication with high likelihood for misunderstanding.

Sharon had recently arrived in the United States from India with her husband, and their three children, the youngest of whom was hearing impaired. In order for Sharon to participate in the parent–child program, she had to attend daily sessions with her hearing-impaired son. Maintaining a household, traveling on public transportation, and assuming such a prominent and public role with her child were new for her. She needed help with some of the duties that had previously been solely her responsibility, but she was reluctant to ask her husband. In time, her husband assumed some of the household and child-care responsibilities and a redefinition of roles emerged. This worked well for the couple, and they were supported in the parent group. However, when her family came for a visit, Sharon was chastised severely for neglecting her wifely responsibilities.

As this couple discovered, previously held cultural expectations may need to be adjusted when there is a hearing-impaired child in the family. The reasons for adopting new behavior patterns need to be explained to other family members without criticism. The more the audiologist is aware of the intricacies of the particular cultural background and expectations, the more helpful their services can be to the family.

In addition to being aware of the differences among cultures, it is imperative that all people are recognized and treated as worthwhile individuals. There are some people who are hearing impaired who believe that there is a specific deaf culture within a larger deaf community. This is a debated point among educators, but what is not debatable is the fact that the larger deaf community can be a valuable resource for families and professionals who interact within the world of those who have hearing impairments.

Single-Parent Households

A large percentage of minority households are headed by females. This fact needs to be considered when we work with children of different cultures. Single parents often need assistance in keeping a balance of their need for self-fulfillment and responsibilities in the care of a hearing-impaired child or children. Since caring for a hearing-impaired child can be overwhelming for one person, particularly in the area of problem solving and decision making, single parents need to have a sense of community as part of their social and educational structure. Work and meeting schedules need to be flexible and considerate of the needs of all potential participants. It is important to consider how these parents will be able to receive needed support. Programs that are effective and flexible are more likely to be attended by single parents than those based on the needs of two-parent households.

At issue, too, is the possibility that single parents may marry or remarry, thus blending more people into the situation. Step-parents, siblings, and grandparents may or may not have the time or interest in becoming actively involved in issues of hearing impairment.

Immigrant Concerns

Newly arrived, often young, immigrant parents frequently feel isolated and unfamiliar in the new world with its culture. Since immigrants are in the process of learning about the predominant American culture, parent groups, audiologists, and other professionals need to be sensitive to the many issues these families must address simultaneously.

For some members of a parent group the reality of hearing impairment may be devastating. To these new members, it is no less devastating but may not be the primary concern. Housing, food and employment are critical for survival and come first,

Many immigrant families come to this country without any family support systems. Frequently, circumstances that brought them to this country were unpleasant and often life-threatening. Contact with family members is sometimes nonexistent and dangerous. They may be wary of discussing their personal lives or accepting help from strangers. Immigrant families' unique experiences contribute to the way they interact with other parents and professionals.

General Minority Concerns

There are many minority families who are not immigrants and should not be viewed as such. Frequently, there is a strong support system within their community but it may not address the feelings and experiences related to having a hearing-impaired child. It is important not to make generalizations about any minority group but to take the time to understand what is important to each family and to learn their ideas about parenting, some of which are culturally based. Certain practices may be common and normal within a particular cultural group but unfamiliar to others. When these practices are discussed in parent groups, there can be misunderstanding and inappropriate judgments of behavior.

I recall a group of parents who were discussing their feelings about not burdening their older daughters with too much responsibility. One of the parents confessed that in her culture, it is the job of the eldest daughter to perform duties that the mother cannot handle, either due to work or other pressures. Her eldest daughter assumed tremendous responsibilities for the household, as she had done.

It is essential for parents and professionals to be aware of their intent when they elicit information from parents of other cultures. The intent may be to change the style of parenting or it may be to understand the parent's approach to parenting based on heretofore unfamiliar cultural roots.

Each person views the process of testing and educating children differently. To some, talking about one's family history and personal issues may or may not be comfortable.

Sharing personal information with strangers, early in a relationship, can be seen as rude and inappropriate by those who are expected to reveal the information. Some people are extremely uncomfortable exhibiting emotion in public or in front of a person of the opposite sex. There are those whose cultural norms prohibit them from speaking without being addressed, talking about personal issues, or both. As a result of language barriers and cultural and socio-economic differences, ethnic minority parents can experience extreme discomfort and feelings of intimidation and alienation in the context of their child's school. If parent support meetings are held in the school, these feelings may carry over in the form of suspicion for those in the group. These feelings become exacerbated in a school for hearing-impaired children, where the specialness and therefore, strangeness, imposes an added barrier for those from a culturally different milieu.

Meetings with minority parents conducted in their own language is an important, worthwhile initial step toward helping these people feel able to take risks and make further contacts with the school and the people associated with the education of their children (Cohen, 1987). Depending on the resources and the services available, conducting parent support groups in one's native language facilitates the participants' expression of their feelings in the language with which they are most comfortable. The ideal is to try to reach families from a variety of backgrounds in their own language. One more added stress in the process of coming to terms with the fact that one's child is hearing impaired, that of having to express oneself in another language, is eliminated. (For a more in-depth review of this topic, the reader is referred to Fishgrund, Cohen, & Clarkson, 1987; and to the Center for Assessment and Demographic Studies, Gallaudet University, Washington, DC.)

PARENT SUPPORT GROUPS

No matter how effectively audiologists convey information and listen empathetically to parents, it is impossible to assume that they know what the parents of children with hearing losses are experiencing. Only other parents of children with hearing losses can come close to understanding, for they have already been through the roller coaster of emotions and confusion discussed by Dr. Van Hecke in Chapter 5. Nobody but these parents empathize with the feelings of observing their children's lack of response to a car horn as they cross the street, or their struggle to communicate with grandparents. Nobody but these parents appreciate the fear and confusion children feel when they are lost and are unable to call home. Only these parents can convey their apprehensions and projections, and share solutions to problems their children must face on a day-to-day basis.

Some of us find it difficult to express and share feelings about our lives. To others, as previously discussed, it is culturally inappropriate to discuss personal matters outside of the family. Even for those of us who do not have personal or cultural constraints, it is hard to communicate feelings of fear, confusion, skepticism, and mistrust even to those who are helping us and our children. It is difficult to complain about a teacher or an audiologist when we are afraid of the impact it may have on our children. We may feel that the children might be ignored or resented and, consequently, not get the support and training that is needed.

Positive Features of Support Groups

Support groups are powerful and valuable influences on parents of hearing-impaired children. Among other things, participants learn that they are not alone. Knowing that some other family is experiencing similar feelings and thoughts is a relief in itself. Although participants begin as strangers, before long they become friends and, to many, a type of family. Struggling through the maze of educational, medical, and philosophical options appears to be safer when it can be navigated with others who have similar concerns.

> Suzanne and James felt like they were the first and only couple to have a hearing-impaired child. None of their friends or family had experienced a "difference in the family," and this young couple felt alone and unsupported. They received family pressure to send their son to a boarding school and to try to have another child, thus building the family they were supposed to have. They were confused about how to raise their son but were certain that they wanted him at home. They joined a parent group for support and direction. Suzanne told the group that she finally understood the meaning of the saying "A shared joy is twice the joy; a shared sorrow is half the sorrow."

Families gain companionship and understanding that emerge naturally from sharing experiences in a support group. Parents, reaching out to help one another, work on solving problems in a nonthreatening context. Since the purpose is to offer parents support and information specific to hearing impairment, friendships develop based on mutuality and similar ordeals. While parents exchange information, they develop confidence in themselves and their children. Slowly they learn to adapt and give meaning to their new role as parents of hearing-impaired children.

Obstacles to Success of Support Groups

The benefits of parent support groups are considerable, yet there are factors that interfere with constant participation and commitment to group involvement. Parents confront practical issues such as attending regular meetings, distance, transportation, and child care. Language and cultural barriers can cause discouragement and irregular attendance. Issues of pride, disappointment, impatience with oneself as a parent, or impatience with parents who are at a different level of adjustment, all impact involvement. Comparing one child's progress to someone else's child can cause discomfort that is best addressed within the group.

Reluctance to face other stress-related matters, such as alcoholism and other substance abuse, abusive child-rearing patterns, and illness, minimize the positive effects the group may have on the parents. Believing that "only the professional knows best" inhibits some participants from valuing other parents' comments.

Despite the obstacles, support groups make a significant difference in the lives of parents and their children. Countless parents report changes in their relationships, in their feelings about themselves and their families, in their understanding of the impact of hearing impairment, and in their manner of communication.

Structure of a Support Group

Each parent support group establishes its own rules, sets its own style, and determines its own content. For more information on group facilitator guidelines that can be helpful when considering support groups, the reader is referred to Dr. Trychin's suggestions in Chapter 10.

When establishing a group, parents need to address the following questions:

- Is the purpose of the group clear to those participating? If the purpose is already established because the group has been ongoing, then participants need to be informed so that they know what to expect.
- Should parent meetings be "educational," "recreational," "administrative" or "emotionally supportive"? The multipurpose approach seems to work best when meetings are clearly designated. Educational meetings are of the lecture and question-and-answer format, while emotionally supportive meetings involve sharing feelings. Recreational events may occur on weekends, at someone's home, a park, or an outing, and the administrative aspects may be attended to in more business-related meetings where parents need to get together to help develop policy for a school or fund-raising event.
- Who leads the group? The purpose of a group leader is to facilitate parent discussion, not to lecture the parents. Some groups function well with the co-leadership of a parent and a professional or two professionals. This can be arranged so that they colead all meetings or they can alternate leadership roles.

The effectiveness of a parent group is dependent largely on the leader. In one particularly successful parent group the leader was a counselor who had studied psychology after she had raised her own hearing-impaired son and his sister. She was hired by the school system and facilitated a weekly support group meeting for parents whose children were in four area schools.

Having someone who is both familiar with the parents and their children and who is experienced in the field of hearing impairment is critical. Someone who is well versed in group dynamics and in fostering and modeling good communication skills is an asset. The group needs to be in agreement about the role of the leader(s).

At one center where I was involved, the first hour of the weekly parent meeting was geared to educational and informational issues about hearing impairment. Parents of similar-age children attended classes taught by teachers of hearing-impaired children. These structured classes focused on speech and language formation, child development, and socialization. During the second hour, the parents attended a support group meeting led by a psychologist. In addition, mothers met in a smaller weekly support group also led by a psychologist. Discussions were free-flowing and topics were determined by the participants. The leader was there to meet the needs of the participants.

Once a month, the parents met for 2 hours to handle administrative issues mostly having to do with fund-raising. They also planned pot-luck dinners, picnics, and outings to encourage the development of social relationships among the families. When the hearing sisters and brothers attended these functions, they met other hearing-impaired children as well as other siblings. The sisters and brothers also participated in "Sibling Days," which will be discussed later in this chapter.

Sometimes an easy, unthreatening social setting provides the atmosphere in which parents can learn how to adapt to life with their hearing-impaired child. Seeing others as models helps in the determination of one's own behavior. At other times a support group is needed so that parents can examine the variety of feelings discussed by Dr. Van Hecke in Chapter 5 and feel better about themselves in a social setting. For other parents, working on a fundraiser may be a means for getting involved. To another person giving time to the fundraiser is "just one more thing to add to an already full schedule."

For all parents, though, learning about hearing impairment and different philosophies of teaching as well as advances in the fields of education and hearing aid and implant technology is invaluable. Some parents, however, cannot "hear" the information because their emotional state of mind prevents them from absorbing the information they need to best serve themselves and their children. Dr. Clark in Chapter 2, and Dr. Martin in Chapter 3 discuss the difficulties of communicating important information when someone appears emotionally blocked or resistant and unable to process the information. Hearing only parts of messages is common, especially when the news is bad. Parents need to be informed of bad news clearly and tactfully, but doing so does not ensure that they have received the information as the professional intended. Previously misunderstood communications can be reviewed safely with other parents. Further discussion of the topic of mixed and missed messages between parents and professionals can be found in the writings of Kroth (1987) and Wolraich (1982).

Success Factors

In addition to the group leadership, orientation, and purpose, other important factors to consider when contemplating establishing a parent group are size, eligibility, attendance, whether sessions will be open or closed, and the number and frequency of meetings.

While assessing the needs of the group, several other factors have to be considered. The group meetings should be easily accessible and comfortable. Where they will be held is important. Possibilities are a school, community hall, church, temple, or someone's home. Somers (1987) underscores transportation as a major problem for low-income families, and this needs to be considered when planning for parent groups that are intended to reach all parents. Another significant item is child care. Costs of babysitters can be prohibitive for some families, particularly for low-income, single parents, so providing child care can encourage attendance.

Most parent groups prefer to meet as parents alone; however, there can be benefit to including teachers and audiologists for a sharing of perspectives. Whether teachers and other professionals are welcome needs to be determined.

Continuity is an essential element of success. Group cohesion and discussion of topics can be affected by whether meetings are weekly, biweekly, or monthly. If the group is open or closed also affects its continuity. There are merits to both orientations. Parents of newly diagnosed children can get hope and guidance from those more seasoned. However, the issues of concern to families who have known for years that their children are hearing impaired may be significantly different from those of the parents who have recently discovered their child's hearing loss.

Interpreter services for the oral hearing impaired, those who use sign language, and foreign language speakers may need to be provided as well, depending on the size, makeup, and nature of the group. If interpreters are used, it is imperative that interpreters be fully qualified. Enlisting a member of the group as the interpreter prevents that person from fully participating and also deprives the person in need of the services of top-notch interpreter assistance.

Meeting the Needs of Participants

Few groups will be able to meet the needs of each member all of the time. The goal should be to continually assess the needs of the whole group as well as the individual members. It is important to understand the various responses of parents in support groups. In spite of our own interpretation, someone who attends the group on a regular basis but is not an active participant may be getting a lot out of the group. The group leader needs to know the community well enough to be able to refer families for outside counseling or specific needs that can be provided by other services (e.g., employment, housing, child care).

Several years ago while facilitating a weekly parent group in California, I observed one mother, Rose, who consistently attended although she never spoke. She appeared sad and angry most of the time and rarely engaged other parents during the coffee break. After 3 years, she told the members of the group that she and her husband had decided to relocate and that the most difficult part of the move was that she would miss the group. Surprised, one mother asked why. Rose replied, "This is the only place where I feel safe, where I know the feelings I have are okay. Week after week, year after year, you all said what I felt inside but could not say. You gave me a voice, and, when I came here, I heard what I needed to say but couldn't. I never felt alone. For months I have tried to talk but I was afraid I would cry; it is a disgrace on the family in my culture to cry in public."

After Rose moved, she kept us informed about her family. After 1 year, she was instrumental in establishing a parent group. Even though Rose never talked, she felt a part of the group, while others mistakenly believed she was apart from the group.

I recall Andrea, a mother of five whose youngest child was hearing impaired. She too never missed a parent support group meeting. However, she rarely spoke until Regina and Todd joined the group. Regina and Todd had a son who had just been diagnosed as profoundly hearing impaired. Andrea welcomed them, and they sat together.

Andrea defined a role for herself as Regina's "friend." By assuming the role of a "supportive big sister," as she liked to refer to herself, Andrea started talking about her own experiences. By talking, she helped Regina and Todd as she had been helped by listening to others discuss their experiences in raising a hearing-impaired child.

There are some families who take a long time to come to terms with a hearing impairment. Their manner of acceptance or adaptation may be difficult for the professionals who work with them to accept. One such family comes to mind.

I met Marta at a weekly parent group. She had three children. One of her baby twins was hearing impaired and this news devastated both her and her husband. Having a son follow in his father's footsteps was important to this family. The father, Jack, whose work required that he be on the road often, found innumerable reasons to stay away even more than necessary. This was difficult for Marta, whose native language was not English, and who was not comfortable driving in the city. Like many mothers, she shouldered the enormous responsibilities of general motherhood and the specifics of mothering a hearing-impaired child single-handedly.

She made many friends while attending day and evening programs. When her husband was in town, he drove her to evening meetings but refused to come into the building. He sat in the parking lot for the whole 2 hours of class. Other parents in the group were upset for her and angry at him for "not assuming his rightful responsibility."

Marta refused to let the other fathers talk to him. For months she repeatedly said, "In his own time . . . " The other parents were outraged, responding, "Marta, you need help! Nobody gave you the luxury of taking 'your own time.'" After several months, one of the couples walked Marta out to the parking lot and the husband greeted Jack. He told him that the following week he would like to keep him company in the car.

In the following weeks, Jack and the other father sat in the car for the 2 hours of our parent meeting. After a couple of weeks, Jack came inside of the room but stayed outside of the circle. He stared at his shoes. By the time he was ready to talk, we were ready to take our summer break!

Marta and Jack did get together with other families, though, over the summer. The other fathers asked him to attend a special planning meeting for the center's yearly fund-raiser. He began to feel accepted and valued. Over the years, Jack continued his involvement at the Center. He was voted president of the Parents' Association and did great work for the Center and for other parents. He was frequently asked and never refused to talk to "new" parents. His attendance at parent groups was constant even when his child was mainstreamed and no longer at the Center!

Each family must come to terms with its own style. Marta coped and adapted to her life without malice. She realized where she needed to go for strength and support and where it was not forthcoming. She loved her husband and felt he was "a good man." Perhaps she knew something none of the rest of us were willing or able to wait for: He was more likely to be a part of her son's life only after he experienced his own reactions in his own way.

Another couple, Joanne and Dennis, discovered that their second child was hearing impaired when she was 10 months old. Their older daughter, a bright, affable child, was very attached to her father and he continued to spend time with her. When their daughter was diagnosed, Joanne became severely depressed and angry. Previously social, she withdrew from her old friends and family. She was convinced that her old friends would not have the patience for her or her hearing-impaired daughter. She feared rejection.

This couple argued frequently and experienced few tender moments. Joanne accused Dennis of purposefully avoiding learning how to work with their daughter. Not unlike many fathers, Dennis threw himself into the business, technological, and informational aspects of deafness. He explored organizations and their philosophies, current research, and conferences. Joanne was not interested. She wanted Dennis at home helping to relieve her burden.

Coincidentally and increasing the stress, both of their businesses were having difficulty and they experienced significant financial strains. Joanne chose not to rebuild her business, opting to stay at home. She told me, "I want to devote my life to my daughter so that she will talk normally."

Other marital and personality incompatibilities that had previously been glossed over became focal point irritants between them. Suddenly, Dennis's optimistic attitude was seen by his wife as immature and irresponsible. Dennis regarded Joanne's serious, perfectionistic style as preachy and tedious. Instead of being supportive of each other, they became nasty, taking out their frustrations, anger, and sadness related to their daughter's hearing loss on each other. Their older daughter exhibited disturbing behavior at school and mistreated the family pet. It appeared impossible for them to have a good time with each other. Dennis felt criticized and Joanne felt she was alone in her struggle. Joanne attempted to attend a parent group meeting but did not feel comfortable participating because "I really can't trust anyone, nobody had it as bad as I do, and I have nothing in common with those people."

There are always other factors that influence the family, the marital relationship, and other relationships. When people asked if they could help Joanne, she replied that nobody could do anything for her. She had to do it all alone. She could not trust anyone to work with her daughter because nobody could do it as well as she. In fact, she may have been right, but their whole world was not made up of her daughter and her bound together by lessons. Sadly, Joanne's sense

> *of isolation and desperation grew. She and Dennis continued to feel alienated from each other. Since they were not getting along, they declined social invitations. Their limited and caustic conversations revolved around their hearing-impaired daughter's education. The older daughter felt ignored and attempted to be the center of attention in a variety of inappropriate ways.*
>
> *This family could have benefited from marital counseling, participation in a parent support group, and individual therapy for the older daughter. The audiologist attempted to introduce them to other families with older, hearing-impaired children as well as to hearing-impaired adults with whom they could meet and ask questions but the family resisted. Their initial reluctance was never challenged again. Although it is discouraging to work with families who have difficulty holding life together, it is not impossible. The audiologist and/or other people involved in the child's world can periodically call the family, send information, or with their permission, ask other parents to contact them. For some families the period of adjustment is longer than others, and additional support services are indicated but not welcome. It is important to keep the lines of communication open even if it appears that they will never be used.*

There are countless individual stories and examples of parent adaptation and of parent groups. The key is to appreciate the individuality of the membership and the dynamic of the group. This dynamic changes when certain people are absent or others attend. If a couple usually attends together, the types of remarks that are made may significantly differ when one of them is absent. The insights gained into relationships resulting from the presence or absence of individuals need to be discussed openly so that the group continues to function well. If there are specific topics that are taboo, the group and its leader must come to an understanding of what is discussable and what is not.

Groups for Parents of Older Children

There are more group programs available for parents of preschool and early elementary children than for parents whose children are in upper elementary or secondary schools. Since parental adaptation to hearing impairment is a cyclical emotional process, it is imperative to have parental support groups for parents of older children coming to terms with peer interaction issues, concerns for independence, and family communication.

There are few support groups for parents of mainstream youngsters. Clearly distance is a contributing factor. But there seems to be an erroneous assumption that if a child is in the mainstream, problems are either solved or insignificant! For me, some of the most poignant meetings I have attended have been with families whose children are "successfully" mainstreamed. These parents crave dialogue with others whose children experience similar kinds of adjustment issues. Access to new information is vital, but having the ability to share feelings about experiences as children grow is also essential.

I disagree with the frequently held view that parents finish their adaptation process when the child is well into a school routine, has formed friendships, and is able to communicate effectively. It is at these times that support groups can be extremely helpful. The concerns have to do more with "life skills and choices," family rules and management, responsibilities, extracurricular activities, after-school jobs, and the complex aspects of social interactions. As children assert their independence, parents continue to address their own feelings. Support groups continue to be a useful forum for parents to address the ongoing issues of raising mainstreamed children.

A mother of a 15-year-old girl was reluctant to talk about her rising anxiety when her daughter began dating. There was no forum where she felt comfortable because she felt her specific concerns had to do with her daughter's hearing loss. Similarly, a father was convinced that his son's biology teacher was going out of his way to make life difficult for him. When he brought these issues to the attention of the principal, he was told that he was being defensive and overly protective. It later became apparent that the biology teacher was not following the suggestions that would have made it possible for his son to have an "equal shot" at the material. Indeed, he tried to make his class even harder for the hearing-impaired boy so that he could have a taste of the real world.

In a group with other parents of mainstreamed youngsters, these parents were able to express their frustration, understand it, and deal with it. They were then more effective in their efforts to manage this and other situations effectively.

Teenage Support Groups

Opportunities for mainstream teenagers to meet and share thoughts and feelings are extremely beneficial. Many teenagers find that support groups are the only forum in which they can share experiences and be understood, since most of their days and nights are spent with hearing people. The value as a productive social outlet is immeasurable.

I have known several audiologists who formed teenage groups for their clients. In some cases, the audiologists who were trained as counselors, served as group facilitators. In others, the audiologist hired a psychologist with expertise in adolescence to cochair the group. The leader needs to feel comfortable with and appreciate adolescents who can prosper from a strong bond with other young people who are hearing impaired.

Just as with parent groups, creativity is necessary to select an appropriate group leader. There are some talented, caring people who can serve as excellent group facilitators, and yet their knowledge about hearing impairment and its impact is minimal.

Fathers' Groups

Some groups are formed specifically to meet the needs of fathers. Among the issues men need to address is their altered self-image. They have fathered a child who is not "perfect" in their eyes. Typically, their dreams for their child and their role as a father are crushed. Many fear that they will not be able to accept the role they must assume. Although these views are not unique to fathers, some men express a reluctance to join with their wives in parent support groups.

Some fathers do not feel comfortable revealing emotions or expressing their discomfort with parenting in front of their partners. They are supposed to be (and frequently have been) the strong ones in the family. Expressions of feelings conflict with the traditional male image, capable of fixing anything. Feeling powerless, many fathers withdraw into their work because they perceive the problem as beyond their control. Helping fathers confront the shattered illusions of life as discussed by Dr. Van Hecke in Chapter 5 can be a valuable contribution of father's groups.

It can also be productive for men to meet together so that they can relate to their partners in more meaningful ways. Intimate concerns about their sexual performance or interest in sex may not surface in a discussion group with their wives or other women present.

Most educational programs for young hearing-impaired children require parental involvement. The involvement often takes the form of "parent as teacher." Some fathers are uncomfortable in the role of tutor. The thought of working closely with their young child in auditory skills or language-learning exercises is outside their traditional perception of a father's role. Men need to develop skills to enter nonoppressive and mutually satisfying relationships with their partners and children. They do not want to feel or appear stupid, unable to manage a situation. They do not want to be in a situation where they have to "learn" something about which they already have ambivalent feelings. Fathers' groups can provide the safe space for the needed learning to occur.

Another benefit of a fathers' group is to help participants build healthy and strong relationships with other fathers of hearing-impaired children. Neighborhood buddies may not understand the impact of deafness on their friend, and may be reluctant to address the problem directly. More commonly, the father may not feel comfortable discussing his feelings, fears, and frustrations with friends or associates. Sharing these feelings with men who are experiencing similar emotions is helpful. Often, fathers' groups serve as excellent transitions to the couples' groups in helping the fathers prepare for discussing their experiences, feelings, and reactions. As an adjunct to the variety of support groups available to the family, national support organizations may have much to offer (Appendix 6–2).

SIBLINGS OF HEARING-IMPAIRED CHILDREN

While parents and audiologists are busy taking care of the myriad concerns related to the hearing-impaired child, one particular group is at risk of being overlooked. The feelings and actions of sisters and brothers may recede into the background when the focus of the family is on the needs of the hearing-impaired child. Researchers in mental health and education have given scant attention to the psychological effects of a hearing-impaired child on a sibling. Research on siblings of children with other types of disabilities indicates that, under certain conditions, nondisabled siblings suffer from psychological problems.

Siblings affect each other in ways that are both positive and negative such as serving as teachers, protectors, confidants, role models, friends, interpreters, sparring partners. Whether positive or negative, there is an interaction. Like all brothers and sisters, hearing and hearing-impaired siblings can exert an emotional, social, and educational influence on each other and other family members. When audiologists and parents recognize and try to foster normal sibling interaction, we are better able to intervene to promote healthy sibling interactions and improved family functioning. Adapting to life with a hearing-impaired brother or sister is a long process involving many stages and changes.

Feelings of the Hearing Siblings

When a hearing-impaired child is present in the family, the interactions of siblings may or may not be mutually satisfying. Frequently, older siblings, particularly sisters, are expected to assume more responsibility than their peers for their younger siblings and for the housework. Interestingly, even when these young people do not have more responsibilities than their peers, self-perceptions are that they do (Atkins, 1982.)

Quite accurately, when they babysit for their younger, hearing-impaired sibling, there may be a higher level of involvement because of that younger child's needs. Communication with a hearing-impaired child requires enormous energy, much more than is required to communicate with a hearing child of the same age. Making oneself understood and understanding a child's message correctly can demand at least twice as much time as with a hearing child (Ogden & Lipsett, 1982). There needs to be more frequent face-to-face contact when there is a child with a hearing impairment, and the hearing siblings feel this difference in how attentive they must be when caring for their charge (Atkins, 1982). This goes counter to what occurs in a family with hearing children, for whom an older sibling can babysit while watching television or communicate by yelling between rooms.

A frequently heard complaint from the hearing child is the amount of attention and time parents give to the hearing-impaired child. That is likely to be true and for very good reasons. However, it also means that the hearing child also needs some individual and quality time from parents, away from the other members of the family. Audiologists can do a tremendous service to the siblings of children with hearing losses by raising parental consciousness of this fact.

Another aspect of sibling relationships often overlooked is that hearing children are also very likely to experience grief resulting from their sibling's diagnosis of hearing impairment. This experience for children is not unlike that of an adult, and the children require the same kind of caring and understanding to cope with a wide range of thoughts and feelings. The positive aspects of having a hearing-impaired sibling in the family seem to be enhanced when the hearing children believe that their parents are available to talk and to listen to them.

Frequently, hearing-impaired children are referred to as "special." They are enrolled in "special education" classes, and brothers and sisters often feel "less special." They, too, are "special" children and are often concerned about the welfare or future of their brother or sister. They frequently feel great love for them. These young people may have to demonstrate inordinate patience with their sibling and should feel proud when they have helped their sibling with an accomplishment. It is imperative that they be told how much their contributions and efforts are appreciated, and that they, too, are special. They need to feel important and special, in their own right, within the family. They have many facets, one of which is their role as a brother or sister.

The feelings of hearing siblings, however, are not experienced in isolation. Feelings of love and pride may be mixed with other emotions that are uncomfortable and unpleasant, including denial, sadness, jealousy, resentment, anger, disappointment, fear, guilt, neglect, confusion, and embarrassment. It is essential that parents are open about their own feelings as a way to encourage brothers and sisters to feel safe and unashamed about expressing their feelings (Atkins, 1987).

Siblings gain a better understanding of the disability if they have access to age-appropriate information on hearing impairment. Audiologists can assist parents in making brothers and sisters feel "special" by including them in discussions and by providing answers to questions on hearing loss that friends often ask. Incorporating video and audiotapes and the actual apparatus that is used in testing helps the siblings understand.

Audiologists, teachers, and parents can sponsor "Sibling Days." At these gatherings siblings can learn about the myths and facts of hearing impairment. Small groups can discuss family adjustment issues and specific coping techniques for individual situations. Children of all ages not only meet other brothers and sisters, but have the experience of interacting with other hearing-impaired people.

Brothers and sisters need to know what will be expected of them and how they can contribute within the family. Explanations take time and need to be repeated and elaborated on as children grow and develop. Books written for and about sibling issues are available, and most audiologists welcome siblings into their clinics and testing rooms so that sisters and brothers can become informed, participate if they care to, and "listen" through hearing aids. (See Appendix 6–1 for suggestions on dealing with siblings.)

When Roger was 10 years old, he had difficulty expressing his feelings of anger and jealousy appropriately. He was afraid of rejection and wanted to be recognized as someone other than "the deaf kid's brother." At school, he was disruptive and unable to control his anger toward other children, particularly when they were in the spotlight. He had trouble waiting his turn and sharing. He frequently visited the nurse because of bad headaches that prevented him from "hearing" anybody.

As a class assignment, Roger wrote a story about his family in which he was the center of attention. He focused on a younger brother with whom he spent hours talking about things, whispering funny stories, and listening to music. He described the endless time he spent alone with his parents, taking walks, and going to the movies. Whenever he wanted anything, all he had to do was ask for it. His brother, on the other hand, had to wait for everything. The story was an elaborate tale of Roger's fantasy.

Roger's mother knew about his difficulties at school. She talked with him about what it must be like to have a brother who demands so much of his parents' attention. She explained that it was tough for her, too. She wanted to plan to have more time alone with Roger, but plans often fell through. She also admitted that not knowing the cause of her other son's hearing loss was painful. She often thought it was the result of something that she had done. She explained that we don't always know why something happens, but she assured him he was not in any danger of losing his hearing.

Roger was quiet and then asked if not liking someone could cause deafness. She said she was sure that couldn't happen but that maybe he asked her for a reason. Roger's relief was apparent when he admitted to his mom that he had been upset when his brother was born 6 years before, because he had gotten so much attention. Roger felt as if he was no longer important. He prayed that something would happen to make his brother go away. When his brother's deafness was discovered a year later, Roger was sure his prayers were the cause. It seemed that nothing Roger did was right, and it seemed that his mom and dad were either angry or sad all of the time.

Also, his mom and brother were together an awful lot. They were always visiting the doctor, the tutor, the special program center, and when they were home, Roger felt that he had to be "extra special good," while his little brother behaved badly. Everyone asked about how his brother was doing and spent time talking to his brother. Nobody spent that much time with him. Everything focused on his hearing-impaired brother. And since Roger wasn't hearing impaired, he began to believe that he wasn't worth the time and attention that his brother got. He felt unloved.

> *Roger's concerns are not unlike those of other brothers and sisters. His acting out in school was a way for him to get the attention he desperately needed but was unable to get at home. He did not think anyone could understand his feelings because, as far as he knew, he was the only boy who had a hearing-impaired brother.*
>
> *Initially, Roger's mother did not have to do anything except listen. Listening lovingly without judgment is a gift that all parents and audiologists can give to one another and to the siblings of hearing-impaired children. After she reflected on the conversation, she explored alternative ways to be with him. She encouraged him to tell her when he felt ignored so that she could become more sensitive to him.*

Psychological Impact on Hearing Siblings

Many brothers and sisters of the children who are hearing impaired feel pressure to do well in school and to achieve great things. Sometimes the motivation for this is to make up for what is perceived as a deficit in the other child. This is not unlike "survivor guilt" in families where a child has died. At times these children work exceptionally hard in school to make good grades, but receive little if any recognition for their effort. They, and sometimes their parents, believe that since they have normal hearing they are capable of doing extremely well because there are no obstacles.

At times, these hearing children are mature beyond their years, appearing to be quite grown up and responsible. Frequently, they refrain from talking about their lives with their parents because they believe that their problems are less significant than those their parents face with the hearing-impaired sibling. They may have difficulty in asking for what they need or want from their parents. Thus, routine concerns, which are very important in other families, may be trivialized in the life of a hearing sibling. Nothing is as bad as not having normal hearing and, since they have that, these young people feel they do not have the right to complain.

These young people can become overly serious and need to be reminded of the importance of making time for themselves and to be with their friends. It is imperative that the responsibility for the hearing-impaired child, whether with regard to lessons or care, does not lie with the hearing siblings. They need to be encouraged to pursue their own interests, and the entire family can be supportive of those pursuits by attending their class plays, basketball games, or band concerts. The hearing siblings' role in the family is as important as any other child in the family. At times, though, when parents are unable to be totally available to each of their children, they can enlist the help of friends or family members who may be eager to help, but may be uncertain of how they can help.

GRANDPARENTS

Since parents of children who are hearing impaired need to develop and rely on a tightly knit support group, grandparents can play a vital role. They help to socialize their grandchildren and are usually excellent resources for family history, values, and traditions. Their perspectives are frequently different from their children's, and grandchildren have the potential to benefit greatly from this exposure.

Grandparents describe feeling as if they are in a paradox when their adult children are in trouble. They care deeply about them and their predicament, feeling sorrow and disappointment. Frequently they want to help. However, they may not offer to help until they are asked. Then they may only be able to help in an indirect or simple way. In times of crisis, adult children are sometimes forced back into roles of semidependency with their parents. Most grandparents, although they have a desire to help their children in time of trouble, resist infringing on their children's independence.

Grandparents also experience tremendous emotional response to the news that their grandchild is hearing impaired. They, too, had dreams and expectations of and about their grandchild. They may feel threatened by the diagnosis, unaware of or unable to express their feelings, needs, and expectations, and unsure of what role they can play in the family. Grandparents, like their children, may feel responsible and wonder whether the hearing loss was inherited.

Roxanne, a 56-year-old grandmother lived in Tennessee, and her daughter and son-in-law lived in Montreal. When she received the letter from her daughter saying that her first grandson was hearing impaired, she cried all night. "What I really wanted to do was bring my daughter and grandson back here to my home and take care of them. I wanted to hold her and try to make things better. I wanted to protect her from all the terrible things that might continue to happen to her. I couldn't call her for two days and I felt guilty because I wanted to be strong for her. I felt sick whenever I looked at healthy babies. Finally, I called her and I think I could have won an award for my acting. I tried so hard to sound optimistic while my heart continued to break inside. Never before in my life did I wish for a lot of money. Now, I wanted money so that I could take trips to Montreal and see my family, call them on the phone whenever I pleased, and help them afford the best doctors if they needed them. All I want to do is help."

Grandparents depend on their children for information about their hearing-impaired grandchildren, yet telephone conversations and letters are seldom adequate. Typically, grandparents who live far from their children will gather information about hearing impairment and send them newspaper and magazine articles. It can be helpful to the family if the grandparent can arrange a telephone consultation with the audiologist to better understand childhood hearing impairments. If this can be accomplished, the parents' responsibility of "informing the world" about hearing loss is eased at a time when they are highly anxious and unable to share information.

Grandparents can be a valued source of emotional support. In addition to providing emotional support, they may be in a position to contribute financially if that is appropriate. Whatever kind of support they offer can help them to feel involved and connected with their family as well as to initiate more frequent communication.

Financial assistance can be received lovingly or resentfully, depending on the nature of the relationship, whether there are conditions related to the gift, and the emotional responsiveness of the parents. The diagnosis of hearing impairment may foster the healing of long-standing family wounds. What parents want and expect from their parents (the grandparents) may or may not be in harmony with what the grandparents are willing or able to give. What each of them needs at various stages of adaptation to the hearing impairment is not always the same. For those grandparents who live close to their children, the possibilities of involvement with their family are endless.

In addition to providing financial and emotional assistance, they can also serve as babysitters, chauffeurs, teachers, and an extra pair of hands. This support, in some cases, enables the family to function. Grandparents deserve respect. They deserve our time and explanations just as parents do.

Life-long patterns of expectations, communication styles, role assignments, and styles of parenting contribute to the creation of a healthy or unhealthy setting in which to rear a family. We each have a desire to be loved by our parents.

Whether we felt we were will affect the nature of the relationship among the adults in the family.

Morris, a 72-year-old grandfather, was shocked when he learned that his granddaughter was profoundly hearing impaired and wanted to learn whatever he could to help her. He did not like the man his daughter had married, and his contact with them was cordial but minimal. When he found out about his granddaughter's hearing loss, however, he decided that he would overlook his son-in-law's deficiencies in an effort to help. He joined a support group for families of hearing-impaired children.

"I felt out of place because I was the only grandparent who attended parent meetings. I was afraid that I inhibited some of the parents from discussing their problems but after awhile I was part of the group. Truly, though, I would have preferred talking to other grandparents. In the presence of my daughter and son-in-law I never felt I could let them know how sad I was. I know that if my wife were still alive she would have known what to do. She would have made it easier for my daughter and for me. I wanted to help my daughter handle everything.

"I cannot make Jenny hear, but I can make life a little easier for my daughter by taking Jenny from time to time. I needed to know that I was talking to her in the correct way, so I had a lot to learn. I felt funny about my accent and thought she might have difficulty understanding me. Her teacher told me that the relationship we were developing was more important than the words. That made me feel good. Also, my English is improving. I have a lot of love to give to her. When I raised my own kids, I was young and very poor. I didn't have a lot of time for them. I do have time for my granddaughter though and I think I can help."

This grandfather, like the grandmother in the previous example, tried to be helpful yet nonintrusive. Both of them defined their roles as that of helper and supporter for their children, yet neither of them specifically talked with their children about how they could be of the most use. Each of them could have benefited from sharing with other grandparents so that they could have received the emotional support that they needed as well.

CONCLUSION

The factors that influence families of children who are hearing impaired are as diverse as the families and the children themselves. An important component of successful adaptation is developing an awareness of the profound "ups and downs" that characterize the experience.

Audiologists are in the unique position to not only facilitate learning about hearing impairment but to provide an atmosphere in which family members can learn more about themselves. An exceptional partnership can develop between the family and the audiologist. Additionally, those who work with the parents, children, brothers, sisters, or grandparents have a rare opportunity to learn about themselves in the process.

Professionals who are unafraid of interacting with families on a personal level can benefit from both the knowledge gained and the experience. Helping families to find a healthy balance in their lives prepares them to face the challenges that they will confront daily. To adequately address those challenges, the families and the audiologists need energy, determination, and patience with themselves and with each other.

REFERENCES

ATKINS, D. (1982). *A comparison of older hearing-impaired and normally hearing children on measures of responsibility and parental attention.* Doctoral dissertation, University of California, Los Angeles.

ATKINS, D. (1987). Siblings of the hearing impaired: Perspectives for parents. 32–45. In D. Atkins (Ed.), *Families and their hearing-impaired children.* Washington, DC: Volta Bureau.

BOOTHROYD, A. (1982). *Hearing impairments in young children.* Englewood Cliffs, NJ: Prentice Hall.

COHEN, O. (1987). Current and future needs of minority hearing-impaired children and youth. Testimony before the Commission on the Education of the Deaf, Washington, DC.

FISHGRUND, J., COHEN, O., & CLARKSON, R. (1987). Hearing-impaired children in black and Hispanic families. *Volta Review, 89* (5), 59–67.

KROTH, R. (1987). Mixed or missed messages between parents and professionals. 1–10. In D. Atkins (Ed.), *Families and their hearing-impaired children.* Washington, DC: Volta Bureau.

MARLOWE, J. (1991, May). Personal communication.

OGDEN, P., & LIPSETT, S. (1982). *The silent garden: Understanding the hearing impaired child.* New York: St. Martin's Press.

PEARLMAN, L., & SCOTT, K. A. (1981). *Raising the handicapped child.* Englewood Cliffs, NJ: Prentice Hall.

RODRIGUEZ, O., & SANTIVIAGO, M. (1991). Hispanic deaf adolescents: A muticultural minority. *Volta Review, 93*(5), 89–97.

SOMERS, M. (1987). Parenting in the 1980s: Programming perspectives and issues. 68–75. In D. Atkins (Ed), *Families and their hearing-impaired children.* Washington DC: Volta Bureau.

WOLRAICH, M. (1982). Communication between physician and parents of handicapped children. *Exceptional Children, 48*(4), 324–329.

RECOMMENDED READINGS

ATKINS, D. (1992). Family involvement and counseling in serving children who are hearing impaired pp. 61–73. In R. Hull (Ed.), *Aural rehabilitation.* San Diego, CA: Singular Publishing Group.

ATKINS, D. (1987). Siblings of the hearing impaired: Perspectives for parents. In D. Atkins (Ed.), *Families and their hearing impaired children* pp. 32–45. Washington, DC: Volta Bureau.

ATKINS, D. (1984). *Sisters: A practical, helpful exploration of the intimate and complex bond between female siblings.* New York: Arbor House.

BANK, S., & KAHN, M. (1982). *The sibling bond.* New York: Basic Books.

BUSCAGLIA, L. (1975). *The disabled child and their parents: A counseling challenge.* Thorofare, NJ: Charles B. Slack.

FEATHERSTONE, H. (1980). *A difference in the family: Living with the disabled child.* New York: Penguin Books.

HARVEY, M. (1989). *Psychotherapy with deaf and hard-of-hearing persons: A systemic model.* Hillsdale, NJ: Erlbaum.

KISOR, H. (1990). *What's that pig outdoors?* New York: Hill & Wang.

LUTERMAN, D. (1979). *Counseling parents of hearing impaired children.* Boston: Little, Brown.

MURPHY, A. T. (1979). Members of the family: Sisters and brothers of handicapped children pp. 352–362. In A. Murphy (Ed.), *The families of hearing impaired children.* Washington, DC: A. G. Bell.

PEARLMAN, L., & SCOTT, K. (1981). *Raising the handicapped child.* Englewood Cliffs, NJ: Prentice Hall.

POWELL, F., FINITZO-HIEKEN, FRIEL-PATTI, S., & HENDERSON, D. (Eds.). (1985). *Education of the hearing impaired child.* Baltimore: Singular Publishing Group.

ROSENBERG, B. G. (1982). Life span personality stability in siblings status. In M. E. Lamb & B. Sutton-Smith (Eds.), *Sibling relationships: Their nature and significance across the lifespan* (pp. 167–224). Hillsdale, NJ: Erlbaum.

SELIGMAN, M. (1983). Siblings of handicapped persons. In M. Seligman (Ed.), *The family with a handicapped child* (pp. 147–174). New York: Grune & Stratton.

STEVENS, J. H., JR., & MATHEWS, M. (Eds.). *Mother/child: Father/child relationships.* Washington, DC: National Association for the Education of Young Children.

APPENDIX 6–1
SUGGESTIONS REGARDING SIBLINGS

1. Let your children know you are available to talk and listen to them.
2. Be open and share your feelings with your children to help them feel safe in discussing their feelings with you.
3. Children need permission to express their feelings and thoughts without threat of feeling judged. You may need to be creative in eliciting these thoughts. By using puppets with young children you can discuss issues that may be difficult for the child to address directly.
4. Admit that you do not have all the answers.
5. Avoid making comparisons among siblings and praise them for helping one another and for helping in the family.
6. Demand the same behavior in the child who has a hearing impairment that you demand from your other children.
7. Responsibilities and chores should be equally divided according to ability and age.
8. Help siblings to develop their own identity and pursue their own interests.
9. Reassure all siblings of their importance in the family by asking for their input and advice in family discussions. Value them.
10. Emphasize the positive interactions that you observe among siblings.
11. Periodically provide your hearing child with correct and age-appropriate information about hearing loss, language, listening, and hearing aids so they will have the information when questioned by friends or strangers.
12. Role-play situations to provide siblings with specific responses they can give when they are asked questions.
13. Allow siblings to watch and to participate in activities designed to help the child with a hearing loss.
14. Reserve time in your schedule to spend with each child alone; let this be consistent and something the children and you can count on.
15. If a decision must be made that inconveniences the hearing siblings in favor of the child who has a hearing impairment, discuss it openly before it happens.
16. Make sure that your hearing children know that they are not responsible for their sibling's hearing loss.
17. Invite the siblings' friends to your home or on outings to see how the child with a hearing impairment functions within your family.
18. Notice if your hearing children are making up for what they perceive as your disappointment in having a child with a hearing impairment.
19. All brothers and sisters have difficulties relating to each other from time to time. Don't confuse normal sibling interaction with behavior related to the hearing impairment.
20. Attempt to keep the lives of all children somewhat separate with regard to toys, friends, special programs so that the individuality of each child can be ensured.

APPENDIX 6–2
NATIONAL SUPPORT PROGRAMS AND ORGANIZATIONS

Alexander Graham Bell Association for the Deaf. 3417 Volta Place NW, Washington, DC 20007. (202) 337-5220.

American Hearing Research Foundation. 55 East Washington Street (Suite 2022), Chicago, IL 60602. (312) 726-9670.

American Society for Deaf Children and National Association of the Deaf (NAD). 814 Thayer Avenue. Silver Spring, MD 20910. (800) 942-2732. NAD: (301) 587-1788.

American Speech-Language-Hearing Association. 10801 Rockville Pike, Rockville, MD 20852. (301) 897-5700.

Auditory–Verbal International (AVI). 505 Cattell Street, Easton, PA 18042. (215) 253-6616.

Family Services of America (FSA). 44 East 23rd Street, New York, NY 10010. (800) 221-2681.

The Family Support Institute. 300-30 East 6th Avenue, Vancouver, BC V5T 4P4. (604) 875-1119.

Gallaudet University. 800 Florida Avenue NE, Washington, DC 20002. (800) 672-6720.

John Tracy Clinic. 806 West Adams Boulevard, Los Angeles, CA 90007. (213) 748-5481.

National Association of Counsel for Children (NACC). 1205 Oneida Street, Denver, CO 80220. (303) 321-3963.

Sibling Information Network (Connecticut's University Affiliated Program). 991 Main Street East Hartford, CT 06108. (203) 282-7050.

Resource Point. Cochlear Corporation, Englewood, CO 80112. (800) 523-5798.

Tripod. Burbank, CA. (800) 352-8888.

chapter seven

Counseling for Pediatric Amplification

Linda M. Thibodeau

The true challenge of audiological rehabilitation arises when the audiologist addresses the amplification needs of young children. Dr. Thibodeau examines amplification for children from both informational and interpersonal counseling perspectives as she discusses the audiologist's role in helping parents and children of various ages to accept and develop responsibility for amplification.

> The shop seemed to be full of all manner of curious things—but the oddest part of it all was that, whenever she looked hard at any shelf, to make out exactly what it had on it, that particular shelf was always quite empty, though the others round it were crowded as full as they could hold.

Lewis Carroll
Through the Looking-Glass

INTRODUCTION

The successful use of amplification for children depends on several factors. Some of these factors are out of the control of the audiologist working with the client, such as the degree of the hearing loss, the personality of the child and parents, and the availability and type of financial resources. Other important factors that impact the successful use of amplification, which are the responsibility of the audiologist, include the evaluation and selection of hearing aids and assistive listening devices, the periodic monitoring of their functioning, and the management of repairs. These technical aspects are not addressed in this chapter because the focus here is on the interaction between the audiologist and the child, family, or significant others. A well-fit hearing aid that allows all of the speech spectrum to be audible, that is electroacoustically evaluated regularly, and that is repaired to specifications when necessary, will not be successfully used if the audiologist has not effectively communicated the appropriate requisite knowledge and established a relationship that facilitates an acceptance of the hearing loss, a development of responsibility for amplification, and an environment for the growth of advocacy roles.

This chapter focuses on two important factors upon which the audiologist can make a great impact and that will influence the successful use of amplification. One of the most important factors is the knowledge of the parents, care givers, teachers, or others involved with the child regarding not only the appropriate operation and care of hearing aids but also the benefits afforded by amplification. The first half of this chapter provides a rationale for the topics to be reviewed in developing the appropriate knowledge base. Because there are several resources that provide factual information about these aspects of amplification, a number of sources are provided in the appendices of this chapter for a review of the actual content to be included in each of these topics.

In contrast, very little has been written about how to get parents to apply this information and eventually become advocates for their child's amplification needs. Thus, the second half of this chapter focuses on techniques to use with parents, teachers, and others who care for the child with a hearing loss, to ensure that amplification is used consistently, maintained appropriately, and modified when necessary. Parents must be able to effectively apply that information at the right times as well as teach the child responsibility for auditory needs.

To illustrate these two factors, consider the analogy of learning to scuba dive as suggested by Abrahamson and Thibodeau (1990). In addition to the prerequisite that one must know how to swim, there is a significant amount of information regarding the equipment operation that must be learned. Interestingly, one may purchase all the equipment including the air tank, fins, and mask, but the air to fill the tank will not be sold until the person has passed a certification class in which one demonstrates that knowledge has been acquired and that it can be applied during actual use. In addition to written and skills tests, the instructor will determine how scuba diving students will react in difficult situations by approaching them from behind and shutting off the air supply. Students are taught to maintain a log book of their dives that are verified by a partner to show to the instructor when purchasing compressed air. If an unusually long time has elapsed since the previous dive, an instructor may choose not to fill a tank with air until a refresher course is completed.

Buying the scuba equipment is much like buying hearing aids or assistive listening devices. Just as instruction is necessary to effectively use the scuba equipment, instruction is needed to use hearing aids. However, information about hearing aid operation and maintenance is not enough. If parents and adolescents with hearing loss do not accept the hearing aids, assume responsibility for proper functioning, and become advocates for hearing needs, they are likely to be in a failure situation like the scuba diver who has been told what to do when the air supply stops but has never actually experienced that situation in a learning environment.

INFORMATIONAL COUNSELING

During the amplification process parents need general background information on the structure and function of the ear, sound characteristics and transmission, perception of speech, and audiograms. The various procedures for the selection of the hearing aid should be reviewed as well as suggestions for facilitating the adjustment to amplification. However, all the information may be meaningless if it is not presented in coordination with information from other professionals, in a conducive format such as a parent group with supportive materials, and at the appropriate time.

Trevor, age 2, was fit with his binaural hearing aids 1 month following identification of his hearing loss. The mother was frustrated by all the information she received, but she reminded herself that it would be her mother-in-law, who cared for him during the day, who would actually use the aids with Trevor. In fact, she expected that by the time she picked him up, he would be too tired to use the aids and she would not have to see him wear them at all. She was relieved that the parent–infant teacher had said she would receive a booklet regarding hearing aids because she realized that she was not following much of the information from the audiologist. The one question dominating her thoughts was "How long would he have to wear these aids?"

This scenario illustrates several important aspects of informational counseling, including who should receive the information and how and when should it be delivered.

Prior to the review of topics to include in informational counseling, these aspects will be discussed. It is easy to deliver lectures regarding hearing aids from prepared outlines. What is more difficult is to convey the information so that parents will understand and retain it. As discussed below, the manner as well as pace of presentation will greatly impact retention.

Aspects of Information Delivery

Information regarding hearing aids should be conveyed to all persons involved with the child. This may include the parents, caretakers, teachers, therapists, or counselors. With today's high divorce rate, the audiologist may actually deal with two sets of parents and must consider that the child of divorced parents may have four sets of grandparents. For simplicity, hereafter this group of persons in contact with the child will be referred to as only the parents. As the children grow, they should also be taught this factual information as they become increasingly responsible for their hearing health care.

It is important that this information be transmitted in a coordinated fashion. Often children receive services from more than one individual. All the professionals involved should work as a team so that the providers do not receive conflicting information regarding hearing aids. Ideally, the audiologists should make home visits, perhaps with parent–infant advisors, to gain an understanding of the family situation. This visit also allows audiologists to be more personable throughout the rehabilitation process and gives them credibility, which is important when asking the parents to conduct home activities.

There are many ways that this information may be conveyed including one-to-one counseling sessions, support group discussions, booklets or home-study guides, videos, and in-service programs. It is important that a variety of methods be used so that information may be reviewed away from the audiologist's office and shared with the extended family if possible. As much time as possible should be devoted to demonstration and practice sessions.

The actual timing of the individual counseling will vary among parents. According to a survey by Martin, George, O'Neal, and Daly (1987), 77% of the parents who responded received information regarding amplification at the time of the initial diagnosis. However, 96% of the parents indicated they would have liked to have received information regarding amplification at the initial diagnosis. In contrast, only 44% of the audiologists who responded indicated that they provide information regarding amplification at the initial diagnosis. The discrepancy may be attributed to the notion that parents will be in a grieving state at the time of the initial diagnosis and unable to really absorb information regarding amplification. It is often advocated that parents be allowed to determine the pace of intervention (Luterman, 1987; Moses, 1983; Bader, 1992). One approach is to ask the parents, "What is it that you want to learn first?" Allowing parents to participate in the direction of the intervention gives them an active role in the process, which will facilitate their eventual acceptance of hearing aids and their ability to assume responsibility for proper functioning. Clark, Morgan, and Wilson-Vlotman (1983) developed a parent education curriculum in which they advocate that the parents be considered as co-workers with the professional. The goal of the professional is to help parents develop autonomy and initiative in order to become effective advocates for their child. They recommend that the professional should be a facilitator and not a teacher.

Tracy was identified as profoundly hearing impaired at 6 months of age when her parents' suspicions led to an evaluation at the speech and hearing center. For the second appointment with the Cardell's, the audiologist had planned to explain the hearing aid selection process, and the types of hearing aids, and to begin the hearing aid evaluation. However, rather than beginning a tutorial of information upon their arrival, she began with a statement that allowed them to initially direct the session and gain some sense that they were capable of determining what information they needed to make decisions for Tracy. The audiologist said, "I'll bet you've been thinking quite a bit about the steps involved in helping Tracy. Tell me what you are thinking." They indicated that they had seen some kids wearing hearing aids that were strapped on their chests and wondered if Tracy would have one like that. The audiologist explained the different types of hearing aids, which led to questions of how one would be selected for Tracy.

> *This example illustrates how parents may be invited to participate in determining the direction of the intervention. By acknowledging that the parents have given the topic much thought, the audiologist is validating their efforts and conveying a sense of confidence that their questions are important to the habilitation process.*

When parents are allowed to determine the information they need, an audiologist will not be able to follow a set outline of general information. However, the following section includes the topics that are considered necessary for parents to understand so they may have effective knowledge of amplification. The order of presentation will change depending on the needs of the parents. Likewise, the necessary time to cover all the topics will vary depending on how much information is desired in a given session.

Background Information

The following information will help parents to understand not only the selection of amplification devices but also the need for adjustments in amplification if the hearing loss changes. More specific information on these topics may be found in Chapter 3. Having acquired this information, they should be especially cautious when their child has an ear infection because they will understand the potential danger of damage to residual hearing. Knowledge of sound transmission and speech acoustics will make them better advocates for their child's amplification needs in the classroom. Encouraging the parents to organize the supplemental handouts in a notebook may prompt review of the material at home and lead to additional questions.

The review of the otological anatomy should be conducted with diagrams, models, and handouts, which are often available from hearing aid manufacturers. It is important to avoid jargon when conveying the key ideas such as the three main parts of the hearing system, the eustachian tube, and the middle-ear muscles. Discussion relative to the anatomy should also include the three types of hearing loss (conductive, sensorineural, mixed), basic testing methods of air and bone conduction, and tympanometry. All terms should be available for review on a handout to facilitate further questions. The importance of avoiding professional jargon cannot be overstressed.

Parents should know the three basic characteristics of sound—frequency, intensity, and duration—which can be easily demonstrated by tuning forks. Concepts regarding transmission to be conveyed include the reduction in sound with increased distance, the degradation of speech through reverberation, and the interference created by background noise. The concepts of frequency and intensity of sound should be related to the audiogram. Symbols should be reviewed, including those designating the right and left ears, air and bone conduction, and aided and unaided results. Sample audiograms may be used to illustrate the different degrees and configurations of hearing loss. In some cases parents might benefit from the opportunity to view their child's audiogram while sitting in the sound booth and hearing the various frequencies at intensities that correspond to their child's thresholds.

The general outline of speech energy on the audiogram is helpful for parents to understand the impact of their child's hearing loss on speech perception. Understanding of speech characteristics is facilitated by playing a recording of male and female speakers with a simulation of hearing loss. (see Appendix 7–6) The audiologist may also demonstrate the visual characteristics of speech by reading along with the tape with no voice when the simulations of the severe and profound hearing losses are played. Many observers are amazed at the improvement in identification they experience when the visual cues are added.

Selection of Amplification

The basic goal of amplification regardless of age is to allow speech to be audible to the child with a hearing loss. This is considerably different from the goal of achieving aided thresholds near normal hearing sensitivity, which is commonly presented to parents (Anderson, 1989). For example, for a child with an unaided threshold of 100 dB HL at 1000 Hz to achieve an aided threshold of 20 dB HL, the hearing aid must provide 80 dB of gain. If the average speech input to this hearing aid is 60 dB HL, then the average output would be 140 dB HL, which may be limited by the hearing aid by peak clipping or compression to about 120 dB HL. Children would receive a speech signal that has been limited in dynamic range, which may result in reduced intelligibility. The Articulation Index, which represents the proportion of the speech spectrum that is audible to a client, is reduced as the speech spectrum exceeds the client's uncomfortable loudness level, which corresponds to reduced speech intelligibility (French & Steinberg, 1947). That is, if the signal is amplified with such high gain that the average speech input is constantly being limited by the maximum output of the hearing aid, the child may not benefit from intensity cues such as those of weaker consonants and the stronger vowels (Boothroyd, Springer, Smith, & Schulman, 1988). Thus, rather than convey to parents that the hearing aid should allow aided thresholds to be below the speech banana (Stone & Adam, 1986), audiograms depicting the unaided and aided thresholds, and level of amplified speech relative to unaided thresholds and tolerance levels, would be more useful, as demonstrated by Ross and Seewald (1990). An example of such an audiogram is provided in Appendix 7–1.

Aspects of the selection process that are important regardless of age include a description of the types of hearing aids, variations in ear molds, batteries, and consumer information such as serial numbers, service plans, and insurance. It is also important to convey information regarding the desirable options on the aids which include telecoil, audio input, compression, and 2-year warranties (Thibodeau, O'Neal, & Richards, 1989). The selection process and decision criteria for these options may vary depending on the age of the child as described below.

Infants. There are many unknowns when fitting a hearing aid on an infant because unaided audiological information is often incomplete, measures of tolerance levels are not possible, and test reliability may be low. It is at this stage where the parents' help in the fitting process, which may take several weeks, is especially important. The audiologist should be honest and convey any uncertainties regarding the selection process to support the significance of the parents' help in monitoring the child's responses to amplification at home. The type and amount of information that the audiologist hopes to receive prior to fitting the hearing aid should be conveyed to the parents so that they have a general idea of the sequence of events during the fitting process. Description of tests to be conducted should be presented, particularly those procedures that were not used during the initial diagnosis such as real-ear evaluation of amplification via probe microphones. Predictions that are made by the audiologist should be brought to the parents' attention so that they have a better understanding as the child develops and as more audiological information is obtained that may result in changes in the amplification. One example is the tolerance level that may be predicted from measures in adults with similar degrees of hearing loss (Skinner, 1988). Charts or diaries may be helpful guidelines to focus the parents' attention to specific changes in behavior they observe during trials with amplification. A sample of a chart is included in Appendix 7–2.

Different opinions among audiologists regarding particular amplification characteristics should be discussed with the parents, including a rationale for the fitting recommended by the audiologist. For example, some audiologists advocate use of an FM system with binaural behind-the-ear receivers as the primary amplification so that the young child receives the best auditory signal possible rather than fitting binaural hearing aids (Madell, 1992). Audiologists will have more credibility if they raise these issues before the parents learn of them from another source. Furthermore, if the audiologist discusses alternate fitting practices with the parents, they are learning that they can participate in the decision process, which will facilitate their development as advocates for their child.

Preschool-age children. Many of the principles for selecting amplification for the infant are also applicable to the preschool child. The parent will still be actively involved in the process and need as much information. As the child learns to respond more in the audiological evaluation, the characteristics of the amplification may be fine-tuned over several weeks of evaluation. If the child was evaluated as an infant, some of the predictions made earlier may be replaced with actual results. For example, Skinner (1988) suggests ways to begin evaluation of tolerance levels in young children with the use of visual analogies of a balloon being blown up until it pops. During the preschool years, parents can be invaluable teachers to facilitate the audiometric examination. They may help by conducting activities suggested by the audiologist to develop localization of sound, familiarity of listening to sound through earphones, routines for play audiometry, and picture associations for speech recognition and tolerance measures.

Parents should be continually informed as more complete audiometric information is obtained. It is important to discuss reliability of results and how this may impact the information on the audiogram so that they can discern true fluctuations in hearing from variability in responses. The variability in thresholds will be different for each child. During the selection process, which may occur over several sessions, the audiologist should point out even the small improvements in performance. For example, explaining to parents that their child conditioned to responding in fewer trials suggests greater attention to sound and is valuable feedback for them even if the final threshold that was obtained did not change from the previous session.

Elementary-school-age children. Although the selection of amplification for the child in elementary school requires active participation by the child, efforts should be made to continue to include the parents in the testing. They may observe testing from the examiner's booth and discuss their expectations regarding the hearing aid selection, which may be influenced by previous hearing aid fittings. However, at this age it is important to request input from children during the selection process, which sends a message to them that they are needed and enhances their self-esteem.

At the elementary level it is necessary to consider how the child's personal amplification may interface with amplification being provided by the school. If the child will be using a personal frequency-modulated (FM) system, the fitting process must involve evaluating the child's hearing aid with the FM system with which it will be used (Lewis, Feigin, Karasek, & Stelmachowicz, 1992). This includes the FM transmitter as well as the FM receiver. If the child will be removing the aids and wearing a basic FM system at school it is still necessary for the FM system to be adjusted to match the amplification characteristics of the personal hearing aids as closely as possible. According to Maxon, Brackett, and Van Den Berg (1991), who conducted a longitudinal survey on the use of classroom amplification, approximately three-fourths of the respondents reported that electroacoustic characteristics of the FM systems were prescribed by an audiologist. However, they reported that only about half their clients brought their FM systems to clinical evaluations. This highlights the need for audiologists to insist on evaluation of the FM system through which the child may listen the majority of the day with the same rigor that is applied to evaluation of personal amplification.

Adolescents. Involvement in the selection of the hearing aids becomes even more critical at the adolescent age. When their opinions are solicited, teenagers develop more of a commitment to wearing amplification because they sense some of the responsibility for the aids. Open-ended questions regarding what they like and dislike about their hearing aids may result in the selection of hearing aids that are more acceptable than those dispensed based solely on what the audiologist thought was best for the patient. Characteristics preferred by the audiologist such as audio input or brightly colored cases may be presented in a question format such as "What do you think about a direct connection from your hearing aid to a stereo system?"

The parents should continue to be involved in the testing. They are usually the ones who know their child the best and can provide insights regarding desires the teenager may not feel comfortable expressing, such as the possibility of wearing in-the-ear hearing aids. The degree of parental involvement may vary depending on the family situation, but at a minimum parents should be included in the final stages of dispensing in order to provide a carryover support system during the adjustment phase.

It is also important to evaluate hearing aids in relationship to the FM system that may be used by the teenager as described above. Adolescents should assume responsibility for taking their FM systems along for evaluation when they are scheduled to see an audiologist. In self-contained classrooms, this may mean that they need to see that arrangements are made with their teachers for loaner transmitters to be used while they bring their system to the evaluation.

Adjusting to Amplification

The adjustment to amplification cannot be described as a single process for all. Some of the factors that influence the ease and duration of the adjustment are the available support system of family, teachers, and peers; age and previous amplification use; the listening environment and related communication demands; and the attitudes regarding amplification of both the parent and the child. It may be assumed that initial adjustment to amplification would be more difficult than adjustment to new hearing aids by an experienced user. However, as discussed below, both periods may be equally difficult.

Initial fittings. The audiologist may provide parents a schedule of expected behaviors during the initial adjustment to amplification. One schedule provided by Northern and Downs (1984, pp. 297–301) includes recommendations for activities to be conducted by the parent during the first 3 weeks of amplification as well as suggestions for overcoming common problems. They recommend that the aids be tried for only short periods of 10 to 30 minutes during the first week when the child is engaged in an enjoyable, but quiet, activity such as a game, reading a book, or coloring. It is important that the aids be removed by the parent before the child becomes tired. Initial trials with the aids may be facilitated also by placing an aid on a favorite doll or stuffed animal. For this purpose manufacturers can supply sample aids with no parts. Such aids may be attached with adhesive velcro and should be inserted during the same routines as those being established for the child. During the second week, Northern and Downs recommend trying the aids for two or three, 1-hour periods a day and drawing attention to sounds such as music, the telephone, or water running. By the third week, the child should sense that wearing hearing aids is part of the dressing routine. The child should wear the aids for longer times in a variety of situations to eventually wearing them all day.

Northern and Downs (1984) also suggest some remedies for common problems. For example, to facilitate cooperation during ear-mold impressions, they advise demonstration first with a large doll and piece of clay or cotton inserted in the doll's ear. For ear-mold retention, a stretch headband may be placed over the aids and ear-molds and around the head in a position that does not block the microphone port. Finally, a program for children who continually remove their aids is suggested whereby the ear-mold alone is inserted at prescribed times, then the aid is added with progressively more volume and for longer periods.

For prelingual children, the initial fitting of amplification may include a discussion of the concept of hearing age (Pollack and Wedenberg, 1970), which is the length of time the child has worn the aid. The way in which this information is conveyed is important.

During the initial fitting of Mandy's hearing aids the audiologist explained to the parents that when she began wearing the hearing aids she would be hearing like an infant. Although she was 2 years old, she would have a hearing age of zero. This information was devastating to the parents, who only heard that their daughter was like an infant. Still upset from the initial diagnosis, they were unable to discuss their feelings with the audiologist and chose to seek services at another facility where they hoped their child's abilities would be recognized.

Parents will not be comforted by building dreams based only on a child's weaknesses. It is important that they be helped to also realize the child's strengths.

Parents' expectations regarding performance with amplification need to be realistic. Once children are fitted with amplification, the parents have dreams of what they will be able to accomplish with the hearing aids. Audiologists may prefer to guide the parents to minimal expectations to reduce the risk of further disappointment. In doing this, the audiologist must allow the parents to rebuild a dream with which they are comfortable. The audiologist may need to help them balance the dream by including the child's strengths in nonverbal areas along with the initial limitations in verbal areas. The concept of hearing age can be very useful as parents guide their child through the adjustment phase; however, audiologists must be sensitive to maintaining a balance between strengths and weaknesses of the child as they discuss the child's reaction to the hearing aid.

Instructions regarding hearing aid use during the first week or two after fitting will also depend on the parents' emotional state. The audiologist may need to ask questions like "How do you think you'll feel when these aids are pulled off and thrown to the floor?" Based on their answers, it may be suggested that the hearing aids be tried only when the child is engaged in a pleasant activity and the parents are not frustrated. Clark et al. (1983) suggest that the same person put the aids on daily at the same location and approximately the same times each day. Ideally, little hands should be occupied to reduce the likelihood of removing the aids. Attachments called Huggies, where one band slips around the hearing aid and a second flexible ring encircles the pinna, may be helpful in keeping the hearing aids in place (see Appendix 7–6). Noise-making toys may be particularly interesting after the child is comfortable wearing the aid in quiet, given that the sound is not so novel it is frightening to the child.

In binaural fittings, parents may try the hearing aid most likely to result in audible speech first. If the child readily accepts the aid during the initial periods, the second aid may be added immediately. If the child has difficulty with the first aid, the second aid should be withheld until the child tolerates the first aid for several hours a day.

It is important that parents emphasize the appropriate hearing aid vocabulary during the adjustment period. The vocabulary will vary depending on the child's age and may include *hearing aid, on, off, in, listen, hear it, earmold, battery, loud,* and *soft.* Adams and Tidwell (1988) found that parents who considered themselves to be successful disciplinarians used techniques involving discussion with explanation in the child's mode of communication. Thus, the adjustment process may be facilitated by consistent use of language.

Once the initial plan of hearing aid use is determined with the parent, some means of evaluating that plan should be provided. Goals for wearing time may be set for each week, and actual time may be recorded in another diary entry or on a chart as shown in Appendix 7–2. Regular follow-up during the adjustment period is critical to maintaining the partner relationship between audiologist and parents. Particularly if the parents are still coping with acceptance of the hearing loss, regular nonthreatening interaction will help to maintain the relationship. Open-ended statements such as "Tell me how things are going with the hearing aid" may be useful.

With older children the adjustment to amplification may proceed more quickly, particularly if they were involved in the decision process. Children should be invited to make daily entries on a hearing aid check chart to facilitate development of responsibility for their amplification needs. Audiologists should respond to entries that suggest difficulty, explore possible solutions, and seek opportunities to acknowledge when these difficulties have been successfully overcome.

Fitting changes. Although young children may not have the cognitive skills to indicate that they detect differences between old and new hearing aids, or between personal hearing aids and an FM system, once they demonstrate discrimination skills they may be expected to be aware of changes in amplification characteristics. There may be a period of readjustment as the child learns to listen to the new sound. Expectations regarding performance may need to be adjusted accordingly. For example, if the child receives high-frequency sibilant information through the FM system at school but not through the personal hearing aid, the parents and teacher should be aware of possible discrepancies in performance, such as responding appropriately to plural information at school but not at home.

The longer a child uses a certain hearing aid the more difficult it may be to adjust to a change in amplification, as reported by Chorost (1990). After wearing the same hearing aids for many years, he found it very difficult to adjust to new hearing aids in college even though they were technically superior to his old ones. The new aids were more powerful and had less internal noise. He described the new sound as if he was hearing through the "aural equivalent of a warped funhouse mirror." He addressed things that may be taken for granted by hearing persons, such as the change in the background noise of the new aid in the absence of auditory input. Because his old aids were noisier, they served as a constant reassurance that he was "on line." With the new, quieter aids he was "straining and failing to hear the noisy texture of silence," which he associated with hearing while at the same time he heard more background sounds than before such as footsteps, fans, and typewriters. Another significant adjustment for him was the sound of his own voice, which was almost unrecognizable with the new aids. It seemed as if his voice were coming from a source 10 feet away. As a result, he found himself talking compulsively in conversations to search for some familiar sound of his own voice.

Chorost recommends that audiologists warn clients that there will be a period of upset and disorientation following a change in amplification. In addition, the way hearing aids sound when fitted is not necessarily how they will sound after a month. He had tried new aids in the past but had always rejected them because he did not realize that the adjustment could take more than a month. He expressed a desire for an objective tool by which to measure his performance over time with the new aids in the real world. Parents may assist in this area by providing feedback to their children regarding their performance with new hearing aids as they observe longitudinal communication changes in similar real-world situations. Chorost (1990) advocates that audiologists make "clients active and knowledgeable partners in solving their own hearing problems" and "abandon the harmful illusion that they are problem-solvers, and embrace, as psychologists do, their powerful reality as consultants."

In order for this to happen, audiologists must guide parents to begin early training with their children regarding their perceptions of their hearing aids. With preschoolers, the early training may involve learning the language necessary to describe sound such as loud/soft, on/off, and clear/fuzzy. Visual aids and a radio may be used to initially convey these concepts by using the volume control to demonstrate the first two pairs of concepts and the tuning control to illustrate the third pair. Elementary and secondary school children should be encouraged to convey their perceptions of sound to the audiologist during each evaluation. When discrimination tasks are learned, they can be asked to compare the sound of their hearing aids to that of the FM system. After the child has worn hearing aids for perhaps a year, tone control settings may be manipulated to determine if they are aware of changes in frequency response and if they have a preference for the current setting. This reaction may be predictive of their ability to identify quality changes in their hearing aids as well as the degree of change they may experience when a change in amplification is made. Training of this type, along with developing responsibility and advocacy for amplification needs, may result over time in clients who are able to effectively convey to the audiologist the psychological aspects of using amplification that should be addressed in counseling the hearing impaired.

Maintenance of Amplification

Parents and older children need the tools and knowledge to not only test their hearing aids but also to repair simple problems such as clogged tubing, dirty battery contacts, or twisted tubing. Recommendations provided to adult hearing aid users in Appendix 9–1 of Chapter 9 are also applicable here. Specific routines for monitoring the hearing aids at home and at school are provided below.

Home.   Parents should have a hearing aid test kit at home. Ideally this kit would be dispensed with the hearing aid to convey the importance of conducting the listening checks. The stethoscope and battery tester should be used to perform listening checks at least twice a day. Bess, Sinclair, and Riggs (1984) found that testing aids in the midafternoon resulted in identification of malfunctioning aids that were functioning properly earlier that morning. Procedures for conducting a complete listening check are provided in Appendix 7–3.

As soon as children are assisting with dressing by pulling on their socks and helping to remove their shirts, they should begin assisting with this daily checking routine by first testing battery voltage. However, parents should be cautioned regarding the serious consequences of accidental battery ingestion, and only children who are not inclined to put batteries in their mouths should be allowed to participate in the battery testing under close supervision. Parents of young children should be informed of the National Button Battery Ingestion Hotline Numbers.[1] When a problem is discovered that alters the sound of one of the hearing aids, the parents should make a special effort to describe the change in sound in simple language while the child listens before and after the problem has been corrected. For example, they might say, "This aid sounds scratchy" and "Now this aid sounds clear."

Parents must also be taught to clean ear molds, which is described in Appendix 9–1 of Chapter 9. A common problem with amplification for young children is feedback. Parents need to understand causes and remedies of acoustic feedback and be told some general guidelines regarding frequency of ear-mold replacement. Other tools to have at home for maintenance include spare batteries, cords, and button receivers if necessary.

When school-age children begin conducting the checks and identify a problem, verbal reinforcement to acknowledge their efforts should be provided. The daily checks should be considered as routine as brushing one's teeth. As children become more active, it may be necessary to introduce measures to protect the hearing aids against moisture. These include wrapping the aid with plastic

---

[1](202) 625-3333 for voice and (202) 625-6070 for TTD.

wrap, applying antiperspirant to the mastoid area, slipping a disposable latex sleeve known as a Super Seal over the aid, and using a drying package known as Dri-Aid when the aids are removed in the evening (see Appendix 7–6 for sources).

School. Unfortunately, according to a survey by Reichman and Healey (1989) of 146 teachers in schools for children with hearing loss across the country, some programs still do not routinely check hearing aids (9%) or FM systems (14%) despite federal regulations that require monitoring (P.L. 94-142, *Federal Register*, 1977, 121a.303). Reichman and Healey considered a minimally adequate monitoring program to include daily visual and listening checks of hearing aids and auditory trainers, hearing aid and auditory trainer loaner programs with 1-day availability, and in-service training. They reported that only 45.9% of the teachers in residential and public day schools combined indicated that their monitoring programs met the minimally adequate criteria. When considering children who are mainstreamed, the situation may be even worse according to Shepard, Davis, Gorga, and Stelmachowicz (1981), who reported that only 2% of the children's aids in the Iowa public schools were monitored by regular classroom teachers. This is alarming considering that 71% of the children wearing hearing aids were in regular classrooms. Recent data reported by Maxon et al. (1991) suggest that the situation may be improving, as they found that half of the FM systems in the programs they surveyed were checked on a daily basis.

These data imply that audiologists must take an active role in the development of school monitoring programs for the children they serve. This is not to suggest that audiologists actually develop the program but rather that they assume responsibility for seeing that an effective one is available or assist in finding the resources to establish one. As emphasized by Dr. Johnson in Chapter 8, communication regarding the amplification monitoring program should first occur with the audiologist employed by the school. However, 14.1% of the programs surveyed by Reichman and Healey (1989) did not have audiological services, in which case the speech-language pathologist may be the most knowledgeable person regarding amplification monitoring. The purpose of contact with these school personnel is to determine who will be responsible for the daily monitoring of hearing aids and if they are in need of any demonstrations or handouts. Information about trouble-shooting equipment and spare parts and batteries may also be conveyed. If possible, the audiologist should encourage the parents of the child with a hearing loss to check on the monitoring program in order to foster the development of responsibility and advocacy for the needs of their child.

INTERPERSONAL COUNSELING

Three important issues impacting how parents will be able to apply the information that has been discussed in the first half of this chapter are acceptance of amplification, assuming responsibility for amplification, and finally becoming an advocate for amplification needs. The interactions among the audiologist, parents, and the child with a hearing loss may facilitate or hinder acceptance, responsibility, and advocacy. The remaining half of this chapter focuses on how to establish these effective interactions.

Acceptance of Amplification

An important aspect of interacting with parents and children during acceptance is the ability of the audiologist to listen. Gatty and Casale (1992) advocate active listening to facilitate communication. This involves conveying a body posture that is relaxed but attentive. As eye contact is maintained, the listener "tracks" the speaker by rephrasing and asking for clarification. The listener also conveys sensitivity to the feelings of the speaker while trying to focus on the speaker and not on solving the problem. An example of this type of listening is illustrated in the dialogue between the parents of a 2-year-old child with a profound hearing loss and the audiologist.

AUDIOLOGIST: "Tell me how your feeling about Megan wearing two hearing aids."

MOTHER: "I can barely keep one hearing aid on her. I just don't see how I can manage two of them. I haven't seen any change in her talking since we put this aid on one month ago."

AUDIOLOGIST: "It sounds like you're not sure if this hearing aid is allowing Megan to hear speech."

FATHER: "I have noticed that she's more interested in her music box when I put her to bed at night. When we were playing on the swings in the backyard, we thought she may have noticed the air conditioner unit come on because she wanted to get out of the swing and sit on my lap."

AUDIOLOGIST: "Megan looks like she really enjoys her time with you. You both seem to consider it very important to spend time with her."

MOTHER: "Yes, but I can't be right with her all the time. After struggling to get the aid on in the morning, oftentimes I'll find it laying on the floor after she's been playing. I'm really afraid we'll lose it and I would really hate to lose two of them."

AUDIOLOGIST: "Let me see if I understand. It's frustrating to you when Megan removes her hearing aid, so you feel that two hearing aids will only create more frustration."

MOTHER: "Yes, do other parents have this much trouble?"

AUDIOLOGIST: "I'm glad you asked that because some members of our parent group who also have two-year-olds are anxious to meet you. Here are their phone numbers if you'd like to call them."

The audiologist in this example believes that the child will benefit from binaural amplification but must work with the parents through active listening as they discuss this possibility. Continued discussion may include questions about what the parents think would be helpful in keeping the aid on the child or how their feelings might change if the aids were covered by insurance.

When audiologists encounter parents who have significant difficulties with amplification, they must resist the urge to provide the solutions. Instead, they must focus on asking questions and actively listening to the parents' answers. This will lead to a trusting relationship that will facilitate solutions to other amplification problems that may arise. As a result of this trusting relationship, parents may develop a sense of confidence that the audiologist will consider their concerns rather than a preestablished schedule of topics to be covered. Dr. Clark presents further discussion of the art of reflective listening in Chapter 2.

Acceptance of amplification may be closely tied to acceptance of the hearing loss. Although the acceptance process differs for parents relative to the child, they both may experience various degrees of acceptance over time. For some it may be a cyclic process where progress alternates with regression. The cycles may depend on the respective peers the parents and children are interacting with in their environment at a given time.

Parents. Most audiologists agree that parents' ability to accept a hearing loss is influenced by the grieving process. Grieving is not only considered acceptable but necessary by some professionals (Bader, 1992; Moses, 1983). The purpose of grieving, according to Bader (1992), is to gather the external resources and the internal strength to deal with the diagnosis. Engaging parents in support groups where feelings about the initial diagnosis and the various stages of grief are shared in a safe environment will facilitate the grieving process (Bader, 1992; Junge & Ellwood, 1986).

The feelings associated with grieving may include guilt, depression, anger, or anxiety. Audiologists should view these feelings as appropriate, healthy, and necessary to reconcile the loss and to lead toward a positive relationship between parent and child. Bader (1992) believes that the acceptance of the hearing loss will be facilitated if the audiologist knows the reason behind each of these feelings and responds appropriately. In addition, it is important for the audiologist not to make assumptions regarding the feelings and attitudes of parents. At least two-thirds of the professionals in the survey by Maxon et al. (1991) reportedly thought that parents were unhappy with FM systems because their child looked different using them. Using the techniques described by Dr. Van Hecke in Chapter 5, the audiologist may explore the parents' feelings about the hearing aids and/or FM systems; for example, "Tell me how you feel when someone notices your child's FM system or hearing aids" or "How do you feel about wearing the FM transmitter when you take your child on an outing?" Knowing how parents feel rather than making assumptions will lead to more effective active listening.

Children with hearing loss. Children who accept their hearing loss and are comfortable with who they are generally have a high self-esteem. The ability of children with hearing loss to accept their handicaps may depend largely on their families' attitude (Loeb & Sarigiani, 1986). If children feel accepted by their families, they can accept themselves. Warren and Hasenstab (1986) found a strong relationship between self-concept of children with hearing loss and parental rejection. Children develop their self-concepts based on how they think others appraise them. If they sense their family considers them to be different and in need of special attention, they will view themselves accordingly.

It is important that children with a hearing loss feel accepted by their families regardless of hearing aid use. When acceptance is contingent upon consistent use of amplification, children learn that hearing aid use is very important for the parent. They may seek a sense of control by rejecting their aids because they know this will upset their parents. If parents display genuine love and affection toward their children, rather than expressing love to reward the child for amplification use, the likelihood of children using their hearing aids to control parents' emotions is reduced.

According to Boothroyd (1982), for very young children hearing aids may become "a pawn in the conflict over independence and control that typically begins between the second and third birthdays" (p. 90). He suggests that parents recognize that the child's need for discipline is similar to that of the hearing child's. The audiologist may show support during this difficult time by allowing parents to verbalize frustrations. They may ask such questions as "What have you tried to do to keep your child from removing the hearing aids?" Responses that highlight inner strengths may be helpful, such as "It sounds like you have given this a lot of thought. You really are concerned that your child benefits from hearing aids."

Acceptance of hearing aids and/or FM systems is often an issue around the teenage years when there are strong desires for peer approval and a struggle for independence from parents. Demands from parents or authority figures regarding hearing aid use denigrate both peer approval and independence. Rather than accept the hearing aids, some teenagers may focus on nonproductive coping strategies.

Jill, who is moderately hearing impaired, was actively using amplification until she reached high school. Her parents became concerned because she never went out with friends, spent long periods of time in her room, and was frequently caught skipping class. Regular meetings with a speech-language clinician were arranged by the school counselor in an attempt to encourage use of the hearing aids at school. Following a thorough hearing aid check to ensure that Jill was receiving benefit from her aids, the clinician arranged a group meeting with Jill and three other hearing-impaired students who were seniors. During these meetings the clinician asked open-ended questions such as "What do you think about your hearing aids?" and "How much do they help you?" During the group discussion, the students developed two goals to improve their auditory functioning. Although Jill did not write a goal related to hearing aid use, she agreed to meet with the group again in 3 weeks to discuss the goals she had written.

The value of peer models and group discussions for teenagers was emphasized by Mann (1992), who is a mental health therapist with a hearing loss. One of the major benefits of group discussions is the support system that may emerge. It is helpful for students to know there are some people with whom they can talk openly and not fear ridicule when students in their classes are making cruel statements. Furthermore, the older students in the group serve as role models to show that one may overcome problems associated with amplification.

An effective peer modeling group was described by Flexer and Wray (1989) in which hearing-impaired college students met with hearing-impaired high school students and their parents. In addition to conveying much factual information about selecting and attending a college, the students shared many of the feelings they experienced throughout the process. Henggeler, Watson, and Whelan (1990) reported that mothers of adolescents with hearing loss believed that their children were less emotionally bonded to their friends than the mothers of hearing adolescents believed of their own children. This suggests that specific efforts may be necessary to build friendships such as those that may occur through support groups.

Discussion of experiences among hearing-impaired students may lead to the development of more realistic goals. When the students are asked to make their own goals, they are more likely to take responsibility for completing them than if they are told they should wear their hearing aids to every class at least 4 days a week. However, if one chooses to allow students to develop goals, they must be accepted even if they do not match the audiologist's goals. Accepting their goals develops trust, which will in turn allow discussion of goals closer to the preferred one. Another advantage of the group discussion with teenagers is the ability to brainstorm for solutions as discussed by Dr. Trychin in Chapter 10. The clinician might say, "Let's think of 20 solutions to Jill's problem" and then ask Jill to pick the three with which she feels the most comfortable. The solution intended by the clinician may be presented by one of the other students and be more acceptable from a peer than from an authority figure.

When group discussions are not possible, the audiologist must develop a communication style with teenagers that reflects openness and a genuine desire to appreciate their views. For example, to convey this attitude one might say, "I can't know what it feels like to wear hearing aids. Could you tell me about it?" It is important to explore the benefit of the amplification system. Mann (1992) advocates one not force teenagers to wear aids if the situation is causing pain or tension within the family. Forcing the use of amplification may cause the teenager to perceive hearing aids as a lifelong enemy and possibly never wear them again.

Peers of children with hearing loss. Although the influence of peers varies with age, the peers of children with hearing loss may have a greater impact overall than peers of hearing children. Children with hearing loss know that they are different and they look to their peers for validation of how important this difference is. One study of peer influence evaluated the attitudes of peers toward children wearing hearing aids. Dengerink and Porter (1984) found that fifth- and sixth-grade children were negatively biased toward their peers who wore hearing aids. Some of this bias may have been learned in the educational environment according to a study by Brimacombe, Danhauer, and Mulac (1983), who found that even teachers have a negative bias toward children wearing hearing aids. However, a recent study by Riensche, Peterson, and Linden (1990) with 4- and 5-year-old children found no negative biases. They suggested that the biases may be developed in the early elementary grades and recommended programs to facilitate classroom peer acceptance of hearing aids.

If information regarding the benefits of amplification can be presented to elementary school children, they may become more accustomed to those who use them. Often the cruel statements made by children are a result of a lack of understanding of the student's needs or reflect uncomfortable feelings the child may have when around someone with a hearing loss. Therefore, the more knowledge they have, the less likely they will feel the need to ridicule the child with a hearing loss. Presentations regarding types of hearing aids including FM systems, function of the ear, and ways to protect ears may be made for regular classes during science or health units. A massive effort will be needed to reach large numbers of children in order for this education plan to have an impact. One way this could happen is for all audiologists to assume responsibility for two presentations a year to elementary classes, perhaps during Better Hearing and Speech Month in May.

Another method to facilitate peer acceptance is to allow hearing peers to participate as role models in one-on-one interactions or in mainstreamed situations. A child with a hearing loss may be paired with an older hearing student who can answer questions regarding a school, difficulty of future classes, or extracurricular activities. Hearing children may share their experiences with their other hearing friends, and consequently the understanding of the children with hearing loss may be fostered. The benefits of mixing the children with hearing loss with hearing children were supported by the findings of Ladd, Munson, and Miller (1984), who conducted a longitudinal study of adolescents who attended a 2-year occupational educational program with hearing students and found that peer ratings of the students with hearing loss improved favorably. Teachers and parents reported improvements in social relations and friendship patterns over the course of the study.

Finally, another method of informing peers about hearing loss involves the use of children's literature. Although many books on hearing loss are available for elementary-school-age children, there are also some appropriate for older children. Parents may encourage school libraries to obtain some of these sources or offer to read some of these to classes at their child's school. A list of children's literature that addresses hearing impairment is included in Appendix 7–4.

Developing Responsibility for Amplification

Parents. Active parental roles in the use and maintenance of amplification may be initiated by including a family goal on the Individualized Education Program (IEP). However, in order for this goal to be seriously addressed parents must feel like an active part of the training program. This naturally occurs in parent–infant training programs where the parents attend the entire session each week with their child because they are the care givers and are in continual contact with the child. Then around age 3, when children enter preschool programs, parents often get the message that they no longer need to be the primary teachers because they are not required to attend the daily sessions. In this situation, carryover of training at home will not be as extensive unless parents remain active in the training at school. Consequently, they may become less involved in monitoring the amplification. In order to maintain a sense of active participation in the child's training, parents may develop a goal for the IEP to attend four sessions per month. Their attendance may be in the form of observing from outside the classroom, but ideally they could be involved within the classroom as teachers' aides on a regular basis.

In some cases where hearing aids are provided by another source, parents may not realize the importance of the aids and use of the hearing aids at home may be sporadic. Getting the parents to assume responsibility for putting the aids on the child each day will require some changes in their behavior. As pointed out by Dr. Trychin in Chapter 10, one way to strengthen desired behavior is to provide positive consequences. Therefore, when parents show some responsibility for maintaining the hearing aids, they should receive verbal reinforcement. The audiologist should not praise the parents, but rather should comment on the parents' actions and feelings. For example one may say, "I can see that you're really happy that your child is wearing the hearing aids all day," rather than "You've really done a great job keeping the hearing aids on all day." Parents need to assume the responsibility as a result of internal motivation, which will be more permanent, and not external praise, which is only possible when in the presence of the audiologist.

School-age children. The need for children to be involved in monitoring their hearing aids was highlighted by the findings of Reichman and Healey (1989) and Maxon et al. (1991) reported above. Developing responsibility for amplification in school-age children should begin naturally at home as the child gradually becomes more involved in the daily monitoring of the aids. Glenn and Nelson (1989) believe that there are seven tools that a child must acquire in order to become a responsible, successful part of society. These tools were discovered as they studied children who failed and then became involved with the criminal justice system or social welfare or who did not realize their potential in school. They refer to the tools as the significant seven, which include the following:

1. Strong perceptions of personal capabilities. "I am capable."
2. Strong perceptions of significance in primary relationships. "I contribute in meaningful ways and I am genuinely needed."
3. Strong perceptions of personal power or influence over life. "I can influence what happens to me."
4. Strong intrapersonal skills. The ability to understand personal emotions, use that understanding to develop self-discipline and self-control, and learn from experience.
5. Strong interpersonal skills. The ability to work with others and develop friendships through communication, cooperation, negotiation, sharing, empathizing, and listening.
6. Strong systemic skills. The ability to respond to the limits and consequences of everyday life with responsibility, adaptability, flexibility, and integrity.
7. Strong judgmental skills. The ability to use wisdom and evaluate situations according to appropriate values. (pp. 49–50)

These principles are especially important for the successful development of the child with a hearing loss who is struggling with a communication system, excessive peer pressure, and adapted educational programs. Audiologists should encourage parents to focus on these areas as they teach responsibility for the care of the hearing aids. Because the perception of capability and personal power are most applicable to caring for the hearing aids, illustrations of these principles will be provided.

One way to develop this sense of personal capability with respect to amplification is to teach the child the task of checking battery voltage. The battery tester that has a contact plate so that only one lead wire must be touched to the battery is easiest for children. The first steps may only involve the child placing the lead wire on the battery. Eventually they may be taught to identify the positive and negative terminals. Training may be accomplished by having the child test a set of batteries including drained ones. The sense of capability may be strengthened as the child is allowed to test the batteries of other children or batteries for other household items.

Mrs. Marshall had been working with Matthew, age 5, for several weeks on checking his batteries by having him complete a chart each morning to indicate the results of his check. Matthew completed the check as part of his dressing routine each morning. One day Matthew was unable to get his tape recorder to work and he brought it to his mother. Rather than replace the batteries immediately, she decided to use the opportunity to reinforce Matthew's sense of capability. She asked him what he thought the problem might be as she opened the battery compartment. After Matthew suggested that it needed new batteries, she asked how they might find out if the existing batteries were good. Matthew gladly got the battery tester and proceeded to test the batteries and confirmed their suspicions. Then he checked the new batteries before inserting them in the tape player. Before going off with his tape recorder he offered to check the batteries in the household flashlights.

Glenn and Nelson (1989) point out that when parents do too much for their children, they may perceive themselves as inadequate and insignificant. Parents must convey the attitude that they need their child's help in testing the aids. This perception of personal capability may also be developed as children are invited to assist in the monitoring of hearing aids of younger children or for the elderly. When children perform a task such as checking battery voltage for someone who is incapable of performing that task, they gain the sense of being able to contribute. Parents may seek opportunities for their child to assist with the hearing aid checks in the classrooms of younger children with hearing loss or in nursing homes. The time invested by the parent to arrange this activity periodically is as important as the time spent on auditory training drills at home.

The perception of personal power or influence over one's life may also be developed through teaching responsibility for amplification. Children need to learn that whatever happens to them is, in part, a result of decisions they make and the effort they put forth. This will help them develop an internal locus of control rather than being dependent on an external locus of control. According to Glenn and Nelson, when children believe that power lies outside themselves, they are highly susceptible to the opinions of others regarding their own self-worth and their potential actions. Thus, in order for children with hearing loss to develop the positive self-image that is necessary to survive the peer pressure they are to experience, they need a strong sense of power over events. They need to see that a correlation exists between what they do and what happens to them. This sense of internal control can be developed as children are taught to identify when their hearing aids are malfunctioning. Initially this must be directly taught. For elementary-school-age children it is easiest to have them listen to their hearing aids several times with and without a battery. Each time they put on the aids, they are to identify whether or not they are working. The parent must lead a discussion of how important it is to tell someone when their hearing aids are not working. On a later occasion the parent may place a dead battery in one of the aids and see if the child reports a problem. When children identify a problem, they should be commended for their excellent listening and responsibility in reporting the problem. To foster the internal locus of control the parent should say something like, "You must really feel good that you are listening so well that you found a problem with your hearing aid." This is better than saying, "I'm so happy you brought your hearing aid to me when it wasn't working," which implies that the child's behavior was appropriate because someone else thought so. To point out the development of responsibility the parent might say, "You are certainly growing up and learning to take care of things for yourself. You'll soon be ready to do some of the things your older brother is allowed to do."

Adolescents. The seven principles underlying responsible behavior also apply to the adolescent. It is important at this age to establish dialogue with the child. The communication should occur in a nonthreatening climate of support and genuine interest and should not necessarily occur just when there are problems. With the fast pace of today's society and the ready access to television and video games, families must make concentrated efforts to practice dialogue. These practice sessions will set the stage for effective skills for when difficult issues must be addressed. To establish a climate of support during dialogue, Glenn and Nelson (1989) suggest that there should be an openness to exploring and respecting other points of view, empathy, which results only from careful listening, genuiness conveyed through warmth and interest, and ownership of personal feelings.

Melody, age 15, came rushing in from school in tears. She had recently changed schools and was not using her FM system yet because she was waiting until her speech clinician had told all of her teachers that she had a hearing loss. When her father asked what was upsetting to her, she said that she had asked a question in her history class that had just been asked by another student and the boy next to her started writing everything the teacher said in large letters and passing it to her.

This created some discussion around her and the teacher asked her if she had material she would like to share with the class because the class seemed interested in what was on her desk. She reluctantly told the teacher that the student was writing down the information the teacher was presenting for her to review. Melody didn't think she could return to that class the next day because she was sure everyone thought she should be in a special education class.

The problem experienced by Melody was a result of not accepting the responsibility of informing her teachers that she was hearing impaired and would be using an FM system. Had she been using the FM system she might not have missed the class discussion and repeated the question.

Glenn and Nelson (1989) would suggest that Melody, in the above example, has to change her perception about the experience and that this type of learning has four levels, which are explored through dialogue. The first level is experience, both positive and negative, in one's life. Melody's father might ask, "Tell me what happened to you today to make you so upset." The next level is identification of what is significant in that experience. So Melody's father might then ask, "What was most important about that experience?" The third level is to analyze certain aspects of the experience to discover why the experience was significant. Questions such as "What made that seem important to you?" or "What caused you to feel that way?" may be asked at this level. The final level is generalization, where one tries to learn something from the experience that may be useful in future situations. Melody's father could ask, "Based on this experience, what would you do differently next time?"

This dialogue process will certainly take longer than perhaps the more natural response of Melody's father, which might have been as follows: "I told you to wear that FM system to each class. You should talk to your teachers yourself. Now tomorrow, I'll take you to school early and we'll find your teachers and you can tell them about the FM system. And don't forget to give them spare batteries to keep in their desk." This response does not allow for Melody to act responsibly by exploring her perceptions about what happened and deciding how she should have reacted. Instead, the answers are given to Melody, her future is directed, and assumptions are made regarding her inability to remember the spare batteries. This type of response creates barriers to dialogue and probably leaves Melody feeling even more insecure.

The problem of limited responsibility for amplification was observed even at the college level by Flexer, Wray, and Black (1986), who interviewed 12 moderately hearing-impaired students at the University of Akron. They found that although these students had used hearing aids for approximately 17 years, most of them could not interpret their own audiograms, knew little about FM systems, or were unable to trouble-shoot their hearing aids. As a result of their findings, an information support group was developed and eagerly attended. Hopefully, students today will begin assuming some responsibility for their own hearing aids as early as preschool such that they will be better equipped when they attend college.

Becoming Advocates for Amplification

It has been said that if we do our job well, we should be out of a job. If parents are dependent on the audiologist to maintain all of the records regarding amplification, to see that the appropriate amplification and monitoring programs are provided by the school, and to remind them when evaluation is needed, children learn that others will take care of them. Not only does this arrangement result in time delays and unwarranted expenses, children with hearing loss do not experience an advocacy model to apply to their own lives as adults. The role of parents as advocates for their child gradually increases following the initial diagnosis and then gradually decreases as they transfer this role to their child. The findings of Flexer et al. (1986) that hearing-impaired college students knew little about hearing aids and hearing loss suggest that students are not being taught advocacy roles. This lack of advocacy may explain why it was 1988 before the first student requested that The University of Texas provide an FM system to facilitate classroom listening. It is somewhat surprising that only four additional systems have been purchased for a campus that serves over 47,000 students, particularly given the fact that there are approximately 300 students over age 50 in a typical semester. Because developing advocacy in students is facilitated by parent models, it is important that audiologists consider this a rehabilitative goal as important as recommending amplification.

Parents. It is difficult for audiologists to draw the line between where their role stops and the parents' role begins in management. It is important for the audiologist to openly acknowledge that they expect parents to become advocates for their child over time. Recognizing that this is a process that occurs over time, the audiologist may discuss with the parents different opportunities for them to develop this role throughout the rehabilitation process. Opportunities that may arise include requesting classroom amplification for their child if not already available, a hearing aid monitoring program including participation by their child, support group sessions for their child with older hearing-impaired students in the same school district, an assistive device at the local library so their child may participate in a story hour, or a swimming teacher at summer camp who uses total communication.

Goldberg, Niehl, and Metropoulos (1989) have recognized the need for parents to be actively involved as advocates for their child and have provided a checklist for parents to follow when evaluating a prospective mainstreamed classroom for their child. Such tools are valuable models for parent groups to use in the development of other resources. Some parents may need the comfort of legislation to back them as they begin advocating for their child. Articles such as those by Herbison (1986) and Williams (1992) may be shared with parents to inform them of the legal rights of hearing-impaired children. Complete references for these items and other resources for parents are included in Appendix 7–5.

Once opportunities for parents to become advocates have been identified and they have been given some tools to use, they will need reinforcement to continue their efforts in an area that may be uncomfortable for them. The audiologist should maintain interest and support in their activities. This is a good time to acknowledge their inner strength as a resource by commenting on their successes. An example of this would be "You must be very happy about the new electroacoustic test equipment that was purchased by Daniel's school. You were very good at presenting information to the administrators to justify your request. Daniel must have noticed all your visits to the school in the past months and feel like you're an active part of his education." When parents receive this recognition, they will begin to realize the importance of teaching this process to their children.

School-age children. Developing advocacy roles in children is the responsibility of the parent and the audiologist. Opportunities to teach this role may be brought to the parents' attention by the audiologist. Beginning in elementary school, children may be encouraged to ask their teachers to keep spare batteries in their desk or provide a chart to record the hearing aid checks as shown in Appendix 7–6. The parents and teachers may brainstorm together to devise contrived situations in which students must assert themselves. These situations should be followed with verbal reinforcement from the parent or teacher. For example, after demonstrating for the child the inappropriate sound that occurs when the FM transmitter microphone is no longer directed toward the mouth, the teacher may purposefully shift the microphone placement to provide an opportunity for the child to request proper placement.

It is important that teachers and parents gradually allow the children to determine appropriate actions in situations to determine maximum hearing rather than to always teach them. This may be done by asking questions such as "How well do you hear the Girl Scout leader at the troop meeting?" or "What might help you hear better in that situation?" Given the opportunity to think about what might be helpful in various situations, the student will be more likely to develop independent thinking. Making requests for amplification needs may need to be practiced through role-playing with hearing peers.

Adolescents. Development of advocacy roles in adolescents is complicated by the peer pressures to conform. Hearing-impaired adolescents may be reluctant to ask for an FM system to be used at the school assembly because they don't want to be different from the other students. Use of older role models may be the most effective teaching resource at this age. A support group may be challenged to evaluate compliance in the community with the Americans with Disabilities Act. (See Chapter 9 for a discussion of the requirements of the American with Disabilities Act.) The students would first have to discuss what facilities needed to comply and how they might do this. Then visits to the facilities could be made to determine more specifically what the assistive needs might be. Finally, a plan must be developed to convey the information to the administrators at each facility. This type of group activity may be better received when students may learn from each other as opposed to teachers assigning specific individual tasks to be completed. Furthermore, the group activity prepares them to participate in other organizations such as university campus groups for students with handicaps or Self-Help for Hard of Hearing People (SHHH). Some students may believe that they function adequately in the hearing world and do not need to participate in such groups. Parents and teachers may need to discuss with them the benefit to other hearing-impaired persons they may provide by being active participants in such groups. It may be brought to their attention that no one is better suited to be an advocate for the needs of hearing-impaired people than those who experience the difficulties firsthand.

CONCLUSION

The role of the audiologist in counseling for pediatric amplification is twofold. One role is to convey a wealth of information to parents in a manner that is sensitive to their ability to receive information at any given time. A second role is to establish a relationship with the parents and child that fosters acceptance of the hearing loss, development of responsibility for amplification, and establishment of advocacy roles for assistive needs. Numerous suggestions to facilitate these two roles of the audiologist were made. In closing, four ideas are presented to facilitate and strengthen all of the principles provided in this chapter:

1. Ask parents to keep a journal. Writing helps one to verbalize thoughts that may otherwise go unspoken and also helps people focus on particular events or behaviors because they know they have to write something down about them. It is important to start the journal for them during a session in which you make observations and then ask them to continue it during the week. Indicate that you will be writing in it when they bring it in. Entries may summarize the activities or discussion that occurred and provide a review for parents when they get home. The journal is also a logical place to begin keeping records regarding hearing aid purchases and repairs, audiometric findings, and school placements. The journals may also be a resource for parent discussion groups to facilitate sharing of information on a particular topic.

2. Periodically ask parents to demonstrate what the child can do and then provide reinforcement. The responsibility for children to receive maximum benefit from amplification is largely that of the parents who must see that the hearing aids are worn consistently and are well maintained. If they are reinforced for their efforts, their behavior is likely to continue.

3. Ask parents to bring questions and then reinforce their efforts when they ask these questions. If the rehabilitation process is to follow the parents' lead, they will need to be encouraged to take that lead.

4. Arrange for parents to communicate with other experienced parents. The value of the support groups for children also applies to the parents. Many times the parents of a child with a handicap lose contact with old friends because of the time commitments required by the training. Bader (1992) believes so strongly in the support group system, that parents are required to attend sessions for couples as well as separate ones for mothers and for fathers. Further discussion of support groups for parents, siblings, and extended family members is provided by Dr. Atkins in Chapter 6.

Many of the concepts presented here are not included in typical audiology training programs. However, as parents and children are taught to become advocates they will demand consideration of these aspects from the audiologists that serve them. In reality, the audiologist may best serve children with hearing loss by accepting the notion that learning is a two-way street with the parents having as much to offer as the audiology professional.

ACKNOWLEDGMENTS

Appreciation is expressed to Laurie Jalenak and Amanda Nevitt for our discussions regarding their experiences with families of children with hearing loss.

REFERENCES

ABRAHAMSON, J., THIBODEAU, L. (1990). *Incorporating coping strategies into hearing aid management programs.* Paper presented at Texas, Speech, Language, and Hearing Association Meeting. Dallas, TX.

ADAMS, J., & TIDWELL, R. (1988). Parents' perceptions regarding the discipline of their hearing-impaired children. *Child Care, Health and Development, 14,* 265–273.

ANDERSON, K. (1989). Speech perception and the hard of hearing child. *Educational Audiology Monograph, 1,* 15–30.

BADER, J. L. (1992). *Helping teachers help grieving parents.* Paper presented at the meeting of the A. G. Bell Association. San Diego, CA.

BESS, F., SINCLAIR, J., & RIGGS. D. (1984). Group amplification in schools for the hearing impaired. *Ear and Hearing, 5,* 138–144.

BOOTHROYD, A. (1982). *Hearing impairments in young children.* Englewood Cliffs, NJ: Prentice Hall.

BOOTHROYD, A., SPRINGER, N., SMITH, L., & SCHULMAN, J. (1988). Amplitude compression and profound hearing loss. *Journal of Speech and Hearing Research, 31,* 362–376.

BRIMACOMBE, J., DANHAUER, J., & MULAC, A. (1983). Teachers' perceptions of students who wear hearing aids: An empirical test. *Language, Speech and Hearing Services in Schools, 14,* 128–135.

CHOROST, M. (1990). An unpublished open letter to Charles Berlin.

CLARK, T., MORGAN, E., & WILSON-VLOTMAN, A. (1983). *The INSITE model: Vol. 2. Parent discussions.* Project funded by U.S. Office of Education, Bureau of Education for the Handicapped, Handicapped Children's Early Education Program, P.L. 91–230, Title IV, Part C.

DENGERINK, J., & PORTER, J. (1984). Children's attitudes toward peers wearing hearing aids. *Language, Speech and Hearing Services in Schools, 15,* 199–204.

FLEXER, C., & WRAY, D. (1989). Hearing-impaired college students reach out to the community. *Volta Review, 91,* 157–162.

FLEXER, C., WRAY, D., & BLACK, T. (1986). Support group for moderately hearing-impaired college students: An expanding awareness. *Volta Review, 88,* 223–229.

FRENCH, H., & STEINBERG, J. (1947). Factors governing the intelligibility of speech sounds. *Journal of the Acoustical Society of America, 19,* 90–119.

GATTY, J., & CASALE, K. (1992). *"They just don't understand me!": A workshop for professionals.* Paper presented at the meeting of the A. G. Bell Association. San Diego, CA.

GLENN, S., & NELSON, J. (1989). *Raising self-reliant children in a self-indulgent world.* Rocklin, CA: Prima Publishing & Communications.

GOLDBERG, D., NIEHL, P., & METROPOULOS, T. (1989). Parent checklist for placement of a hearing-impaired child in a mainstreamed classroom. *Volta Review, 91,* 327–332.

HENGGELER, S., WATSON, S., & WHELAN, J. (1990). Peer relations of hearing-impaired adolescents. *Journal of Pediatric Psychology, 15*, 721–731.

HERBISON, P. (1986). Legal rights of hearing-impaired children: A guide for advocates. *Health and Social Work, 11*, 301–307.

JUNGE, M., & ELLWOOD, A. (1986). Parent information and support groups. *Infant Mental Health Journal, 7*, 146–155.

LADD, G., MUNSON, H., & MILLER, J. (1984). Social integration of deaf adolescents in secondary-level mainstreamed programs. *Exceptional Children, 50*, 420–428.

LEWIS, D., FEIGIN, J., KARASEK, A., & STELMACHOWICZ, P. (1992). Evaluation and assessment of FM systems. *Ear and Hearing, 12*, 268–280.

LOEB, R., & SARIGIANI, P. (1986). The impact of hearing impairment on self-perceptions of children. *Volta Review, 88*, 89–100.

LUTERMAN, D. (1987). *Deafness in the family*. Boston: College Hill Press.

MADELL, J. (1992). FM systems as primary amplification for children with profound hearing loss. *Ear and Hearing, 13*, 102–107.

MANN, M. (1992). Adjustment issues of hearing-impaired adolescents. In J. Feigin & P. Stelmachowicz (Eds.), *Pediatric amplification: Proceedings of the 1991 national conference*, pp. 173–182. Omaha, NE: Boys Town National Research Hospital.

MARTIN, F., GEORGE, K., O'NEAL, J., & DALY, J. (1987). Audiologists' and parents' attitudes regarding counseling of families of hearing-impaired children. *Asha, 29*, 27–32.

MAXON, A., BRACKETT, D., & VAN DEN BERG, S. (1991). Classroom amplification use: A national long term study. *Language, Speech, and Hearing Services in Schools, 22*, 242–253.

MOSES, K. (1983). The impact of initial diagnosis: Mobilizing family resources. In J. A. Mulick & S. M. Pueschel (Eds.), *Parent–professional partnerships in developmental disability services* (pp. 11–34). Cambridge, MA: Academic Guild Publishers.

NORTHERN, J., & DOWNS, M. (1984). *Hearing in children*. Baltimore: Williams & Wilkins.

POLLACK, D., & WEDENBERG, E. (1970). *Educational audiology for the limited hearing infant*. Springfield, IL: Charles C Thomas.

REICHMAN, J., & HEALEY, W. (1989). Amplification monitoring and maintenance in schools. *Asha, 31*, 43–45.

RIENSCHE, L., PETERSON, K., & LINDEN, S. (1990). Young children's attitudes toward peer hearing aid wearers. *Hearing Journal, 43*, 19–20.

ROSS, M., & SEEWALD, R. (1990). Hearing aid selection and evaluation with young children, pp. 190–213. In F. Bess (Ed.), *Hearing impairment in children*. Parkton, MD: York Press.

SHEPARD, N., DAVIS, J., GORGA, M., & STELMACHOWICZ, P. (1981). Characteristics of hearing-impaired children in the public schools (Part I, demographic data) *Journal of Speech and Hearing Disorders, 46*, 123–129.

SKINNER, M. (1988). *Hearing aid evaluation*. Englewood Cliffs, NJ: Prentice Hall.

STONE, P., & ADAM, A. (1986). Is your child wearing the right hearing aid? Principles for selecting and maintaining amplification. *Volta Review, 88*, 45–54.

THIBODEAU, L., O'NEAL, J., & RICHARDS, N. (1989). A review of desirable features of children's hearing aids. *Journal of Academy of Rehabilitative Audiology, 22*, 74–81.

WARREN, C., & HASENSTAB, S. (1986). Self-concept of severely to profoundly hearing-impaired children. *Volta Review, 88*, 289–295.

WILLIAMS, J. (1992). What do you know? What do you need to know? *Asha, 34*, 54–61.

APPENDIX 7–1
SAMPLE AUDIOGRAM

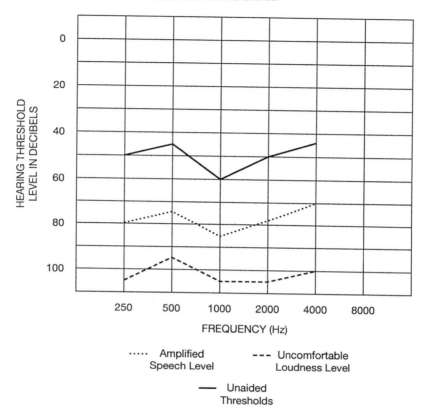

..... Amplified
Speech Level

- - - Uncomfortable
Loudness Level

—— Unaided
Thresholds

APPENDIX 7–2
AMPLIFICATION ADJUSTMENT CHECKLIST

	MON.	TUES.	WED.	THURS.	FRI.	SAT.	SUN.
Receptive Behaviors							
Awareness of environ-mental sound	____	____	____	____	____	____	____
Awareness of voice	____	____	____	____	____	____	____
Localization	____	____	____	____	____	____	____
Discrimination	____	____	____	____	____	____	____
Indentification	____	____	____	____	____	____	____
Expressive Behaviors							
Crying	____	____	____	____	____	____	____
Babbling	____	____	____	____	____	____	____
Acceptance of Aid							
Child	____	____	____	____	____	____	____
Parents	____	____	____	____	____	____	____
Special Problems							

Usage Summary

APPENDIX 7–3
DAILY HEARING AID CHECK

This procedure should be done each day before the hearing aid is put on the child at home and/or at school.

1. **Visually inspect the hearing aid**. Scan the aid visually for any obvious problems such as cracks in the case, earhook, tubing, transducer, or cord.

2. **Check the battery**. Remove the battery and test; replace if needed. Notice the battery contacts; they should be free of dust, dirt, and corrosion. Dust and dirt in and around the battery compartment can be removed with a typewriter brush. If you notice corrosion, rub the contacts gently with a cotton swab dipped in vinegar, ammonia, or baking soda. Remove excess moisture with a dry cotton swab.

3. **Inspect the earmold**. Make certain that the sound bore is free of wax and dirt. Any debris may be removed with a pipe cleaner. The earmold can be washed in warm water with a mild dishwashing liquid. Be sure to detach the earmold from the transducer on body aids and the earhook on ear-level aids before washing. Be sure the earmold is completely dry before putting it back in the ear; it is best to wash it in the evening so that it may dry completely overnight.

4. **Perform a feedback check**. Turn the aid on and the volume control to its full on position. Place your finger over the sound bore of the earmold; the feedback should stop. If it does not, disconnect the earmold and place your finger over the transducer on body aids or the earhook on ear-level aids. If the feedback stops, then there is sound leaking out from the tubing or earmold itself and one or the other will need to be replaced. If the feedback does not stop, there is a problem with the casing or the internal parts of the hearing aid. At this point, the aid will need to be professionally repaired.

5. **Listen to the hearing aid**. Connect the aid to a hearing aid stethoscope and gradually increase the volume to the recommended setting for the child. Check to see if the aid gets louder as the volume control is rotated. It will never be linear, but there should be no "dead spots" as the volume is increased. For body aids, take the cord between your thumb and index finger and run your fingers down the cord. Wiggle the cord at both ends and listen for breaks in the sound. If the sound is intermittant at any point during this check, the cord will need to be replaced.

6. **Say the Ling 5 sounds**. With the stethoscope attached, say the following sounds slowly and at approximately the same intensity:

   /a/ as in f*a*ther
   /i/ as in f*ee*t
   /u/ as in f*oo*d
   /sh/ as in *sh*oe
   /s/ as in *s*o

   It will be necessary to subjectively determine if any of these sound distorted to you. After a short time, you will begin to feel comfortable with how the aid should sound and you will notice distortion if it occurs. Remember that each hearing aid will sound differently, so it becomes important to be very familiar with your child's hearing aids.

APPENDIX 7–4
CHILDREN'S LITERATURE DEALING WITH HEARING LOSS

Preschool and Elementary

A Button in Her Ear (1976) by Ada Litchfield
Albert Whitman & Company, Niles, IL

Anna's Silent World (1977) by Bernard Wolf
J.B. Lippincott Company, Philadelphia

Claire and Emma (1976) by Diana Peter
John Day Company, New York

Ear Gear (1986) by Carole B. Simko
Gallaudet University Press, Washington, DC

Hearing Aids for You and the Zoo (1984) by Richard Stoker and Janine Gaydos
Alexander Graham Bell Association for the Deaf
3417 Volta Place, NW
Washington, DC 20007-2778
(202) 337-5220 (TDD/Voice)

Lisa and Her Soundless World (1984) by Edna Levine
Human Sciences Press, New York

My Friend Leslie: The Story of a Handicapped Child (1983) by Maxine Rosenberg
Lothrop, Lee and Shepard Books, New York

Now I Understand (1986) by Gregory S. LaMore
Gallaudet University Press, Washington, DC

Tim and His Hearing Aid (1975) by Ronnie, Eleanor & Jean Porter
Alexander Graham Bell Association for the Deaf
3417 Volta Place, NW
Washington, DC 20007-2778
(202) 337-5220 (TDD/Voice)

We Can! (1980) by Robin R. Star
Alexander Graham Bell Association for the Deaf
3417 Volta Place, NW
Washington, DC 20007-2778
(202) 377-5220 (TDD/Voice)

Adolescents

Chelsea: The Story of a Signal Dog (1992) by Paul Ogden
Time Warner Co., Boston

How the Student with Hearing Loss Can Succeed in College: A Handbook for Students, Families and Professionals (1990) by Carol Flexer, Denise Wray, and Ron Leavitt
Alexander Graham Bell Association for the Deaf
3417 Volta Place, NW
Washington, DC 20007-2778
(202) 377-5220 (TDD/Voice)

Silent Night (1990) by Sue Thomas and S. Rickley Christian
Alexander Graham Bell Association for the Deaf
3417 Volta Place, NW
Washington, DC 20007-2778
(202) 377-5220 (TDD/Voice)

What's That Pig Outdoors? A Memoir of Deafness (1991) by Henry Kisor
Alexander Graham Bell Association for the Deaf
3417 Volta Place, NW
Washington, DC 20007-2778
(202) 377-5220 (TDD/Voice)

APPENDIX 7–5
PRODUCTS TO USE WITH HEARING AIDS

Super Seals, available from many hearing aid accessory suppliers

Dri-Aid Packages, available from many hearing aid accessory suppliers

Huggies, available from Huggie Aids TM
837 NW 10th Street
Oklahoma City, OK 73106, (405) 232-7848

RESOURCES TO USE WITH FAMILIES

A Difference in the Family, Living with a Disabled Child (1981) by Helen Featherstone
Penguin Books, New York

A Hug Just Isn't Enough (1980) by Caren Ferris
Gallaudet University Press, Washington, DC

Amy: The Story of a Deaf Child (1985) by Lou Ann Walker
Lodestar Books, E. P. Dutton, New York

Broken Ears, Wounded Hearts (1983) by George Harris
Gallaudet University Press, Washington, DC

The Deaf Can Speak (1985) by Pauline Shaw
Alexander Graham Bell Association for the Deaf
3417 Volta Place, NW
Washington, DC 20007-2778
(202) 377-5220 (TDD/Voice)

Deaf Like Me (1978) by T. Spradley and J. Spradley
Random House, New York

Deafness in the Family (1987) by David Luterman
College Hill Press, Boston

Family to Family (1980) by Betty Griffin
Alexander Graham Bell Association for the Deaf
3417 Volta Place, NW
Washington, DC 20007-2778
(202) 377-5220 (TDD/Voice)

Growing Together (1991) National Information Center on Deafness
Gallaudet University Press
800 Florida Avenue, NE
Washington, DC 20002

Hearing Aids: A User's Guide (1991) by Wayne Staab
512 East Canterbury Lane
Phoenix, AZ 85022

Hearing Aids: Who Needs Them? (1991) by David Pascoe
Big Bend Books, St. Louis, MO

Hearing Impaired Children—A Guide for Concerned Parents and Professionals (1988) by
Richard C. Bevan
Charles C Thomas, Springfield, IL

How to Get the Most Out of Your Hearing Aid (1981) by Joan Armbruster and Maurice
Miller
Alexander Graham Bell Association for the Deaf
3417 Volta Place, NW
Washington, DC 20007-2778
(202) 377-5220 (TDD/Voice)

Language Says it All (video) (1991)
Tripod Grapevine
2901 North Keystone Street
Burbank, CA 91504

Learning to Listen: A Book by Mothers for Mothers of Hearing-Impaired Children (1981)
by Pat Vaughn
Alexander Graham Bell Association for the Deaf
3417 Volta Place, NW
Washington, DC 20007-2778
(202) 377-5220 (TDD/Voice)

Legal Rights of Persons with Disabilities: An Analysis of Federal Law (1990)
(Supplement, 1992) by Bonnie Tucker and Bruce Goldstein
Alexander Graham Bell Association for the Deaf
3417 Volta Place, NW
Washington, DC 20007-2778
(202) 377-5220 (TDD/Voice)

Once Upon a Time (video) (1991)
Tripod Grapevine
2901 North Keystone Street
Burbank, CA 91504

Negotiating the Special Education Maze: A Guide for Parents and Teachers (1990) by
Winifred Anderson, Stephen Chitwood, and Deidre Hayden
Alexander Graham Bell Association for the Deaf
3417 Volta Place, NW
Washington, DC 20007-2778
(202) 377-5220 (TDD/Voice)

*94-142 and 504: Numbers That Add Up to Educational Rights for Handicapped Children:
A Guide for Parents and Advocates* (1989) by Daniel Yohalem and Janet Dinsmore
Childrens Defense Fund
122 C Street, NW
Washington, DC 20001-2193

Parents in Action: A Handbook for Experiences with Their Hearing-Impaired Children
(1978) by Grant B. Bitter
Alexander Graham Bell Association for the Deaf
3417 Volta Place, NW
Washington, DC 20007-2778
(202) 377-5220 (TDD/Voice)

Parents' Guide to Speech and Deafness (1984) by Donald R. Calvert, Ph. D.
Alexander Graham Bell Association for the Deaf
3417 Volta Place, NW
Washington, DC 20007-2778
(202) 377-5220 (TDD/Voice)

Raising Your Hearing-Impaired Child: A Guideline for Parents (1982) by Shirley
McArthur
Alexander Graham Bell Association for the Deaf
3417 Volta Place, NW
Washington, DC 20007-2778
(202) 377-5220 (TDD/Voice)

Talk With Me (1988) by Ellyn Altman
Alexander Graham Bell Association for the Deaf
3417 Volta Place, NW
Washington, DC 20007-2778
(202) 377-5220 (TDD/Voice)

When Your Child Is Deaf: A Guide for Parents (1991) by David M. Luterman and Mark Ross
Alexander Graham Bell Association for the Deaf
3417 Volta Place, NW
Washington, DC 20007-2778
(202) 377-5220 (TDD/Voice)

APPENDIX 7–6
CHART FOR HEARING AID MONITORING

	MON.	TUES.	WED.	THURS.	FRI.	SAT.	SUN.
Visual Inspection							
Case and earhook	____	____	____	____	____	____	____
Earmold and tubing	____	____	____	____	____	____	____
Earphone and cord	____	____	____	____	____	____	____
Battery Check							
Contacts	____	____	____	____	____	____	____
Voltage	____	____	____	____	____	____	____
Feedback Check	____	____	____	____	____	____	____
Listening Check							
Loudness	____	____	____	____	____	____	____
Consistency	____	____	____	____	____	____	____
Ling 5 sound	____	____	____	____	____	____	____

chapter eight

Educational Consultation: Talking with Parents and School Personnel

Cheryl DeConde Johnson

As stressed by Dr. Johnson, there is a need for audiologists to abandon their individual prejudices as they help parents to make wise educational decisions for themselves and their children. Her empathic approach to this task can greatly help parents, first, to understand, and then, to advocate for the educational needs of their children. In this chapter, Dr. Johnson also discusses ways for noneducational audiologists to interact effectively with education professionals as advocates for children with hearing loss.

> . . . things cannot be expected to turn up of themselves. We must, in a measure, assist them to turn up.
>
> Charles Dickens
> *David Copperfield*

INTRODUCTION

This is an appealing chapter for me to write, as I have perspectives both as a professional and as a parent (personal connections seem common in our field). As a mother, I felt little respect from the medical and audiological personnel I had to deal with and as a result sought information on my own, eventually leading to my degree in audiology. Accurate diagnosis of my daughter's hearing impairment took 3½ years after raising the question with my pediatrician when she was 1 year old. I continue to hear similar sagas today, 20 plus years later. In this chapter I hope to share what I have learned about communication between parents and professionals through many years of both parental and professional experiences.

Effective communication is most critical to the counseling process. We all know that the best professional expertise or advise can be wasted if presented poorly. Communication skills are much harder to teach than content and technical skills, yet preprofessional course work in many degree programs rarely offers training in this area. Some individuals have naturally good communication skills, while others do not. Those who do not achieve good communication skills must themselves be counseled out of the interactive part of audiology.

Effective counseling with parents demands the provision of accurate information, honoring the opinions of those involved, and achieving credibility within the local professional community. This chapter includes critical information on federal laws and their audiological implications within the educational arena, suggestions for working with educational audiologists and other school personnel, and ideas for working with parents so that a strong and supportive network among the audiologist, the school, and the family can be established and maintained.

UNDERSTANDING THE SCHOOLS' ROLE IN PROVIDING AUDIOLOGY SERVICES

Audiology services in public schools have been slowly evolving since the mid-1960s. However, special public and private residential and day schools for the deaf have included audiology as a part of their programs since much earlier. Even though audiology flourished as a result of a need to rehabilitate servicemen who lost or damaged their hearing during combat, the medical alliance of audiology has often created a perception of a profession that carries more of a medical than rehabilitative connotation. The rubella epidemic of the 1960s probably drove the need for audiology and hearing services within local school systems more than any other factor. The numbers of children with significant hearing impairment grew quickly and dramatically at that time. With the desire to educate those children within local school systems, programs for children with hearing impairment sprung up in cities with concentrated populations. As programs developed, the need for audiology was apparent, just as it had been in residential and special day schools.

Federal Legislation

Momentum for educational audiology (the term used to describe the focus of audiology as practiced in the school setting) was spurred with the passage of the Education for All Handicapped Children Act (P.L. 94-142) in 1975. The Rules and Regulations for Implementation of the Act specifically detailed the responsibility of public education with regard to audiology services. The stage for this legislation was set by earlier laws that authorized grants to state agencies to educate children with disabilities in state-operated or supported schools and institutions (P.L. 89-313, 1965) and subsequently at the local school level (P.L. 89-750, 1966). The Bureau of Education of the Handicapped was also established in the 1966 law and charged with administering all U.S. Office of Education programs for children and youth with disabilities. Centers and services for deaf-blind children were established through 1968 legislation (P.L. 90-247) in order to further supplement and support specific services to this population. Section 504 of the Rehabilitation Act of 1973 prohibited discrimination of individuals with disabilities, particularly with respect to accessibility in public facilities. For deaf and hard-of-hearing children in the schools this possessed implications for access to information and warnings presented auditorily (fire alarms, verbal communication, etc.).

Even as the children who contracted rubella were getting older, other early childhood disorders and problems began to attract additional attention. With more children surviving high-risk births due to medical advancements, the characteristics of the population of children with hearing impairment have changed. Diagnosis has often been comprised of more than one problem, which individually may be less severe but collectivly affect a greater multitude of abilities. Due to the complex nature of many of these disorders, communication efforts among agencies and individuals involved has become critical.

Under pressure to enact early intervention legislation to improve services for infants, toddlers, and preschool children, the Education of the Handicapped Act Amendments (P.L. 99-457) was passed in 1986. This law extended services to children with disabilities down to age 3 as identified in P.L. 94-142 as well as offered incentives and guidelines for services from birth through 2 years (Part H). Part H, the infant and toddler program of P.L. 99-457, included the charge to develop and implement "comprehensive," "coordinated," "multidisciplinary," "interagency" services commencing in programs that are family centered (rather than child centered as defined in P.L. 94-142) and driven by an Individual Family Service Plan as compared to an Individualized Education Program (IEP). Infants and toddlers with identifiable handicaps or delays, or children at risk for significant delays are eligible for services. Early intervention services may include audiometric testing, case management, family training/counseling/home visits, certain health and medical services, nutrition, occupational therapy, physical therapy, psychology, social work, special instruction, speech-language pathology, and transportation.

The law also defined "qualified personnel" as persons who meet the highest requirements in the state for that profession or discipline. Further legal clarification came with the passage of additional amendments in 1990. P.L. 101-497, the Education of the Handicapped Act Amendments, changed the title to Individuals with Disabilities Education Act (now referred to as IDEA) and all references to "handicapped children" were changed to "children with disabilities."

Audiological Implications

The result of all of this legislation as it relates to hearing impairment is that every school system must have a process to "seek out and identify" (called Child Find in most states) children, birth through age 21, who may be hearing impaired. Suspected children are entitled to a hearing screening and subsequent audiological evaluation at no charge to the family. Public schools must ensure access to or provide this evaluation as well as an individual, multidisciplinary assessment if the child is found to have a significant hearing impairment. For children who are age 3 or older, with documented hearing impairment, schools must additionally provide free and appropriate services as defined by the IEP. State education agencies have developed regulations and plans that drive these services in individual school districts that are approved by the federal government; states must monitor the schools to ensure that the intent of the federal and state laws are met. For Part H of P.L. 99-457, individual states may determine who will be the lead public agency for directing these efforts. Part H also requires an implementation and monitoring plan. The federal government provides funds to each state to supplement the cost of these programs and services. If, through the monitoring process, schools are found to violate the established state regulations, funds may be withheld until the school system has corrected the compliance issue.

What then is the specific impact of this legislation for audiology? The regulations of P.L. 94-142 [34 CFR 300.13(b)(1)] mandated that schools provide access to a full range of audiological services at no charge to families. It is essential that every audiologist involved with children know the public schools' precise responsibilities regarding audiology. Those mandatory services are:

1. Identification of children with hearing loss
2. Determination of the range, nature, and degree of hearing loss, including referral for medical or other professional attention for the habilitation of hearing
3. Provision of habilitative activities, such as language habilitation, auditory training, speech reading (lip reading), hearing evaluation, and speech conservation
4. Creation and administration of programs for prevention of hearing loss
5. Counseling and guidance of pupils, parents, and teachers regarding hearing loss
6. Determination of the child's need for group and individual amplification, selecting and fitting an appropriate aid, and evaluating the effectiveness of amplification

These same regulations (34 CFR 300.303) also state that: "Each public agency shall ensure that the hearing aids worn by deaf and hard of hearing children in school are functioning properly."

Several states have developed specific guidelines for how they provide audiology services according to the federal definition. Unfortunately, a survey that I conducted for the Educational Audiology Association found that there is a great deal of variability among states in the interpretation of the law (DeConde-Johnson, 1991). Some states in fact still do not recognize their need to provide audiological assessment. This has raised significant concern among educational audiologists across the United States, and as a result the American Speech-Language-Hearing Association (ASHA) agreed to update its "Audiology Services in the Schools" position paper of 1983 to reflect current interpretation and to provide guidelines for state education agencies in developing audiology programs in the schools. Specific responsibilities of the educational audiologist as suggested by ASHA (1992) are outlined in Appendix 8–1. Most important to recognize is the complex nature of the assessment and management of children with hearing impairment in the schools, which commands that professionals work together as a team with families if the outcome is to be productive.

There appears to still be significant concern among audiologists in private practice and in speech and hearing clinics that schools will take over the pediatric population limiting their ability to provide clinical services. The opposite has occurred; increased identification programs have increased referrals for treatment and hearing aid fittings. Audiologists outside the school environment can develop a complementary working relationship with the educational audiologist by supporting the school efforts through consistent communication, taking time to understand the schools' process, and providing good care to the child and family. In fact, clinical audiologists' efforts will be enhanced by the schools' support in the hearing aid fitting process, orientation to the use of the hearing aids, and monitoring of hearing aid function. The habilitative activities of the school program should result in a more positive use of hearing aids by the child. The best care is achieved when all parties work together.

Current Educational Issues

It may be helpful for audiologists outside the school setting to be aware of some of the issues facing audiologists who work in the schools. I discuss these topics because parents will often ask a variety of professionals, including the audiologist, for their opinions, as they themselves are searching for information to understand their child's hearing problem.

Credibility.   Although not a parent issue, credibility is a concern that affects the services audiologists are trying to provide in the schools. Credibility is the biggest obstacle audiologists face, and it is shared across work environments within the profession. How do we market audiology so that it becomes a routine, integral part of health care, and, for children, education care? Funding shortages have made it even more difficult to advance the critical importance of hearing disorders because of the priority taken by other, more life-threatening conditions.

In the schools, the audiologists' position and responsibility may be undermined by administrators who neither recognize nor understand the importance hearing plays in the learning process. As audiologists, we must focus on this critical role of hearing as well as the impact of hearing impairment. Administrators recognize the implications of deafness; however, when a child can speak and communicate orally, the associated learning problems are more difficult to justify. Educational services are usually available in the schools, while audiological services may not be. Yet without adequate identification programs, many children are not receiving the services they may be entitled to.

Certainly the first of the National Education Goals, that "By the year 2000 all children in America will start school ready to learn," has enormous implications for children with hearing impairment. Without adequate hearing, language does not develop normally; without adequate language skills, children cannot learn like their typical hearing peers. We must capitalize on the education reform movement to advance the understanding of the critical role hearing plays in learning, and hence the importance of audiology in education.

Accessibility. "Acoustic accessibility" is very often overlooked with regard to handicapped children. Physical barriers to children's mobility are obvious; barriers caused by hearing problems, inattention, and poor acoustics are invisible. Educational audiologists are working to help administrators and teachers understand the implications of high-background noise levels, poor classroom acoustics, and weak teachers' voices for hearing and learning. These problems can even affect hearing children's accessibility to information. For hearing children who have language and learning problems, acoustic variables should also be considered.

When children with compromised hearing and language abilities are integrated into regular classrooms, noise levels and distance from the teacher neccessitate modifications of the classroom structure and environment. The high incidence of otitis media and resulting fluctuating hearing levels in the preschool and primary years, and in children with other handicaps, adds to the acoustic accessibility problem. Amplification options such as classroom and personal frequency-modulated (FM) systems can provide significant improvement for the hearing and learning of hearing-impaired as well as non-hearing-handicapped children. Even for children with attention and processing problems who are not handicapped (re P.L. 94-142), these devices may be required to meet accessibility regulations as determined by Section 504 of the Rehabilitation Act of 1973.

Inclusion and mainstreaming. Mainstreaming is a now familiar term that has been used to describe the process by which students with a disability join the regular classroom for a selected portion of their school day. Mainstreaming may occur for academic and/or social reasons and usually implies that the student is managed more by special education than regular education.

Inclusion means that students with disabilities are members of the regular classroom with all of the same opportunities for participation as their typical peers. Adaptations are made and support provided within the regular classroom whenever possible to maintain the student in that setting. Specialized instruction is provided in another environment only when the student cannot benefit from instruction in the regular classroom. Through inclusion the student is part of the regular classroom and leaves only when absolutely necessary to receive support services, while through mainstreaming the student often starts each day in the special classroom and is then integrated with the regular classroom when it is beneficial. I address this issue because the inclusion movement is powerful. It was primarily promoted for children with mental, physical, emotional, and learning disabilities who had traditionally been educated separately from their nondisabled peers.

The inclusion philosophy is often not appropriate for children who are deaf. For these students, the regular classroom environment may be more restrictive than a special classroom due to communication barriers, regardless of the communication mode. For children whose primary communication mode is manual, there are usually so few signing peers that information is obtained primarily through an interpreter, which is hardly a normal communication situation. For students who use oral/aural communication, the rate with which information is presented in the regular classroom usually far exceeds their ability to understand, process, and respond accurately. The appropriateness of the social and learning environment must be considered when placement is determined for deaf and hard-of-hearing students. When parents ask the audiologist if their child will be successful in a regular school, we must help them understand how complex the issue is and to see the potential problems and barriers that hearing impairment can create.

American Sign Language versus manually coded English. We have another controversy within education of the deaf regarding the language/culture issue. American Sign Language (ASL) is one language, and manually coded English is another language. Which system should be taught as the child's first language? Many thoughts abound on both sides with no clear answer except for deaf children of deaf parents where the language of the parents, usually ASL, should naturally be the child's first language. Unless some intense interest has been taken in this area, I would recommend deferring to specialists in education of the deaf when parents ask this question.

Services to the nondisabled student. Although audiology services in the schools are funded with federal and state monies earmarked for special education, programs for prevention of hearing loss open the door to support "hearing" in a more general sense. Certainly all audiologists could market the importance of hearing, but within education our job is even more crucial due to the auditory-verbal structure of the classroom.

The assistive listening devices that are now available have the potential to provide assistance to a variety of students with auditory and attention impairments that may not be significant enough to handicap the child auditorily but that do create an accessibility issue under Section 504. The audiologist must be a promoter of the use of this technology when it is appropriate for a student. Appropriateness must be determined by a reasonable trial period with the device (that goes beyond the novelty stage) and careful documentation of improved listening performance. If an accessibility problem is determined, the student's school may be responsible for providing the listening device. Classroom FM amplification systems have been found to benefit all students in the classroom. The implications for audiologists in promoting these devices and for the children using them are exciting: There are fewer parts to break down, children do not have to wear a device that makes them appear different, and every student in the room benefits. However, the audiologist must work with the schools to establish the cost-effectiveness of these devices in terms of student outcomes.

CONNECTING WITH THE SCHOOLS

The Audiologist

It should be obvious by now how important it is for the clinical and school audiologists to work together. Some specific situations of how this collaboration might work are examined below.

Audiological assessment. Routine clinical evaluation establishes an audiological diagnosis. When a parent, school nurse, or teacher receives an audiogram and accompanying report (often only an audiogram is provided) that only states the audiometric findings (e.g., a moderately sloping high-frequency sensorineural hearing impairment bilaterally), the implications of that hearing impairment for the child for a variety of instructional and listening situations is unknown. Our recommendations usually include a statement regarding amplification, perhaps preferential seating (although without clear guidelines), and when to return for follow-up.

Missing from audiological reports are the specific implications in functional terms, such as the student may not hear some of the consonant sounds like /s/ and /f/, or may have difficulty hearing when background noise is present, or may experience fatigue and attention problems due to the extra concentration required for listening. Also missing are recommendations such as maintaining proximity and visual contact with the student or checking for understanding of information presented. Unfortunately, I find this situation is more the rule than the exception. It is particularly a problem in rural school districts, where there is limited, if any, access to an educational audiologist. Special education directors rarely have the knowledge of audiology to evaluate the appropriateness of the assessments they are paying for. They are usually satisfied that they are meeting the spirit of the law by just paying to have the testing completed. I feel the schools are being short-changed by being given assessments that are not meaningfully interpreted for the teacher and school staff. Appendix 8–2 contains a list of suggestions from which appropriate implications and recommendations may be determined for a particular student depending upon the hearing impairment. It is helpful to individualize recommendations as much as possible within the report that can then be supplemented by a handout containing more general suggestions (see Appendix 8–3).

Assessment of hearing ability when hearing impairment is present must also include information regarding the impact of noise, distance from the speaker, and visual cues on comprehension of auditory stimuli. Ying (1990) has suggested a Functional Listening Paradigm, in which skills are assessed in a classroom to replicate a more typical listening situation. As an example, a phonetically balanced (PB) word recognition list is presented via live voice in eight different modes: close/ quiet, close/noise, distance/quiet, and distance/noise for auditory input only and repeated with the addition of speech reading. Audiologists should make more attempts such as this to obtain data that are more reflective of the situations that the listener experiences.

Auditory skill development should also be evaluated for children with significant hearing impairment. The Test of Auditory Comprehension (Trammell et al., 1976) is a good measure that is normed for a variety of hearing levels. Sound booth assessment needs to include speech in noise measures (usually at 50 or 55 dB HL at +5 dB S/N in sound field) when a functional paradigm such as suggested above is not used. For students who wear hearing aids, the measures should also be done in aided conditions. Justification for the need and value of FM amplification can also be determined from evaluations such as these.

Another concern I have with the assessment process is the lack, or poor level, of sign skills among audiologists. Those in the business to help the hearing impaired need to make their services accessible by learning sign or hiring an interpreter. Explanation of results, discussion of hearing, and other counseling interactions can be severely hampered when communication is belabored and tedious. Many individuals who are deaf do not like audiologists because they think they are always trying to "fix" their hearing. They may be correct, and it is probably because some audiologists' intentions were poorly communicated. Audiologists need to get off to a positive beginning with deaf children by talking with them about their feelings of deafness, offer options, and respect their opinions and decisions.

Suggestions

1. Work with educational audiologists to establish what their assessment protocols include; determine which tests might be done outside the school and which through the school.
2. Children with hearing impairment are assessed at least annually in the schools. Consider the child's time and the audiologist's time; it might be better for all hearing assessment (after initial diagnosis) to be done through the school to avoid duplication.
3. Establish a process to share results so that both the school and the clinic sites have current information.
4. When the clinical audiologist is conducting the assessment for the school, provide as much functional information as possible; always include a written report with the audiogram.
5. Respect deafness; learn sign or hire an interpreter for deaf students.
6. Most importantly be professional and current on pediatric practices. If working with young children is not an area of expertise, seek assistance or refer to a pediatric audiologist. Do not try to muddle through; parents do not need incorrect or conflicting information.

Amplification. Personal amplification is usually selected and dispensed by the clinical audiologist. Although schools must ensure that the students' hearing aids are functioning properly, schools do not pay for repairs or earmolds except in special circumstances where that may be the only amplification available to the child. Hearing aids must be selected so that they are compatible with FM systems and should routinely include direct audio input.

Colored hearing aids and earmolds are very popular with children, yet most audiologists do not even offer them as an option. Interestingly, the parents' level of acceptance of their child's hearing impairment may be reflected in their color choice for the hearing instrument (DeConde, 1984).

I remember a situation where I asked a dispenser to order a child's hearing aids in orange; he thought I was referring to a code for the tone or output and could not believe that I would think of putting orange hearing aids on a child. I have even had children choose the colors of their favorite professional football team. I always show children the colors available and let them choose, rather than the parents (unless the child is too young).

Color choice gives children some ownership in the selection of their aids and earmolds and can enhance the overall attitude and acceptance of the aids. Other advantages of colored hearing aids include greater ease of locating instruments when dropped or lost and greater ease in distinguishing one student's hearing instruments from another.

FM amplification for school should be routine for nearly every child with hearing impairment. I even recommend FM systems for use in the home with many toddlers. Although some problems arise with the wearability of some of the instruments on young children, I think it is because we have been spoiled with ear-level aids. To add a body-style arrangement now seems cumbersome. The advantages of the FM signal are well established, leaving cost as the primary factor limiting more widespread use, whether at home or at school. When considering an FM system for home it is important to evaluate the parents' motivation to use it, the potential benefit to children based on their hearing and developmental ability, the structure and noise levels of the home environment for communication, and the financial resources available. If the child is in a day-care or preschool setting, the FM system might be even more necessary. As with any amplification, a strong habilitation program must accompany the fitting; amplification is of little value if the child does not learn how to use the input that is received. We all need to strongly advocate for FM use, at least during school.

Classroom amplification systems are also becoming more widely used. They are particularly beneficial for minimal or mild impairments where hearing aids may not be appropriate, or where students refuse FM systems. Care should be taken so that the significance of the hearing impairment and need for hearing aids or personal FMs are not minimized by suggesting this arrangement. While classroom amplification is appropriate to suggest as an option, it is critical to know the schools' position, criteria for use, and availability of this type of system before providing the information to parents.

Suggestions

1. Always check with the educational audiologist or whoever is responsible for FM systems to see what type of systems are used in order to properly interface the FM system and hearing aid.
2. Work with the educational audiologist to coordinate hearing aid orientation and habilitation efforts. A particularly effective method is to invite the educational audiologist to join a session with the parents and child during the hearing aid fitting process.
3. Always order hearing aids for children with direct audio input.
4. Advocate colors.
5. Routinely discuss FM systems with parents, recommending their use, when appropriate, to parents and to the school.
6. Consider FM amplification for the home environment.
7. For children, birth through age 2, establish contacts with local early intervention programs to coordinate habilitation efforts.
8. Know the school's position regarding classroom amplification.

Central auditory processing disorders.   Assessment of central auditory processing function in children is controversial among audiologists. The issues of reliability and validity must be considered when conducting an assessment and interpreting results. Rather than to get into a discussion of what a central auditory processing disorder (CAPD) is, how to assess it, and how to treat it, I would like to emphasize that in most situations for children it is more of an educational issue than a medical one. Therefore, the problem should be dealt with in the context of the school environment or as part of a comprehensive educational assessment rather than in the isolation of a clinical audiology practice. I think that school audiologists have a responsibility to at least consider a CAPD and have a process for dealing with it.

Suggestions

1. If parents request CAPD testing, encourage them to take their concern to their child's teacher and school and contact the school audiologist.
2. If there is no school audiologist, discuss with the special education team at the school or for the school district how you can best interface with their assessment plan. Be prepared to be involved in a staffing, or meeting with the child's parents, possibly the child, and the educational team at the child's school to describe implications and to integrate the results into the child's overall functioning profile. Be prepared to make recommendations that are functional for the child and to give guidance to the school for implementation. Be prepared to reevaluate the status of the child's CAPD skills at 3-year intervals or sooner if considered appropriate by the educational team.

Other School Professionals

Myriad personnel and services in the schools have evolved to complement and support teachers, and some were also mandated with P.L. 94-142. Each offers a unique perspective to the complex nature of children with and without handicaps. The ability to conduct a multidisciplinary and multifaceted assessment within the education setting promotes the consideration of all aspects of a child's development to determine how the problem affects the whole child rather than an isolated function. For children with hearing impairment, I find the outcome of such an assessment results in the development of plans and goals that address not only academics, hearing, and speech and language development, but also cognitive ability, learning style, social-emotional function, health concerns, and family, cultural, and environmental issues. Often hearing impairment is present with other problems that affect development and learning. Regardless of the concomitant conditions, appropriate services can only be determined once the interaction of all of these variables is analyzed. For most audiologists in clinical settings, the opportunities to be involved with this type of process are limited. Attendance at preassessment meetings, postassessment debriefings, staffings, and review conferences are time-consuming, yet representative of the communication and planning process necessary to develop successful programming for children.

Typical team members of multidisciplinary assessments may include psychologists, counselors, social workers, speech-language pathologists, nurses, occupational and physical therapists, interpreter-tutors, teachers of the deaf and hard of hearing, special education teachers from the areas of learning disabilities, emotional disturbance, and vision, regular classroom teachers, school principals, and special education administrators. Decisions regarding which of these individuals might be involved in the assessment of a child are usually determined in a preassessment conference based on the available information about the child's situation and functioning levels. If this sounds a little intimidating or overwhelming, it can be, especially for parents. The support of the clinical audiologist can help alleviate some of the stress and fear for parents by providing accurate information and follow-through.

Suggestions

1. Know the referral and assessment process for the school system.
2. Try to meet as many of the school support personnel as possible so that a bridge is established for communication. If the school district has a center-based program for its students with hearing impairment, this effort is even more critical and will go a long way to establishing a respectful rapport with those individuals.
3. Never leave the educational audiologist out of the communication loop; that individual will be able to provide most of the necessary information as well as access to the other personnel.
4. Develop an array of services with the educational audiologist so that both audiologists have a defined role in providing services for the child.
5. Be respectful of educators' time. When included in meetings be prompt.
6. Be caring, and be willing to help with follow-through and management of recommendations made.
7. Try to be realistic with expectations (put yourself in the parents' or teacher's place).
8. Be a team player, and be careful not to leave an impression of superiority.

Professionals within the Community

In addition to school personnel, involvement with other community agencies is often necessary when working with children with hearing loss. The concept of interagency networking is popular because it is effective. These efforts reduce duplication of services as well as improve cooperation among agencies.

I diagnosed a mild sensorineural hearing impairment in a 3-year-old boy. His behavior was immature, noncompliant, and peculiar in a way I could not readily define, and I suspected some other developmental problem that typically would not be attributed to that degree of hearing impairment. However, the family had been questioning the cause of their child's behavior problems and the hearing impairment provided the concrete and treatable evidence that they could accept. My recommendations for further developmental evaluation were generally ignored, and the parents told their son's preschool teacher that I said he would be better now that he could hear with his new hearing aids. Through discussion and cooperation of the preschool teacher, we jointly continued to confront the parents with the need for further assessment until finally, when 9 months later the behavior issues had not subsided, the parents were willing to seek further evaluation. An organic-based, autistic-like disorder was diagnosed, and appropriate treatment was finally initiated.

Communication among professionals is essential and helps deter some of the manipulations that families can do with agencies.

Common agencies to consider when networking include community deaf services, vocational rehabilitation, mental health services, Social Security disability, and handicapped or crippled children's funding programs. Social service agencies might also be involved if documented or suspected neglect or abuse exists. I have made referrals to social services for medical neglect when families do not follow through on obtaining medical treatment recommendations. These referrals are not comfortable to make because it usually damages the client–audiologist relationship. One particularly memorable referral to social services that I made for medical neglect resulted in a bullet hole in my bedroom window that evening!

Programming for infants and toddlers usually involves services outside the school. Hospitals, speech and hearing centers, rehabilitation centers, and private speech-language pathologists are among the community service options that need to be considered, while also keeping the school district apprised of the status of the child. I have a particular bias in favor of home intervention programs that are family centered and operate under the philosophy that parents are the primary care provider and therefore should be taught the essential elements of effective communication to be used with their young children. Child-centered therapy is usually not as effective or appropriate at this age level.

Suggestions

1. Always work with the schools when making referrals to any outside agency. The problem or need may also be apparent to others and might have been addressed or dealt with in another manner. The additional support of school personnel might also result in more rapid action.

2. Choose the battles for referrals that might be construed as negative, carefully considering how it might jeopardize the relationship that has been established with the family.

3. Keep the school district informed of any infants and toddlers who have hearing impairment even if it is not having a perceivable impact on the child's development. It is helpful to have the school district conduct periodic speech and language screenings to ensure that development is on target.

WORKING WITH PARENTS

The parent–audiologist partnership is a trust relationship that is necessary for every successful habilitation process with children. Because hearing impairment sometimes is considered to be an uncommon disorder, parents are really at the mercy of the physician and audiologist for initial diagnostic and treatment information. Unfortunately, diagnosis is very often still delayed longer than necessary. Even with the use of auditory brainstem response and cortical-evoked potentials, it may be difficult to establish an accurate hearing diagnosis when other neurological impairments are present. And because of the controversial status of communication philosophies among educators of the deaf, parents can easily be confused and misled as to their habilitative options.

Parents, who are vulnerable as a result of the loss, feel frustration and often helplessness after being told that their child has an impairment. It is critical they be given accurate, straightforward guidance. They need and want professional advice so that they can make their own choices. If audiologists can help with case management and guide parents as they investigate their options, they will probably earn the respect and credibility needed to influence parents when changes need to be made in treatment and habilitation.

An ineffective audiologist can impair the process of helping children more than facilitate it. We must recognize our own strengths and weaknesses. If talking with parents about their child's hearing impairment is uncomfortable, the parent will probably sense the uneasiness, jeopardizing the parent–audiologist credibility that needs to be established. We cannot afford to gamble with this most critical time in the habilitation process. Sometimes the best advice to give parents is to refer them to an audiologist who is highly respected and who specializes in working with young children and their families. If one is unsure about the quality of services that is provided, feedback, using a questionnaire or written evaluation, may provide the audiologist with helpful information and suggestions.

Cooperation with families may also be dependent upon the parents' level of acceptance of their child's hearing status. As discussed by Dr. Van Hecke in Chapter 5, the grieving process is never really over but is rather a series of stages that change as the child grows. Each stage in a child's development represents a new loss, hence another grief. Parents often hear what they want to hear as a result of how they understand and accept their child's impairment.

In a recent review staffing, a mother with whom I have been involved for 15 years was blaming the school because her 18-year-old deaf son could not read. I remembered when the preschool teacher and I went to the home when the child was 3 years old and just diagnosed as deaf, to teach sign language to the mother. Although she had many opportunities over the years to improve her signing skills, she never went beyond the basic level of instruction she initially received. She communicates with her son by writing words on paper and doesn't understand the correlation between reading and exposure to language (sign language for this student). She also denied any responsibility in needing to provide support at home for his studies. The boy now holds a grudge against his mother because he has interpreted her lack of signing as not having enough desire to talk with him to want to learn to sign. And because she used to take him to a healer every summer, he still had held out hope for himself that his deafness might be cured.

This parent never accepted the deafness of her son. As a result she never heard what the school personnel told her every year about her son's progress and how that was affected by her inability to communicate with him. Unfortunately, at times we must recognize our limitations to change situations and be satisfied that we have done our best with the problem.

Parental support is absolutely the most critical component in the successful development of children with hearing impairments. Parenting classes to learn behavior management strategies, home intervention programs that educate family members and guide communication development, and family support groups to share experiences are common activities that may help encourage the positive growth of parental involvement.

Communicating with Parents

As a parent, I think the most important aspects of parent–audiologist rapport are credibility and empathy. Credibility is based on abilities such as providing quality assessments of pediatric patients, communicating and networking effectively within the community, and following through on what one says one will do. Empathy includes listening to and showing genuine interest in the concerns expressed by parents, being committed to assisting families, and trying to understand the situations that make a particular family unique.

Is it possible to be empathetic when a person has not shared the same experience? Of course. As discussed by Dr. Clark in Chapter 2, by practicing reflective listening, asking appropriate questions, and interacting in a nondomineering and nonjudgmental manner, it is possible to identify with the feelings, thoughts, and attitudes of parents. Knowing when to listen and knowing when to talk can be difficult. Effective communication is all part of the guidance process, which should occur naturally with parents throughout the diagnostic and habilitation stages of treatment. Realistically, there are times in clinical practices when scheduling constraints do not allow the time needed for this type of communication to be successful. Time issues need to be recognized so that appointments are scheduled when time is not a pressing issue and also when both parents (when there are two) are available to attend. The inclusion of grandparents, siblings, and other family and/or friends who are part of the support structure is also helpful. Home intervention programs are successful many times because the professional "joins" the family and becomes part of the support structure. This process allows the home interventionist to guide and advise the family in a way that is nonthreatening and, in the end, empowering. Audiologists who truly want to be a part of the habilitative process with children should try some home intervention techniques or refer families to a program that provides home intervention.

How much information should be given to parents? How often? Each parent has a different perspective and set of needs for each situation. We must be able to sense how much the parents need, and how often, by the questions they ask and the intensity of their concern, balanced with the urgency to begin treatment. Most parents recognize the need for immediate amplification, particularly if the child is over the age of 3 or 4 months. As age increases, the diagnosis usually confirms what the parents have suspected, so that relief is felt as much as despair.

For infants identified at birth, I feel it is certainly appropriate for the parents to have some time to bond with and enjoy their child before the hearing aid fitting is conducted. Often 1 to 2 months is sufficient for parents to come to acknowledge the need to get on with habilitation. During this time contacts should continue as often as parents would like; it might be every other week or once per month. I think it is helpful for parents to have access to the audiologist whenever they have questions, or at least to be told to jot questions down between office visits.

Once the hearing aid fitting has occurred, follow-up needs to be regularly scheduled either with the audiologist or coordinated with the home intervention or habilitation program. Written materials are extremely helpful to parents, parceled out over the diagnostic and hearing aid fitting period and continuing through habilitation. Reading materials need to be geared to the degree of hearing loss so that parents of a child who has a moderate hearing impairment are not reading about deafness, and vice versa.

For children with severe and profound hearing impairments, it is important to include materials about a variety of communication options, although parents should never be pressured to make decisions before they are ready. They must also understand that no decision ever has to be permanent. As the habilitative process continues it is very helpful for the parents to visit different programs and preschools to experience for themselves some of the options available to them that they have read about.

As discussed by Dr. Atkins in Chapter 6, it is also very helpful for parents to have an opportunity to meet other parents who have been through similar circumstances with their own child. Matching experienced parents with parents of newly identified children can be facilitated through the educational audiologist. We must provide parents with the information for them to make an informed decision about the habilitative option they want for their child; we cannot and should never make that decision for the parents.

Suggestions

1. Explain to parents how we hear and include a diagram of the ear.
2. Give parents an audiogram interpretation (frequency and intensity) with the child's loss graphed on an audiogram that shows various speech and nonspeech sounds.
3. Show parents how hearing aids operate; give realistic expectations of amplification; every parent should have a stethoscope and be taught to do daily listening checks (include written instructions for how to check and what to listen for).
4. Establish for parents a hearing aid orientation program including charts for recording when hearing aids are worn until full-time usage is established.
5. Use recorded simulation of various degrees of hearing impairment to build parental appreciation of hearing impairment.
6. Give parents a list of resources within the community and state that provide support and financial assistance to families of children with disabilities, specifically hearing impairment.
7. Give parents a reading and resource list of materials that can be mail-ordered, including articles and books written by other parents about experiences with their children and hearing impairment. (*Parent–Infant Communication* [Infant Hearing Resource, 1985], the *Parent Resource Catalogue* [House Ear Institute, 1992], and the Gallaudet University Press catalogue are excellent resources.)
8. Educate parents about normal speech and language development and potential effects of hearing impairment.

What about noncompliant or dysfunctional families? Obviously not all families we work with are willing and able to follow through on the recommendations that are necessary for the child. In fact, I find that nearly half of the families I am involved with have significant financial, cultural, or priority differences that make diagnosis and treatment a real challenge. These situations particularly benefit from the community interagency structure that should be in place to support families and children. When working together, it is possible to arrange transportation and to have someone accompany the family or mother and child to the audiologist for testing, to the physician for treatment, or to the hospital for surgery. I do not recommend transporting children without a parent present. However, if a parent is unwilling to follow through, social service involvement is necessary.

For children under age 3, habilitation efforts in the home are probably the most fruitful, since the high incidence of missed appointments tends to create a problem for many clinics. However, in spite of not having transportation to get to appointments, it is amazing how often some people are away from home at the scheduled visit with the home intervention specialist. Some families test the professional's patience, yet they know the children have a right to services and deserve the same opportunities as other children; it is no fault of the children that their parents' priorities are elsewhere.

For children over age 3 early childhood programs in the schools should provide transportation to preschool or other appropriate services. In these cases, it is probably most efficient for the educational audiologist to provide the majority of hearing evaluations, hearing aid monitoring, and habilitation services, since these can be conducted while the child is at school. One of the biggest difficulties with these children is consistent hearing aid use outside and in school.

When and how do audiologists convince parents to change what they are doing when it is not working for the child? When the audiologist is an integral member of the treatment team and/or has the confidence of the family, the recommendation for trying different methods or therapies can occur rather naturally as parents raise questions or discuss current progress and concerns. For audiologists not directly involved, it may be better to approach the habilitation specialists to address these concerns.

Treatment changes should be considered when progress has plateaued or been limited. Careful and consistent monitoring of vocabulary and language abilities and behavior is necessary to make these decisions of change and should occur every 6 months during the child's preschool years. Habilitative changes may include the addition of an FM system to improve the speech signal, more opportunities for language activities between the child and peers or parents, and assistance for the parents in how to structure language activities to facilitate growth.

The addition of signs may be necessary to accelerate language growth. One must be cautious, however, when discussing sign language. Manual communication should never be presented as a method that is used when oral/aural communication has failed. When failure is implied, this often generates more feelings of guilt.

Sign language should be presented as another communication system, without judgment, but with respect to what is realistically suited to a child's hearing ability and learning style. This chapter is not the place for a discussion of the pros and cons of communication methodology, but I do need to say that this is one area I feel we have really created a guilt issue for parents. Audiologists have to be realistic with parents, sharing the limitations of hearing aids, particularly for profound hearing impairments. Significant aided gain does not equate with adequate amplification for the development of language and speech through the auditory channel for most children. I think it is appropriate to discuss primary communication channels as part of the habilitation process. But only after considerable time and opportunities for the child to develop audition skills might it be possible to project whether the child will be likely to use hearing to augment manual communication, or use manual communication to augment oral/aural communication or use them equally. Even then, it is still possible that skills will change. Certainly technological advances in cochlear implants, hearing aid technology, and visible speech therapy tools will facilitate the development of speech for some deaf children.

What Should Parents Know about School Services?

This text has addressed the importance of knowing when and how much information to provide parents at different stages of the diagnosis and treatment process. The main rule of thumb I use is to always provide some materials (written for and often by, parents) that are appropriate to the given degree of hearing impairment. If a school discussion has not come up sooner, it is necessary to begin talking about available school services by the time the child is 2 years old. These discussions may occur over a period of time as parents bring up questions, or time may be scheduled specifically to address school programs. Each family situation must be considered when deciding how to provide information, just as education programs are adapted to each child's needs. It is obviously important to get parents connected with the education system if the situation warrants long-term involvement with special education. At this point the audiologist should decide if a joint meeting with the educational audiologist and the parents (if it has not already occurred) would best facilitate the presentation of information or if the audiologist possesses enough information to get the parents started. The process that results in the smoothest transition for the parents and child between the various phases of treatment should be chosen.

Within this process parents need to understand the following:

1. General parental rights according to state and federal laws, including the services that the school can and legally should provide (this may mean the family will choose to have the school provide their child's audiological services other than hearing aid repairs) emphasizing
   a. that decisions about education and therapy are never final so that at any time parents may ask for a meeting with all school personnel involved with their child to discuss concerns or progress
   b. that services must reflect the individual and unique needs of each child because there is no one correct way to educate children with hearing impairment
   c. the amplification responsibilities of schools
2. The importance of structure and consistency when planning how to integrate preschool/school, day-care, home, or other environments
3. That eclectic use of communication methodologies is acceptable because children will sort out themselves the mode which is most functional in a particular situation
4. How to access services and the key contact person in the school system
5. How to evaluate available services regarding appropriateness for their child and where to go for support when they do not feel the school is responsive to their child's needs

CONCLUSION

Successful education experiences are built in the same way that the patient–professional partnership in the audiology practice is built. Audiologists must respect the families they work with and honor their feelings. They must know when to listen and when to talk. They must provide accurate information and be clinically sound with their judgments. They must find a balance between guidance and persuasiveness. Most important, audiologists must give parents the tools, the support, and hence the power, to make reasonable decisions for themselves and their children.

REFERENCES

AMERICAN SPEECH-LANGUAGE-HEARING ASSOCIATION. (1983). Audiology services in the schools position statement, *Asha, 25*(5), 53–60.

AMERICAN SPEECH-LANGUAGE-HEARING ASSOCIATION. (1993). Guidelines for audiology services in the schools *Asha, 35,* Supplement 10.

COLORADO DEPARTMENT OF EDUCATION. (1992). *Effectiveness indicators for audiological services.* Denver.

DECONDE, C. (1984). Children use colors to flaunt their new hearing aids. *Hearing Instruments, 35,* 22.

DECONDE-JOHNSON, C. (1991). The "state" of educational audiology: Survey results and goals for the future, *EAA Monograph, 2,*(1), 71–79.

HOUSE EAR INSTITUTE. (1992). *Parent resource catalog.* Los Angeles.

INFANT HEARING RESOURCE. (1985). *Parent–infant communication.* Portland, OR.

TRAMMELL, J., FARNER, C., FRANCIS, J., OWEN, S., SHEPHERD, S., WITLEN, R., & FAIST, L. (1976). *Test of auditory comprehension.* North Hollywood: Foreworks.

YING, E. (1990). Speech and language assessment. In M. Ross (Ed.), *Hearing impaired children in the mainstream* (pp. 45–60). Parkton, MD: York Press.

APPENDIX 8–1

Suggested Responsibilities of Audiologists Who Are Employed in the Schools

- Provide community leadership to ensure that all infants, toddlers, and youth with impaired hearing are promptly identified, evaluated, and provided with appropriate intervention services.
- Collaborate with community resources to develop a high-risk registry and follow-up.
- Develop and supervise a hearing screening program for preschool and school-age children.
- Train audiometric technicians or other appropriate personnel to screen for hearing loss.
- Perform follow-up comprehensive audiological evaluations.
- Assess central auditory function.
- Make appropriate referrals for further audiological, communication, educational, psychosocial, or medical assessment.
- Interpret audiological assessment results to other school personnel.
- Serve as a member of the educational team in the evaluation, planning, and placement process. Make recommendations regarding placement, related service needs, communication needs, and modification of classroom environments for students with hearing impairments or other auditory problems.
- Provide in-service training on hearing and hearing impairments and their implication to school personnel, children, and parents.
- Educate parents, children, and school personnel about hearing loss prevention.
- Make recommendations about use of hearing aids, cochlear implants, group and classroom amplification, and assistive listening devices.
- Ensure the proper fit and functioning of hearing aids, cochlear implants, group and classroom amplification, and assistive listening devices.
- Analyze classroom noise and acoustics and make recommendations for improving the listening environment.
- Manage the use and calibration of audiometric equipment.
- Collaborate with the school, parents, teachers, special support personnel, and relevant community agencies and professionals to ensure delivery of appropriate services.
- Make recommendations for assistive devices (radio/television, telephone, alerting, convenience) for students with hearing impairment.
- Provide services, including home programming if appropriate, in the areas of speechreading, listening, communication strategies, use and care of amplification, including cochlear implants, and self-management of hearing needs.

Source: From American Speech-Language-Hearing Association (1993). Reprinted with permission.

APPENDIX 8–2

SUGGESTED IMPLICATIONS AND RECOMMENDATIONS*

Consider the effects of the identified hearing impairment for each of the following skills when describing the implications of the hearing status within audiological reports to school personnel:

- Consistency of speech or auditory signal (due to fluctuating hearing levels)
- Speech recognition
- Hearing and speech recognition in presence of background noise
- Distance hearing
- Locating sound source
- Detection versus comprehension
- Speech reading
- Fatigue due to concentration required for listening
- Attention
- Language command (receptive, expressive)
- Use of amplification (hearing aids, FM systems, etc.)
- Cognition (thinking, reasoning)
- Social/emotional state
- Suspected or diagnosed auditory processing complications
- Primary language mode
- Academic achievement and school performance

Consider the following needs relative to the identified hearing impairment when making recommendations for a child or student:

Amplification Alternatives

- Personal (hearing aid, cochlear implant, tactile device)
- Personal FM system (hearing aid + FM)
- Auditory trainer (utilized without hearing aid)
- FM system only (Walkman-style)
- FM speaker system (sound field)

Communication Modifications

- Seating to facilitate hearing and listening (e.g., front row, end seat with better—right or left—ear to class and away from noise sources) that is flexible for different situations
- Attention obtained prior to speaking with child/student
- Limited auditory distractions

---

* *Source:* Adapted from Student Staffing Checklist for Hearing, *Effectiveness Indicators for Audiological Services*, Colorado Department of Education (1992).

- Ease with which to see face and lips for speech-reading cues (avoid hands in front of face, mustaches well trimmed, no gum chewing)
- Information presented in simple, structured, sequential manner
- Teacher to check for understanding of information presented
- Clearly enunciated speech
- Extra time for processing information
- Limited visual distractions

Physical Environment Modifications

- Noise reduction (carpet, room location, ventilation)
- Specialized lighting
- Room design specifications
- Flashing fire alarm
- Telecommunication device for the deaf (TDD) (more recently known as text telephone (TT))

Instruction/Material Modifications

- Visual supplements (overhead, chalkboard, charts, vocabulary lists, lecture outlines)
- Captioning or scripts for television, movies, filmstrips
- Buddy system for notes, extra explanations/directions
- Checking for understanding of information
- Down time/break from listening
- Extra time to complete assignments
- Materials at appropriate reading levels

Supplemental Services

- Instruction in speech, language, pragmatic skill development
- Instruction in auditory skill development
- Instruction in speechreading skill development
- Interpreter (oral, manual)
- Tutor
- Note taker
- Instruction in hearing aid use, orientation, maintenance
- Instruction in social skills, responsibility, self-advocacy
- Instruction in sign language

Personal and Family Services

- Medical attention
- Financial assistance
- Counseling
- Community resources
- Vocational rehabilitation
- Ear protection

- Sign language instruction
- Family support
- Recreational opportunities
- Assistive devices
- Independent living skills
- Career/job exploration
- Deaf peer interaction opportunities

APPENDIX 8–3
GUIDELINES FOR THE CLASSROOM TEACHER*

Serving the Child with Hearing Impairment

1. *Classroom Seating.* Children with hearing impairment should be assigned seats away from hall or street noise and not more than 10 feet from the teacher. Such seating allows the child with hearing impairment to better utilize residual hearing, the hearing aids, and visual cues (speechreading, gestures, etc.). Flexibility in seating—movable desks and group arrangements—better enables the child to observe and actively participate in class activities.

2. *Look and Listen.* Children with even a mild hearing loss function much better in the classroom if they can both look and listen.

3. *Check Comprehension.* Consistently ask children with a hearing loss an occasional non yes/no question related to the subject under discussion to make certain that they are following and understanding the discussion. Many children smile and nod yes when they do not understand.

4. *Rephrase and Restate.* Encourage children with hearing impairment to indicate when they do not understand what has been said. Rephrase the question or statement, since certain words contain sounds that are not easily recognized by either speechreading or defective hearing. Also, most children with hearing impairment have some delay in language development and may not be familiar with key words. By substituting words, the intended meaning may be more readily conveyed.

5. *Pretutor Child.* Have children with hearing impairment read ahead on a subject to be discussed in class so they are familiar with new vocabulary and concepts, and can thus more easily follow and participate in classroom discussion. Such pretutoring is an important activity that the parents can undertake.

6. *Involve Resource Personnel.* Inform resource personnel of planned vocabulary and language topics to be covered in the classroom so that pretutoring can supplement classroom activities during individual therapy.

7. *List Key Vocabulary.* Before discussing new material list key vocabulary on the blackboard. Then try to build the discussion around this key vocabulary.

8. *Visual Aids.* Visual aids help children with hearing impairment by providing the association necessary for learning new things.

9. *Individual Help.* The child with impaired hearing needs individual attention. When possible provide individual help in order to fill gaps in language and understanding stemming from the child's hearing loss.

10. *Write Instructions.* Children with hearing impairment may not follow verbal instructions accurately. Help them by writing assignments on the board so they can copy them into a notebook. Also, use a buddy system by giving a hearing classmate the responsibility for making certain the child with hearing impairment is aware of the assignment made during the day.

11. *Encourage Participation.* Encourage participation in expression activities such as reading, conversation, storytelling, and creative dramatics. Reading is especially important, since information and knowledge gained through reading help compensate for what is missed because of the hearing loss. Again, parents can assist the child through participation in local library reading programs and modeling in the home.

---

* *Source:* From Matkin and Sturgeon University of Arizona (1980). Reprinted with permission.

12. *Monitor Effects*. Remember that children with impaired hearing become fatigued more readily than other children because of the continuous strain resulting from efforts to keep up with and compete in classroom activities.

13. *Inform Parents*. Provide parents of children with hearing impairment in your class with consistent input so that they understand the child's successes and difficulties.

14. *S-P-E-E-CH*. The following mnemonic device entitled SPEECH has been found helpful by teachers and parents when communicating with children with hearing impairment:

    State the topic to be discussed.

    Pace your conversation at a moderate speed with occasional pauses to permit comprehension.

    Enunciate clearly, without exaggerated lip movements.

    Enthusiastically communicate, using body language and natural gestures.

    Check comprehension before changing topics.

15. *Monitor Hearing Aids*. Many children with impaired hearing are wearing hearing aids that are in poor repair. The school audiologist or speech language pathologist can give you information about how the hearing aid works and guidance for checking its daily function. Ideally, a battery tester and a hearing aid stethoscope will be available for the daily hearing aid check. Also, a small supply of fresh batteries should be kept at school.

chapter nine

Hearing Aid Acceptance in Adults

Dean C. Garstecki

In this chapter, Dr. Garstecki goes beyond the factors audiologists must consider when helping others accept and adapt to hearing aids and assistive listening devices. He also provides a valuable overview of the Americans with Disabilities Act and how this legislation may impact the counseling audiologists provide to patients and to the community. As Dr. Garstecki stresses, audiologists can be instrumental in providing their patients not only with information on the use, care, and maintenance of personal amplification and assistive devices, but also on the intricacies and impact of recent legislation.

Everything in life is unusual until you get accustomed to it.

L. Frank Baum
The Marvelous Land of Oz

INTRODUCTION

Hearing loss affects one in nine individuals living in this country. Greater than one in four adults ages 65 to 74 years and almost two in every five adults ages 75 years and older report experiencing handicapping hearing loss (Shewan, 1990). By the year 2030, aging adults with self-reported hearing loss will number approximately

21 million (Fein, 1984). If the past is any indication of the future, in this group, incidence of hearing loss will be exceeded only by arthritis, high blood pressure, and heart disease (Goozner, 1990). The majority of these people will experience hearing loss that is medically nonrestorable—hearing loss of cochlear origin. The most usual recourse is amplification: hearing aids and assistive listening devices (ALDs). Electromechanical sound-amplifying prostheses increase low-intensity auditory signals thereby improving signal intelligibility for many hearing-impaired individuals. These instruments enable individuals who might otherwise be linked to the world visually to effectively engage in interpersonal, auditory-oral communication, to navigate through everyday activities guided by auditory warning and alerting signals and to enjoy the pleasure of sound (Weinstein, 1991).

While audiologists can praise the potential benefit of hearing aid use, many hearing-impaired individuals simply do not accept hearing loss or admit that hearing aids are a logical solution. Hearing aids are rarely the preferred means for addressing hearing loss, even though their use makes communication easier. The perceived reasons for avoiding amplification are many and varied.

Clinical observation suggests that it is common for hearing-impaired adults to experience feelings of lowered self-esteem with realization that their hearing loss is a permanent condition. Projected lifelong dependence on amplification is often difficult to accept. In addition, there are immediate frustrations to deal with in manipulating hearing aids and dealing with the hearing aid delivery system. Part of the difficulty relates to adjusting to a device that only partially restores hearing to "normal." In addition, in and of itself, hearing-aid-amplified sound suffers in quality compared with what is heard naturally without hearing loss. Some component of the auditory signal remains distorted or lost, even with the most appropriate hearing aids and the best earmold-hearing aid fitting. Some sound reception capability is gone forever with hearing loss. Clearly, then, the new hearing aid or ALD user encounters a special adjustment process. Audiologists, have an obligation to ease this transition while optimizing the hearing-impaired individual's sensory capability. They must fit the most appropriate amplification system in a program of client-centered professional care emphasizing individualized attention, careful instruction, an "empathetic ear," and steadfast encouragement to succeed in what some perceive to be a near-herculean task.

The purpose of this chapter is to address the audiologist's role in helping adults adjust to acquired hearing loss through successful use of amplification. Ideally, we would like the new user to approach this process with the same attitude and motivation as demonstrated by Mr. Finklestein, an elderly gentleman who, when asked why he enrolled in Northwestern's adult aural rehabilitation program after experiencing longstanding hearing loss, said, "I know I have a hearing loss. I want to know what I can do about it!"

Before we review ways to help others like Mr. Finklestein, it is important to recall (a) how hearing loss impacts on everyday communication and psychosocial function; (b) the scope of the unmet need for use of amplification systems; (c) factors determining candidacy for the use of hearing aids and ALDs; and, (d) factors relating to rejection or nonuse of amplification systems.

THE IMPACT OF HEARING LOSS

How does acquired hearing loss impact on lifestyle and communication? By its nature, with increasing hearing loss, people become increasingly less aware of available auditory stimuli. Alerting and warning signals—such as doorbells, automobile horns, emergency vehicle sirens, elevator bells, smoke alarms, train whistles, telephone bells, barking dogs, buzzing hornets, clanging alarm clocks, crying children—lose their emphasis. Radio and television broadcasts, public address announcements, telephone messages, and interpersonal conversation may be understood by the hearing-impaired individual only with concerted effort, great difficulty and ambiguity, or not at all. Audio entertainment, music, news and information opportunities such as those found in radio documentaries, televised programs, lectures, theater and movie presentations, opera, taped guided tours and the like, all may be inaccessible to hearing-impaired individuals.

Hearing-impaired individuals live in a sound-filtered world. Given this circumstance, it is common for negative behavior inherent in all healthy adults to be exacerbated by acquired hearing loss, resulting in what the professional literature refers to as stereotypical behavior. That is, it may be common, particularly in the early stages, for someone to deny the onset or significance of hearing loss. Some may "buy time," pretending their loss is not debilitating while they contemplate the future. They blame others for communication failure and accuse others of mumbling or not speaking up. Blame also may be placed on interference from environmental factors such as background noise. Some hearing-impaired adults become embittered and angry at having access to their world gradually whiled away by this insidious condition. Ultimately, anger gives way to depression, to a desire to shut out the external world and to question the importance of one's existence. Depression subsides as personal energy is channeled toward understanding that while hearing loss exists, its problems are resolvable, adjustments *can* be made, and life goes on (Combs, 1986; Rezen & Hausman, 1985). Focusing on what is positive in one's life and concentrating on personal strengths and accomplishments help minimize the impact of self-perceived hearing handicap. Optimizing sensory capability through the use of amplification cannot help but accelerate positive psychological adjustment to hearing loss.

HEARING AID CONSUMPTION

It is standard clinical practice to manage medically irreversible hearing loss with amplification, yet estimates of the number of individuals who elect to use hearing aids are alarmingly low. Fewer than one out of every five hearing-impaired individuals elect to use hearing aids (Gallup, 1980; Ries, 1982). Comparing hearing loss prevalence rates to estimated hearing aid use rates, the unmet need exceeds 85% (Goldstein, 1984). Moreover, this need is considered to exist almost entirely among the adult population. Kochkin (1991) estimated the number of hearing-impaired nonusers of hearing aids at 18.4 million people.

Why don't more hearing-impaired individuals use hearing aids and ALDs? What can audiologists do to increase the likelihood of successful acceptance of hearing loss through adjustment to amplification? The answers to these questions, in part, are outside of the dispensing audiologist's direct control. The potential user must be psychologically ready to accept use of a prosthetic device. Acceptance can be fostered by a strong social support system. The hearing-impaired individual's family, friends, and co-workers can facilitate hearing aid acceptance through their recognition and positive reinforcement of successful use of hearing aids. It may also help for the audiologist to demonstrate how much more visible *hearing loss* may be than *hearing aids*. That is, missed communication and the resulting frustration and embarrassment may be more obvious to others than the fact that an individual is wearing hearing aids. It also helps if an individual can develop a sense of humor about hearing aid use and, in this way, help put others at ease when they notice the hearing aids and may not know how to react to the hearing-impaired individual. The overall process of adjustment to hearing aids can be expedited when they are comfortable to wear and cause no special problems for the user. If communication performance is noticeably improved, amplification not only will be accepted, but should be welcomed, if not demanded.

Self-perceived benefit in everyday conversation, telephone communication, social interaction, communication on the job, listening for pleasure, and in instances requiring detection of auditory warning signals will lead to acceptance and use of hearing aids. Those whose unique hearing loss characteristics predispose them to successful use are likely to depend on hearing aids.

HEARING AID AND ALD CANDIDACY

Successful use of hearing aids or ALDs is dependent on a multitude of interrelated factors. First, consideration must be given to degree and type of hearing loss—the impaired ear's sensory capability. Pure-tone and speech audiometric data reveal the degree and type of hearing loss and provide an indication of the impact of hearing loss on speech recognition. If the loss is unilateral, for example, an attempt may be made to fit a hearing aid on the impaired ear to restore hearing symmetry. However, the greater the loss and the poorer the speech recognition ability, the less likely the benefit from this approach (Mueller & Grimes, 1987). Most often, hearing aid candidates, especially those whose loss is due to the normal process of aging, demonstrate symmetrical bilateral sensorineural hearing loss ranging from mild to profound degree with falling or broad-band audiometric configurations. Current ear-mold hearing aid technology successfully accommodates these losses. It also is common for those with only islands of hearing, left-corner audiograms, and no measurable change in hearing sensitivity with amplification to report benefit from hearing aid use. For example, Mr. Roscoe, an automobile accident victim suffering bilateral temporal bone fractures, preferred not to give up his hearing aids for a cochlear implant even when no benefit could be measured.

Personal motivation is a key factor in successful hearing aid use (Mueller & Grimes, 1987; Reber, 1989). The hearing-impaired individual must *want* to use a hearing aid. If use of amplification in social communication, on the job, or with family members results in the desired benefit, the system will be used. Motivation among adults in the work force may be higher than in other population sectors, as might be expected. Motivation may change with the onset of a more sedentary lifestyle. For example, Marrer and Garstecki (1985), in a study of hearing care preferences among 200 adults over age 55, reported that only 8% of those who failed a hearing screening elected to participate in a free follow-up hearing aid evaluation. The majority were unwilling to explore possible benefit from hearing aid use. They minimized the importance of improved hearing.

Vanity remains an inhibiting factor among candidates for amplification (Mueller & Grimes, 1987). And while many have abhorred the appearance of hearing aids, ALDs tend to be even less accepted. "Hearing hardware" perceived to be "unsightly" generally will not be accepted and worn, regardless of its benefit in amplification. Size and visibility of the earmold-hearing aid system contributes to the "hearing aid effect" described by Johnson and Danhauer (1982), stereotypical negative reaction to hearing-impaired individuals because they wear hearing aids.

To be accepted, amplifying systems must be well fitting and comfortable. They must be able to be used independently and with ease. It is important for control markings on the instrument to be readable by the user. Switches and battery compartment doors must be manipulable at will and with ease. Earmolds hearing aids must be able to be inserted in the ear and independently operated and maintained by the user.

Consideration also must be given to personal ability to use desired ancillary equipment, such as direct audio input accessories for behind-the-ear (BTE) and some in-the-ear (ITE) hearing aids. For some, consideration must be given to interest in and ability to use hearing aids alone and in conjunction with frequency-modulated (FM), infrared, or inductive loop personal and group amplification systems. Consideration must be given to selection of telephone amplifying and/or decoding systems, television amplifying and/or captioning systems, as well as the most effective signal format (i.e., auditory, visual, or tactile) to use in home and office alerting and warning systems.

In summary, personal acceptance of amplification is associated with self-perceived improvement in basic sensory capability, everyday communication, and overall psychosocial function. If the user communicates more efficiently with the device than without it, the device will be accepted. However, even though communication can be facilitated, a significant number of hearing-impaired individuals do not take advantage of current technology. Knowing why hearing aids and assistive devices are not used and/or are rejected will lead to more effective preventive care and, hopefully, greater hearing aid/ALD consumption.

NONUSE OR REJECTION OF AMPLIFICATION SYSTEMS

There are no definitive answers to why so many hearing-impaired individuals choose not to use hearing aids or ALDs. It is likely that nonuse and rejection are based on some combination of psychological, economic, physical, experiential or marketing/health care delivery system factors.

Psychological Factors

Probably no factor is more compelling than the potential user's attitude. Stephens and Goldstein (1983) addressed the issue of attitude and attitude typing in reference to self-management of hearing loss. Essentially they suggested basing the prognosis for self-management of hearing loss on acceptance and use of amplification. Stephens and Goldstein labeled individuals as having a Type I attitude when they are highly motivated toward self-management and consider the audiologist to be an important resource for addressing whatever has to be done to maximize compensation for hearing loss. These individuals see an opportunity to minimize difficulty in self-management of hearing loss through consultative-instructive interaction with the audiologist, as well as with other hearing-impaired individuals in a clinical setting.

Mr. Day represents a Type I attitude with a high level of motivation toward self-management. During the trial-use period with his first hearing aids, this older gentleman purposely engaged in conversations with family members and strangers in quiet and noisy conditions with and without his hearing aids. He listened to radio and television programs, attended lectures and concerts, and participated in small group meetings. He listened to his favorite recordings, speech and music. In all instances he kept a log noting differences in listening ease and clarity with and without his hearing aids.

Mr. Day's daily log of listening experiences proved to be an important reference for orientation and counseling during the trial period. It helped him realize the benefit of hearing aid use.

A Type II attitude (Stephens & Goldstein, 1983) refers to individuals possessing generally the same qualities as a Type I with the exception of a negative, complicating factor. For example, this person may lack an encouraging support system. Spouses may be embarrassed by their partner's hearing loss and dependence on use of hearing aids, or perhaps this person had a negative experience in a community lip-speechreading class.

Mr. Marigold, an older gentleman with a history of multiple ear surgeries and progressive, severe to profound hearing loss, exemplifies a Type II pattern. While motivated to self-manage his hearing problem, it became increasingly more difficult to fit him with an earmold and ear-level amplification system that would accommodate his surgically altered ear canal and rapidly progressing hearing loss. In addition, his wife, while being supportive enough to arrange audiological care and accompany him to the clinic, refused to take an active role in accommodating his communication needs. She believed her husband would be better served by arming himself with strategies necessary to survive everyday communication on his own rather than by using her as a "communication crutch."

A person with a Type III attitude (Stephens & Goldstein, 1983) essentially is not interested in using amplification. However, preconceived notions about the limitations of hearing aid use may be reversed by introducing this person to the benefits of amplification indirectly through communication training and interaction with others who are already well-adjusted amplification users.

A good example of a Type III attitude is provided by Mrs. Cars, a middle-aged mother of two with a progressive sensorineural loss and an active lifestyle. She was referred to our clinic by her dispensing audiologist for counseling in acceptance and use of hearing aids. Mrs. Cars refused to wear her new aids. She came to our clinic looking for lip-speechreading lessons to improve her communication skills so she could "get by" without having to wear them. Gradually, she was introduced to use of a pocket amplifier, an ALD worn in the pocket, resembling a small radio and used with earphones. She loved it! She looked like the hundreds of other people she observed everyday listening to their favorite music while being "tuned out" to other sound (and people) in the environment.

Through this experience, Mrs. Cars gradually realized that the importance and benefit of amplified sound outweighed any self-consciousness experienced in wearing hearing aids. She gradually accepted full-time use of binaural hearing aids and became an advocate for public access for hearing-impaired adults—a true success story.

A Type IV attitude (Stephens & Goldstein, 1983) is demonstrated by individuals with strong negative attitudes toward hearing aid use or any formal program in self-management of hearing loss. These individuals are not ready to confront hearing loss and its management. However, it may be beneficial to introduce these individuals to the range of devices, services, and information available for them when they are interested. Inviting them to a group rehabilitation session, providing an opportunity to share their hearing loss experience with other hearing-impaired individuals, or providing written information relating to hearing loss may lead these individuals closer to accepting responsibility for self-management of hearing loss.

Obviously, greatest effort is directed toward working with those in the Type II and III attitude categories. Examples of problems confronting the audiologist in working with such people are gleaned from comments made by older hearing-impaired adults surveyed by Smedley and Schow (1990). In this survey, respondents were asked to discuss concerns they had with hearing aids and audiologists/hearing aid dispensers. Their reactions are typified by the following statements:

"I can hear as plainly with my hearing aid as without it."
"I would rather not hear than wear these aids."
"These aids are a damned nuisance."
"These aids make my wife feel I hear her better."
"Hearing aids are no good; I've tried them all."

These individuals complained about the attention drawn to their hearing loss and/or advancing age by wearing hearing aids. Audiologists may need to remind them that hearing aids may be less "visible" than behaviors commonly demonstrated by hearing-impaired individuals. Also, it may be beneficial to remind some that there are many young hearing-impaired individuals and many older adults who have normally functioning hearing ability. So hearing aid use cannot be tied directly to advanced age. An empathic exploration of patient complaints through a cognitive counseling approach as discussed in Chapter 1 may help patients place their experiences into a more constructive perspective.

Other complaints included negative reaction to interference created by background noise, hearing aid style, failure of a new aid to exceed the performance of an older aid, and being "suckered" by clever advertising. Background noise may be suppressed by some hearing aid circuitry. Whether or not such a system would otherwise be appropriate, the audiologist can be instrumental in helping patients to learn ways to control the influence of noise on signal reception by reducing noise-generating sources in a room (e.g., shutting off running water, turning down the volume on a television set, etc.) and by moving to quieter places within the room or leaving a room for a quieter place. Hearing aid style may be dictated by amplification requirements. Also, it can be demonstrated that hearing aid size does not always correlate with hearing aid visibility (i.e., in-the-ear aids may be more visible than larger-sized behind-the-ear aids). A new aid may not appear to function as satisfactorily as an old aid used to because one's hearing loss has progressed, not because the newer aid is an inferior product. Finally, prospective purchasers of hearing aids should be guided toward reputable dispensers to increase the likelihood of a positive purchasing experience. Some individuals indicated that their hearing aids were purchased under pressure by a spouse, employer, or other family member. Whether this is an individual's perception or a reality, it suggests that hearing loss has become a burden to all who interact with the hearing-impaired person and this person should be positively reinforced for taking steps to minimize difficulties related to hearing loss. If others did not care about interacting with the hearing-impaired person, they would not be suggesting that a hearing aid be considered.

Are the complaints of hearing aid users supported by hearing aid dispensers? Yes. Hearing aid dispensers maintain that the longtime negative stigma associated with hearing aid use continues. Potential consumers reportedly continue to suffer from problems of personal vanity. They lack awareness or desire to admit hearing loss. They lack motivation to hear better (Kochkin, 1991). This also supports the earlier view of Franks and Beckmann (1985), who reported that many aging adults consider hearing loss to be an unacceptable human condition.

Economic Factors

Regardless of the actual dollars spent in acquiring hearing aids, including the cost of otological and audiological evaluation, ear molds, hearing aids themselves, as well as anticipated long-term repair, battery use, and eventual aid replacement costs, hearing aids are perceived to be expensive. A common complaint listed in consumer surveys is that hearing aids *cost too much*, no matter what portion of the overall expense may be covered by third-party reimbursement (Fino, Bess, Lichenstein, & Logan, 1992; Gallup, 1980; Libby, 1990). Excessive cost was the most common reason for hearing aid rejection reported in the Franks and Beckman (1985) survey of retired adults. No matter what percentage of an individual's discretionary income may be required for hearing-aid-related costs, the amount is considered to be greater than the perceived benefit. Cost was listed among the top four categories of complaints about hearing aid use in Smedley and Schow's (1990) survey where respondents indicated they paid from $200 to $1,000 per aid. In addition, it is not only consumers who have complained about cost; dispensers consider hearing aid cost to be too high for aging adults living on fixed incomes (Kochkin, 1991).

Alternately, cost was *not* a primary reason for rejection in a New York League for the Hard of Hearing survey (Madell, Pfeffer, Ross, & Chellappa, 1991). However, retired respondents over age 71 were more likely to return their hearing aids following a trial period than those who were employed. Goldstein (1984) reported there actually were increases in hearing aid sales during the recession of the early 1980s—a time when third-party reimbursement decreased by 25%. He also cited low takeup rates in countries where hearing aids are distributed without direct charge to the consumer.

Audiologists need to be cognizant of the fact that cost may be a real factor in hearing aid rejection or nonuse for some individuals. Audiologists and manufacturers need to explore means of making hearing aids more affordable to those who would use them if cost was not a prohibiting factor. They also need to help potential consumers understand hearing aid costs. Skafte (1992) reports that hearing aid costs hold steady (rather than drop) because of economic factors associated with the relatively small market. A small market keeps manufacturing industries from being able to effect savings through mass purchases and, in turn, pass these savings on to the consumer. Also, hearing aid assembly procedures are complicated and labor-intensive. Because many hearing aids are custom made, repairs and warranty maintenance costs are high. Manufacturer overhead costs continue to rise. Product research and design and development of product standards add to the cost of each instrument. There are significant retail costs as well. Dispenser costs include the expense of setting up an office or clinical facility and conducting a professional business. Funds are needed for rent, taxes, insurance, staff salaries, special equipment, supplies and dispensary consumables, advertising, and a profit margin for self-support. These costs may not be readily perceived by the hearing aid consumer.

Physical Factors

Another factor potentially contributing to rejection of amplification is the sensory capability of the impaired ear. For example, problems in discriminating the sounds of speech may be exacerbated by the use of amplification in adults with retrocochlear involvement. Unilateral loss may obviate the need for amplification except under select listening conditions. With mild hearing loss, and in instances of marginal functional residual hearing, hearing aids and assistive devices may be of questionable benefit. In some cases, it may be advantageous to consider the combined use of a hearing aid and an ALD, particularly in noisy situations where either direct audio input or use of an ALD may help enhance aided signal-to-noise ratio.

Fitting Factors

Among those who *are* able to benefit from amplification, there are other inhibiting factors. Again, Smedley and Schow's (1990) survey reveals complaints about earmolds and hearing aids not fitting properly after repeated attempts to remedy known problems. Some complained that the aids were difficult to put on or to use with a telephone. Others complained about feedback created by head motion and wearing tight-fitting head gear. For some, earmolds and hearing aids made their ears sweat, and sweating ears resulted in malfunctioning hearing aids. Several complained about the difficulty separating competing noise from primary signals when using a hearing aid. One person indicated the hearing aid "wore a sore on her head." Another indicated her canal aids "flew out of her ears whenever she blew her nose."

To increase the likelihood of hearing aid and ALD acceptance and use, audiologists must ensure that any recommended instrument can be worn comfortably. Skill and care in taking an earmold impression and fitting the device are critical. Amplified sound levels must be within the tolerance limits of the hearing-impaired individual's ear. The device's saturation sound pressure level (SSPL) must be set to within user limits (Davis & Mueller, 1987). When there is an option, hearing aids with unidirectional microphones should be selected over those with omnidirectional microphones. Unidirectional microphones help enhance the signal-to-noise ratio in noisy conditions (Davis & Mueller, 1987). Binaural fittings, when feasible, are preferred over monaural fittings. Binaural fittings are superior to monaural fittings in regard to improvement of speech recognition, sound localization, loudness summation, and suppression of background noise (Davis & Mueller, 1987). It is important to provide careful instruction in how to wear an aid to derive maximum benefit without the problem of acoustic feedback. Finally, the hearing aid/ALD user may need to be instructed regarding circuitry options, attachments, and strategies for managing problems relating to noise interference.

It is important that new users form realistic expectations when attempting to benefit from an amplification system, particularly under conditions of adverse humidity and noise or in telephone communication. In addition, the natural course of aging may impact on upper body strength, range of movement and manual dexterity, as well as tactile sensitivity and thus make it difficult to manage hearing aid insertion and removal, battery insertion and removal, and manipulation of hearing aid controls and battery compartment doors.

Experimental Factors

Ignorance or lack of experience may contribute to nonuse or rejection of amplification systems. The audiologist may need to dispell common myths associated with the use of hearing aids (Combs, 1986). One myth suggests that hearing aids do not help those with sensorineural hearing loss, when, in fact, the majority of hearing aid users demonstrate hearing loss of cochlear origin. Another myth is that hearing loss is exacerbated by the use of hearing aids. There is no evidence supporting this contention in instances where aids are properly fitted. Finally, there are individuals who have failed to use hearing aids successfully who suggest to others that amplification systems may not be helpful. Such myths can be dispelled with proper fitting and instruction in the use of amplification systems and counseling in the benefits and limitations of hearing aid use.

Madell et al., (1991) surveyed ITE hearing aid users and found that more inexperienced than experienced users rejected their hearing aids. Similarly, Kochkin (1991) reported that hearing instrument dispensers blamed lack of hearing aid acceptance on undereducation of potential consumers. Garstecki (1990) reported that only 25% of the aging adults surveyed in his study believed that hearing loss could be helped by hearing aids; 60% disagreed on the importance of binaural amplification and 40% were undecided about associating hearing aid cost with benefit. Implications drawn from this study included the need to educate the general aging population in regard to potential impact of hearing loss and the benefits of amplification.

Marketing Factors

Goldstein (1984) described problems with the hearing aid delivery system. For example, in order to obtain a hearing aid, the consumer must pass through the "medical funnel." While there are advantages to medical evaluation and treatment in preparing for an earmold impression and it is agreed that medical-surgical treatment may obviate the need for amplification, most aging hearing aid candidates do not have a hearing *health* condition. Most potential adult hearing aid and assistive device users are not ill. Goldstein refers to acquired hearing loss occurring within the normal process of aging as a mere "life-cycle event"—not a disease or an illness. In fact, by requiring a medical evaluation for purposes of hearing aid fitting, it is speculated that management of hearing loss may actually be slowed or halted by physicians who remain skeptical regarding benefits to those with sensorineural hearing loss.

Goldstein also commented on the personal influence of audiologists on decisions to use amplification. Skepticism among some audiologists regarding the cost of hearing aids and ALDs or the cost-benefit ratio may suggest to the consumer that it may be prudent to wait for technological advances and possibly lowered costs before investing. Some audiologists reportedly recommend use of ALDs over hearing aids only for purposes of cost savings. Franks and Beckmann (1985) reported that their survey respondents felt that instrument dispensers were interested primarily in financial gain and that deceptive sales practices and high-pressure sales techniques were used to increase personal income. Hearing aid consumers surveyed by Smedley and Schow (1990) complained about the quality of hearing aid construction, attitudes of hearing aid dispensers, misleading and false advertising, and insufficient time spent in hearing aid orientation by the hearing aid dispenser. Kochkin (1991) reported that hearing aid dispensers perceived consumers as having a negative image of the dispenser community and that poor fittings have resulted in negative word-of-mouth advertising. Marketing, then, remains as an area for improvement to promote greater acceptance of amplification.

In summary, there are a number of factors that singly or in combination contribute to poor acceptance of hearing loss and the use of amplification systems. Our attention to these factors, as audiologists, should improve upon this situation. The next section reviews ways in which we can address these factors in clinical practice.

ACCEPTING HEARING LOSS BY ADJUSTING TO AMPLIFICATION

Hearing loss will be *accepted* only when it is minimally limiting—when those who suffer hearing loss can function essentially as effectively as those with normal hearing. The onus is not only on the hearing-impaired individual to optimize sensory capability and to learn to manage problems relating to hearing loss, but on society at large. Public consciousness must be raised regarding the importance of hearing, its preservation, diagnosis and treatment of hearing disorders, and accommodating those with impaired hearing. Meeting the special needs of hearing-impaired individuals is federally mandated.

The Americans with Disabilities Act

On July 26, 1990, President George Bush signed the Americans with Disabilities Act (ADA) into law (P.L. 101-336). This new law is intended to eliminate discrimination against all individuals with disabilities. It provides a federally enforceable standard for addressing discrimination in regard to hearing loss. The ADA is intended to guarantee equal opportunity for individuals with disabilities in employment, public accommodations, transportation, state and local government services, and telecommunications. In order to understand this law and how audiologists may be involved in its implementation, we should be familiar with each of its components or title areas.

Title I—Employment

Title I protects qualified individuals with disabilities from discrimination in all aspects of employment from the time of application through hiring, orientation, advancement, and dismissal (Equal Employment Opportunity Commission, 1991). Under Title I, employers are allowed to inquire about an applicant's ability to perform job tasks, but may not rightfully ask if an applicant has a disability or attempt to screen out individuals with disabilities in the employee selection process. For example, an employer may not ask if an applicant has a hearing impairment, but may ask if an applicant can efficiently manage interpersonal or telephone communication.

Employers are expected to provide reasonable accommodation to individuals with disabilities. This involves making existing facilities and/or equipment accessible and usable. A hearing-impaired person may require a telephone amplifier, interpreter, or visual alerting device, for example. Reasonable accommodation also applies to job and work schedule modification. However, employers do not need to provide accommodations that impose undue hardship or expense on the employer.

In the regulations governing Title I, hearing loss is listed as a potentially disabling physical impairment. An individual with hearing loss is regarded as having a physical impairment regardless of mitigating measures, such as satisfactory use of hearing aids or ALDs. However, a hearing-impaired individual is not regarded as disabled until it is determined that hearing loss substantially limits one or more of life's major activities, such as telephone communication. If telephone communication can occur effectively with hearing aids and/or telephone amplifiers or decoders, the hearing-impaired individual will not be considered disabled under Title I.

In implementing the ADA, an audiologist may need to demonstrate to potential employers how a hearing-impaired job candidate may be able to perform essential job functions with or without assistive devices. For example, if a job requires face-to-face interaction with others, the employer needs to be aware of FM, infrared, or loop induction personal communication systems to enhance message reception in noise. Also, if a job requires telephone communication, consideration should be given to use of visual (light) alerting devices, telephone amplifiers, and strategies that can be used by third parties to relay information to hearing-impaired persons.

Title II—Public Services

This component of the ADA protects qualified individuals with disabilities from exclusion or denial of services, programs, or activities sponsored by a public entity. Qualified individuals are defined as those with disabilities who are eligible for services or participation in programs and activities that may require modification of rules, policies, and practices, or removal of architectural, communication, or transportation barriers, or provision of auxiliary agent services to do so. A public entity is any state or local department, agency or other instrumentality of a state or local government, Amtrak, and any commuter rail authority (Department of Justice, 1991a).

Title II guarantees that auxiliary agent services will be made available to ensure communication access. These services include any means of accessing information through use of telephone amplifiers, ALDs, hearing-aid-compatible telephones, text telephones (TTs), telephone relay services, public address systems, transcription services, written notice, and closed and opened television message captioning. Under this legislation, the audiologist has a new and vital role to play in selection, fitting, and orienting others in the use of devices to accommodate individuals with hearing disability.

Title III—Public Accommodations

This section of the ADA ensures nondiscrimination toward individuals with disabilities in the employment of goods, services, facilities, privileges, advantages, and accommodations of any public entity as of January 26, 1992 (Department of Justice, 1991b). Auxiliary aids and services must be provided to hearing-impaired individuals unless undue burden would result. In determining level of burden, the cost and nature of required action, overall financial resources of the providing facility, overall size of the business, and number, type, and location of facilities are considered.

Audiologists involved in implementing Title III regulations will need to consider the types of assistive devices and related services that would guarantee access to places of lodging, exhibition or entertainment, public gathering, sales or rental establishments, stations used for public transportation, places of public display, places of recreation, places of exercise and education, and social service establishments.

In public accommodations equipped with audible emergency alarms, the alarm signal must exceed prevailing sound by 15 dB or the maximum sound typically occurring in an area by at least 5 dB. Audible alarms having a periodic element to their signals, such as a single stroke bell, may be easiest for a hearing-impaired person to hear. Continuous and reverberant alarm signals should be avoided. Public accommodations are required to modify policies, practices, and procedures to allow the use of service animals, such as guide dogs trained to provide assistance to disabled individuals. A hearing-ear dog, for example, will need to be accommodated in public places visited by hearing-disabled individuals.

Under Title III, telephones must be hearing-aid-compatible. Telephone amplifiers must allow for a signal intensity increase ranging from 12 to 18 dB. If an automatic volume control reset feature is provided, the 18-dB limit may be exceeded. Telephones equipped with amplifiers must be identified by a sign depicting a telephone handset with radiating soundwaves (see Figure 9–1). Text telephones used along with pay telephones must be permanently affixed to the

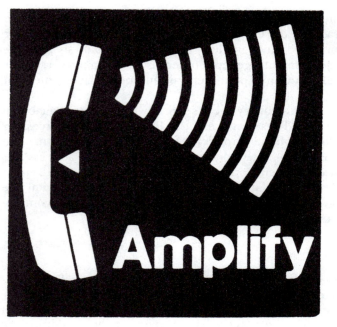

FIGURE 9–1 Symbol Used to Identify Amplified Telephone Handsets in Public Places. (*Source:* C. L. Compton [1989].) Used with permission.

telephone enclosure. Text telephones are required to be identified by the international telephone communication device for the deaf symbol (see Figure 9–2).

Places of lodging and hospitals providing televisions in five or more guest rooms are required to provide a television decoder for hearing-disabled individuals. Hotels also should provide a text telephone to take calls from guests who use text telephones in their rooms. Hotels providing 1 to 25 sleeping rooms must equip a minimum of one room with devices for hearing-disabled individuals, such as visual alarms and amplified or text telephones. Visual alarms should be located and oriented so they spread light signals and reflections throughout a space or raise overall light level sharply.

Title III also ensures that no individual is discriminated against because of absence of auxiliary aids and services, unless it can be demonstrated that taking such steps would result in undue hardship. For example, if a listening system is to serve individuals in fixed seating, seats must be located within a 50-foot viewing distance of a target area. In areas where permanently installed assistive listening systems are required, the availability of such systems must be identified with signage that includes the international symbol of access for hearing loss (see Figure 9–3).

Title IV—Telecommunications

Title IV of the ADA amends Title II of the Communications Act of 1934 by making available to all individuals a rapid, efficient, communications service. Under Title IV, the Federal Communication Commission (FCC) ensures that

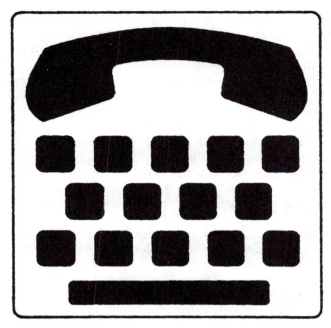

FIGURE 9–2 International Text Telephone Symbol. (*Source:* United States Architectural and Transportation Barriers Compliance Board [1991].)

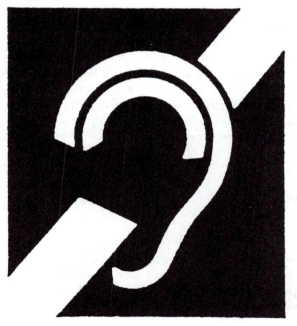

FIGURE 9–3 International Symbol of Access for Hearing Loss. (*Source:* United States Architectural and Transportation Barriers Compliance Board [1991].)

inter- and intrastate telecommunication relay services are available that enable a speech- or hearing-impaired individual to communicate by wire or radio in a manner functionally equivalent to that of someone without a communication impairment (Federal Communications Commission, 1991).

Telecommunication relay system providers are responsible for supplying communication assistants (CAs) who are trained to meet the specialized needs of individuals with speech or hearing disabilities. The CA must demonstrate skill in typing, English grammar usage, oral and written communication, interpretation of American sign language, and familiarity with the culture, language, and etiquette of speech- and hearing-disabled individuals. Audiologists may play an important role in educating CAs to understand hearing loss, its effects on communication, how to overcome speech understanding problems related to hearing loss, and the influence of hearing loss and deafness on everyday psychosocial functions.

Overall, implementation of the ADA should foster development of new relationships between audiologists, hearing-impaired adults, and society in general. The ADA provides an opportunity to extend the scope of audiological practice well outside the confines of hearing clinics and well beyond compensation for hearing loss with hearing aids and ALDs. It will become increasingly more common for audiologists to carry their practice to the community at large, providing informational counseling to acoustical engineers, architects, transit authority officials, employers of hearing-disabled individuals, assistive device manufacturers and distributors, telecommunication service representatives, proprietors of businesses serving individuals with hearing disabilities, and attorneys. It is also likely that with implementation of the ADA, audiologists will assume the responsibility of "case worker" in championing the rights of hearing-disabled individuals to access the community and workplace.

Having considered the impact of acquired hearing loss and relatively low interest in use of amplification, and having reviewed factors that contribute both to successful candidacy and nonuse or rejection of amplification, what can we do to promote acceptance of hearing loss through use of amplification systems? The next section reviews factors for the audiologist to consider when providing counseling on the amplification and assistive device needs of hearing-impaired adults, the preselection process, the introduction to the use of amplification systems, and maintaining adjustment to the use of hearing aids and assistive devices.

ACCEPTANCE AND USE OF HEARING AIDS AND ALDS

General Considerations

Matters relating to personal style. Individuals who take a "proactive" (Morgan, 1990) stance toward health care are likely to approach the prospect of using hearing aids like today's personal computer buffs approach the use of new computer equipment. They will consider the audiologist to be a professional resource for advice they are already collecting on hearing aids or ALD selection and use. They want to know the benefits and limitations of available systems before committing to use of the system most appropriate for and acceptable to them. They want to know how use of selected system(s) might be enhanced. They may even request participation in classes providing them with practical information and controlled exercises to introduce them to the range of listening experiences they might encounter while wearing hearing aids and strategies for overcoming communication difficulty. For these individuals, the audiologist facilitates and guides an adjustment process that is client driven.

Next, there are those who take the "faithful patient" (Morgan, 1990) approach. These individuals will dutifully follow the audiologist's advice in selection and fitting, but not with the same self-initiative as demonstrated by the proactive adult. They are likely to believe it is in their best interest to take advantage of available technology for compensating for hearing loss. While they may not challenge the audiologist to optimize their sensory capability, they exhibit a positive attitude toward use of hearing aids and ALDs and welcome all effort by the audiologist to improve upon their hearing-loss condition and its related problems. For these individuals, the audiologist directs and controls the adjustment process.

There also are the "optimists"—those who truly believe that their hearing-loss-related problems will be overcome with minimal personal effort (Morgan, 1990). They may not accept any form of hearing prosthesis until all hope from anticipated advances in medicine and/or hearing aid and assistive device technology wanes. Optimists may express an interest in information concerning latest developments in medicine and in the hearing aid industry, but only for the sake of internalizing a plan for addressing their hearing problem.

> Mr. Robinson was one such person. Mr. Robinson "hung around" the senior activity center when presentations on hearing aids and assistive devices were scheduled. However, he rarely committed himself to participate in such programs in advance. He would never register for such a presentation. He would update his knowledge of hearing aid benefits and limitations by quizzing the presenter outside the context of the scheduled program and conclude by rationalizing that "new developments" were on the way and only when they arrived would he invest in hearing aids or an assistive device.
>
> *In dealing with the optimist, the audiologist can only hope to facilitate the process leading to a positive decision regarding hearing aid use by continuing to provide appropriate advice and counsel.*

Finally, there are "disillusioned" (Morgan, 1990) hearing-impaired persons, those carrying a grudge or "chip on the shoulder" over the fact they are burdened with hearing loss. They feel their life's dreams have fallen. They have no hope that hearing aids or assistive devices will be of benefit. Disillusioned individuals may also distrust members of the hearing aid/ALD delivery system, particularly because they had hoped for better results for their investment in medical or surgical care or the purchase of hearing aids and assistive devices. For these individuals, the audiologist's best efforts might be directed toward informational counseling or public education.

Optimists and disillusioned hearing-impaired individuals can present a true counseling challenge to the audiologist. Both types recognize their hearing difficulties but are either not ready or are unwilling to address the concomitant communication problems their hearing losses present. It is important for the audiologist to help these patients realize that their decision to ignore their hearing problems may impinge greatly on their spouses or other significant people in their lives. At the very least, coping and communication strategies (Chapter 10, Appendix 10–1) should be provided to the spouses of optimistic and disillusioned patients. In addition, advising patients that classes for coping with hearing loss are a possible alternative solution to amplification may help them to gain exposure to others who have successfully accepted and adjusted to amplification.

In summary, adjustment to hearing loss through acceptance of hearing aids and ALDs is a process that requires some incentive on the part of the hearing-impaired individual to improve upon the status quo. Psychologically, some hearing-impaired individuals are internally controlled; they drive the adjustment process. Some are more externally controlled; they are more comfortable letting the professional direct the adjustment process. Some wait for conditions to improve, and others choose to minimize the importance of improved hearing.

Matters relating to professional service. Smedley and Schow (1990) suggested guidelines to follow in professional interaction with hearing aid/ALD candidates. A key factor is employment of a client-based strategy in selection of amplification systems. Beyond addressing the appropriateness of a system for a given hearing loss, the match between hearing function and electroacoustic properties of earmold amplification systems, consider the personal preferences of the potential user, particularly in regard to ease of use and personal vanity. Facilitate adjustment to amplification through early use rather than waiting until hearing difficulty reaches crisis proportions. It is easier for the aging adult to adjust in the early, less innocuous stages of hearing loss than in later stages when benefit from amplification may diminish. Individualized counseling is a critical component of the adjustment process, particularly for aging adults. Audiologists need to help new users develop realistic expectations from amplification and to feel comfortable and appropriately assertive in "stage-managing" communication situations as discussed in greater detail by Dr. Trychin in Chapter 10. Smedley and Schow also indicate that frequent postfitting follow-up visits contribute to successful adjustment. While the mechanism for postfitting contact may vary by individual and clinic, the importance of this process for patient satisfaction cannot be overemphasized (see Appendix 9–1).

Matters relating to professional business. Business practices associated with hearing aid/ALD dispensing may impact negatively on the adjustment process. While no longer required by FDA regulation, a 30-day trial period is recommended for new hearing aid users as standard business practice. If a fee is charged for the trial, those concerned should be informed well in advance. The dispenser should clarify how much of a trial fee may be refundable and explain how changing aids during the trial period influences the trial schedule and associated costs. Finally, be sure to credit days lost from the trial period due to manufacturing or fitting problems (Shimon, 1992). In summary, the new hearing aid user is entitled to a full trial with each hearing aid.

While most manufacturers are prepared to accommodate the audiologist's interest in providing a trial period in hearing aid fitting, the same cannot be said of ALD manufacturers. The best procedure for handling assistive device trials is to inquire about possible support from manufacturers with a history of developing products for the hearing impaired. In general, it is better practice to allow potential device consumers to become acquainted with available products in the clinic under the audiologist's supervision than independently in another setting. This trial can be incorporated into a traditional aural rehabilitation program or offered as a separate service. Unfortunately, experience suggests that when assistive devices are loaned to potential consumers for trial use they are likely to be misused, and they are more likely to require mechanical or cosmetic refurbishing than is typically the case with hearing aids. It is recommended, therefore, that adjustment to use of assistive devices be accomplished by trial in the clinic in a setting simulating everyday-use conditions.

FDA regulations provide a 1 year warranty to cover defects in workmanship and malfunction resulting during normal use of hearing aids (Shimon, 1992). A warranty is not an insurance policy, and the new user should be apprised of what is covered by the manufacturer's warranty, especially concerning whether an aid will be replaced if lost, stolen, or damaged beyond repair. Also, if there is a charge for the warranty or an extended warranty, these charges should be made known at the outset. Hearing aid insurance and the option of adding insurance for hearing aid replacement to a homeowner's policy should be considered by the new user. While there are no comparable regulations applying to warranties for assistive devices, they are available from device manufacturers.

As part of the adjustment process, it is helpful for hearing aid/ALD consumers to understand their legal rights and limitations under available warranty agreements. Warranties may be canceled or not honored if problems result from abuse such as may occur during attempted self-repair or exposure to extreme heat or moisture (Shimon, 1992). It is helpful for those seeking warranty service to realize that when an instrument needs to be returned to the manufacturer, repairs may take several weeks, and a loaner aid may be desired in the interim period. If the hearing aid is out of warranty, repairs may be made at the owner's expense. Most hearing aids used by adults under normal everyday conditions will function satisfactorily for at least 5 years, and those that are properly cared for will last longer (Shimon, 1992). However, even though the hearing aid may continue to function for an appreciable period of time, changes in hearing aid fit may occur requiring either that they be recased or replaced. Besides possible changes in external ear size or shape, changes in hearing loss characteristics may require that more appropriate hearing aids be fitted before the current aids wear to the extent of requiring replacement.

In every instance, information relating to the sale and use of amplification systems, their warranties, and insurance policies should be presented honestly, completely, and in a way that promotes clear understanding of realistic expectations from the product, manufacturer, distributor, and dispensing audiologist (Smedley & Schow, 1990).

Preselection Considerations

The need for amplification is evident from audiometric data and/or self-report. Essentially, as long as some evidence of functional hearing can be demonstrated, there is potential for benefit from use of amplification. Once it is decided that amplification may appropriately be considered, then consideration should be given to the advantages of binaural fittings and fittings that allow for enhancing benefit from combined hearing aid/ALD use. For example, those who routinely need to communicate in noisy situations may benefit from noise-attenuating hearing aid circuitry, aids with extended microphone-direct audio input capability, aids coupled to pocket amplifiers (via T-coil/neckloop transmission) with external extended microphones, and other customized hearing aid and/or assistive device arrangements.

Preselection of assistive devices should be determined by observation, self-report, and/or clinical assessment. This process may be expedited by use of interactive product locator software (Palmer, 1992; Palmer, Garstecki, & Rauterkus, 1990). At a minimum, the following questions should be asked when an interest is expressed in improving telephone communication:

1. Can standard telephone equipment be used efficiently without amplification?
2. Is amplification desired and beneficial?
3. Is a text telephone desired and beneficial?
4. Is a telephone relay system required?
5. Does the potential user have adequate visual skills for independent use of telephone equipment?
6. Does the potential user have adequate manual dexterity and mobility for independent use of telephone equipment?
7. Will systems under consideration be used both by hearing as well as hearing-impaired listeners and, if so, are any special adjustments necessary?

Questions to be asked in preselection of television devices include the following:

1. Can a standard televised message be understood efficiently without amplification?
2. Is amplification desired and beneficial?
3. Is a caption device desired and beneficial?
4. Does the potential user have adequate visual skills for independent use of television equipment?

5. Does the potential user have adequate manual dexterity and mobility for independent use of television equipment?

6. Will systems under consideration be used both by hearing as well as hearing-impaired listeners and, if so, are any special adjustments necessary?

Finally, in assessing appropriateness of home warning and alerting systems, the following questions should be addressed:

1. Do existing warning and alerting systems (e.g., telephone bells, doorbells, etc.) need to be modified?

2. Are amplified warning and alerting systems desired and expected to be beneficial?

3. Are visual warning and alerting systems desired and expected to be beneficial?

4. Does the potential user have the auditory and/or visual skills required for independent use of warning and alerting system?

5. Does the potential user have the manual dexterity and mobility required for successful use of warning and alerting system?

Perhaps the most dramatic circumstance under which a comprehensive assistive device evaluation might be conducted is in the instance of sudden deafness.

One night, Mr. Williams, a middle-aged security guard with a history of sudden unilateral deafness, noticed that sound had all but disappeared during his nightly rounds in a large department store. He called out and couldn't hear his own voice. Weeks later, he appeared in our clinic with an elderly uncle who complained that since this episode Mr. Williams had lost all hearing; he resigned himself to his apartment, covered his windows with newspapers, and depended on relatives to bring him food. His family was concerned about his loss of interest in living, personal safety, loss of independence, and loss of livelihood.

Mr. Williams wanted privacy. His landlord would enter his apartment without warning, while he was there, to check on Mr. Williams's safety. A doorbell-flashing light system was installed to help give him privacy. A text telephone helped him to stay in contact with his sisters. A television caption device helped him keep abreast of events of the day. Finally, a hearing-ear dog helped to provide safety and companionship. We worked with Mr. Williams and his relatives to understand his need for various types of assistive devices. Selected devices were purchased by different family members who took it upon themselves to learn how to use the device, teach Mr. Williams how to use it, and see that he did, in fact, benefit from its availability.

This example demonstrates the importance of assistive devices, particularly for individuals suffering sudden, severe, or profound hearing loss. It also demonstrates the value of maintaining a clinical stock of representative devices. In addition, it illustrates how family members may play a key role in the selection and use of assistive devices.

Finally, during the preselection process, consideration also must be given to an individual's potential for using selected devices independently. Are the candidates likely to be able to insert and remove earmolds, set volume and tone controls, balance binaural input, use attachments (e.g., neckloops, silhouette adaptors)? Will they be able to insert and remove batteries, troubleshoot and remedy problems that may occur, and be able to install devices that require installation? How will devices be paid for, and will the consumer be able to maintain the cost of maintenance and use? These questions need to be resolved before concluding the preselection process (Garstecki, 1988).

Orientation

Coupling the amplification system to the user's ear. Successful independent use of hearing aids or ALDs is facilitated thorough orientation. The new user must learn to insert and remove the earmold-hearing aid from the ear. This requires upper arm strength and mobility, fine motor control, and coordination. It requires the ability to follow verbal directions and to see switches and controls and the ability to read and understand written instruction. Earmold removal also requires practice and skill, and a routine must be developed for "unlocking" the ear mold from the pinna. Initially, the audiologist may guide ear-mold insertion and removal by demonstration and verbal instruction, and it may be helpful in some instances to teach these maneuvers to someone close to the new user who may be called on to assume this responsibility on a daily basis as needed.

Unlike most hearing aids, many ALDs incorporate the use of muff-type receivers that allow them to be used by almost anyone without instruction or practice. These include headphones, earphones, earbuds, infrared system receiver bars, and the like. Other ear-coupling systems may include neckloops and silhouette T-coil adapters. Also, some BTE hearing aids and ALDs allow direct audio connection to telephones, televisions, radios, audio cassette players, and the like, as well as allow for the attachment of hand-held and conference microphones.

Setting the volume control. With the hearing aid/ALD in place in the ear and ready to be turned on, the user must decide where to set the volume control for the greatest amount of consistent benefit under typically fluctuating listening conditions. The best practice is to begin adjustment to sound at the "just-on" position. The user should proceed by increasing volume to a level just below where the incoming signal is perceived to be uncomfortably loud. Any nonlinearity in gain with increasing volume control rotation should be noted by the audiologist in advance of suggesting a procedure for determining an optimal-use setting. Some telephone amplifiers, for example, demonstrate relatively little change in gain from 50% to 75% volume wheel rotation. In such instances, the user should be informed of what to expect in terms of change in gain with increase in volume control rotation. When the volume control cannot be set voluntarily, standard clinical procedures for predicting and measuring aided gain level may be used (Pascoe, 1990).

When a system provides binaural input, the user will want to experience balanced sound, each ear perceiving sound equally. This is accomplished by having the user develop a sense of when sound appears to be at midline or the center of the head. Assuming independent control over volume level into each ear, a useful procedure according to Pascoe (1990) is to set the level of input into the better ear just below what it would be if an amplification system was to be worn monaurally. Then set the input to the poorer ear to the level where it is just perceived in that ear. Finally, lower the volume setting in the poorer ear until sound is perceived at midline or equidistant from each ear.

Presently, there are no international standards regulating electroacoustic assessment or fitting of ALDs. There are no universal clinical guidelines to direct ALD assessment and fitting. Few device manufacturers routinely provide electroacoustic specification data. In addition, there are only a small number of published clinical research reports demonstrating the need for and desirability of measuring the electroacoustic properties of ALDs.

In guiding ALD users, the ideal practice would be to electronically monitor volume control linearity and frequency response characteristics as part of the usual clinic routine. When this is not feasible, audiologists may need to rely on amplified sound field data and self-report of improved function with use of a device. Self-report scales such as those developed by Cox and Gilmore (1990), Newman and Weinstein (1988), and Walden, Demorest, and Hepler (1984) provide a useful guide to determining self-perceived benefit from amplification.

Setting other controls and attachments. Some hearing aids and ALDs are equipped with tone controls to shape amplifier frequency response characteristics. Tone controls essentially serve to filter the instrument's normal frequency response to accommodate "nonlinear" hearing loss. For example, it may be desirable to emphasize high-frequency information and allow low-frequency information to pass without amplification in systems used primarily by individuals with sloping, high-frequency hearing loss. Systems equipped with tone control adjustments may enable this to occur without risk of overamplifying and distorting low-frequency information.

Some hearing aids and loop induction receiver units are equipped with copper coils (telecoils and T-switches) that enable electromagnetic transduction of auditory signals. Signals transmitted electromagnetically do not suffer from the same type of acoustic masking that occurs when attempting to understand speech in open field, as ambient noise is not amplified. This enhances telephone communication and understanding in noisy lecture halls for individuals who have this listening option. In adjusting to the telecoil option, users will need to be familiar with appropriate hearing aid or loop induction receiver settings and possibly how to manage noisy situations, neckloops, and silhouette adaptors. In summary, comprehensive, client-based care involves instruction and practice in dealing with all switches, settings, and attachments on all amplification systems of interest in a comprehensive aural rehabilitation program.

Managing acoustic feedback. One common source of frustration and irritation for users of personal amplification systems is acoustic feedback. This high-pitched squeal may be a source of embarrassment and frustration to the user. Acoustic feedback occurs when there is an opening or obstruction in the line from the hearing aid microphone to the user's eardrum. A break may occur whenever an earmold or other ear-coupling transducer (e.g., headphones, earbuds) is ill fitting, allowing the system to amplify its own signal. As Pascoe (1990) notes, the more powerful the amplifying device, the tighter the required fit in the ear canal. Feedback also may occur when an ear canal is plugged with cerumen or when the user cups a hand or wears a cap over the microphone. Feedback may also indicate an internal malfunction in the amplifier, or loose-fitting or cracked earmold tubing or hearing aid earhooks.

It is beneficial to the hearing aid user not only to recognize potential sources of acoustic feedback, but to understand how to remedy these problems as well (see Appendix 9–2).

Ms. Bell, an elderly longtime behind-the-ear hearing aid user encountered a feedback problem associated with a cracked ear-hook late one Friday evening. Facing the possibility of a weekend without an aid, she found a dispenser who informed her that her aid was beyond repair and needed to be replaced. Ms. Bell insisted that such a decision would only be made in consultation with her "regular" audiologist. She was provided with a loaner, but found it unacceptable and returned it the following day. At that time she was presented with a "reconditioned" aid and given the opportunity to purchase it if she found it acceptable. Ms. Bell wore the reconditioned aid to her Monday morning appointment with her regular audiologist. She indicated that she would like to proceed with purchasing the reconditioned aid. When her audiologist found this to be an appropriate fitting, Ms. Bell's files were checked and it was determined that the reconditioned aid was actually her own aid and that it had been repaired by the dispenser merely by replacing the cracked earhook.

Problems associated with this experience could have been avoided if Ms. Bell would have been aware of what repair problems could be managed by her or the audiologist and which problems require repair by the manufacturer.

Batteries. Cell batteries are the usual power source for hearing aids and most ALDs. Battery size is specified by the hearing aid or device manufacturer. While some battery types may be used interchangeably (e.g., silver oxide, zinc air), the user will need to know how different battery types will impact differently on device performance. Battery size (e.g., 675, N, AAA) can be only as specified by device design. Because of battery size, particularly for some hearing aids, Pascoe (1990) suggests that the act of battery replacement be mastered before the new user leaves the dispenser's office. Small batteries may create difficulty for individuals with low vision and/or fine motor coordination problems. Also, it is common for new hearing aid/ALD users to question how long batteries should last or how they can determine when they should consider replacing their battery.

Batteries contain chemicals that may become harmful if swallowed.

Therefore, they should be stored away from children and pets in a way that they cannot be mistaken for pills. They should be discarded whenever they show any sign of leakage, and they should not be incinerated because of danger of explosion. When a battery is ingested, the individual should be rushed to a hospital emergency room and the National Battery Hotline called (collect) at (202) 625-3333 (Shimon, 1992). All of the above should be discussed in the hearing aid orientation period.

Battery cells used in hearing aids are available from pharmacies, grocery stores, radio supply stores, and hardware stores, as well as from hearing aid dispensers and hearing clinics. Battery cells used in ALDs generally are available from the same sources. Essentially, all personal, wearable hearing aids are powered by battery cells, including rechargeable cells. However, some assistive devices may draw power from their host appliance (e.g., telephone or television).

In counseling individuals in managing this aspect of hearing aid/ALD maintenance and use, we need to provide information regarding different types of batteries, their appropriateness for different systems, how to maintain battery function in humid conditions, how to use battery testers, and how to prevent unintentional battery drainage.

Protection from abuse.   New users should be encouraged to protect their hearing aids by inserting and removing them over soft surfaces to guard against accidental damage if they are dropped. Hearing aids and ALDs should be kept dry. Contact with extreme heat, water, creme, oil, or hair spray should be avoided. These substances may clog the microphone grid and/or cause internal components to malfunction.

Maximizing opportunities during the trial period.   During the trial period, new hearing aid/ALD users are encouraged to obtain maximum benefit from their amplification system, resting only when nervous or fatigued. In general, they should not remove hearing aids/ALD that they are enjoying and they should not wear a system that causes discomfort. New users should be encouraged to compare the quality of amplified sound and ease of listening in difficult situations with and without the new amplification system. Keeping a log of these observations will facilitate decisions regarding benefit and help the new user to make informed judgments concerning use and/or modification of amplification during the clinical trial. Such a log should contain information regarding amount of use, situations in which systems were used, listening ease, listening accuracy, problems encountered, and battery life.

It is important for the audiologist to maintain contact with the new hearing aid user during the trial period. At a minimum, new users should be encouraged to contact the audiologist when problems occur. It is helpful to set up a weekly telephone reporting schedule during the trial period. In some instances, weekly clinic sessions for small groups of new hearing aid users and family members may assist in developing trouble-shooting skills as well as provide an opportunity to provide information regarding self-management of hearing loss and to develop improved aided communication skill (see Appendix 9–2). Such sessions are particularly helpful in the early days of hearing aid adjustment when some new users need encouragement to take a calm, collected, and objective approach to hearing aid problem solving.

At the conclusion of the trial period, new users should be encouraged to keep the hearing aids if they are satisfied and return them if they are dissatisfied. If a major alteration or adjustment is required, the trial period should be reinitiated or extended and the term of a new trial should be specified in writing. Every effort should be made to avoid the sale of an instrument that will not be accepted and used.

Maintenance

Ideally, after a decision is made to accept the hearing aids, the experience of the trial period will have adequately prepared the new user to successfully manage recurring concerns relating to the use of amplification. New listening circumstances will create new challenges for those who depend on amplification. Changes in hearing ability and improvement in amplification system design and function will more or less ensure continuing attention to hearing loss and use of amplification.

While most new hearing aid users will not require audiological intervention beyond initial adjustment to amplification, some will benefit from an extended hearing aid orientation program or participation in a comprehensive aural rehabilitation program. Others may find it helpful to participate in meetings of hearing-impaired consumer groups, such as Self Help for Hard of Hearing People, (SHHH), an organization by and for hearing-impaired individuals to educate themselves and others in the causes, characteristics, problems, and possible remedies to hearing loss.

It is important for the audiologist to remain in contact with hearing aid users to provide an opportunity to assist with any problems or concerns relating to use of amplification. Scheduling annual hearing tests and regular hearing aid maintenance (e.g., electroacoustic check, visual and listening inspection, tubing changes, and battery contact and sound port cleaning) provides an opportunity to ensure continued adjustment to the use of amplification. It also is helpful to maintain contact by newsletter or periodic mailings of announcements of new products, assistive devices, improved hearing aids, and legislation or community events of particular interest to those with hearing loss.

CONCLUSION

Successful adjustment to the use of hearing aids and ALDs is a process in which the audiologist must be armed with knowledge of how hearing loss, acquired hearing loss in particular, impacts on an individual's ability to communicate and compete for and maintain personal independence in today's fast-paced society.

Bringing such a person to the point of accepting amplification may be easier than convincing that person to continue the self-adjustment process beyond a formal trial period, as so many candidates choose not to use amplification. However, knowledge of the personal characteristics of those who do succeed and of the reasons why professional recommendations to use amplification fail should better prepare audiologists to increase the probability of amplification system acceptance and use. Knowledge of newly mandated opportunities for access to communication under the Americans with Disabilities Act should encourage more hearing-impaired individuals to accept and use hearing aid and assistive device technology than has been our past experience. Finally, by understanding individual differences in the approach to hearing care delivery and by applying standard ethical business practices and highest-quality, client-centered professional services in the preselection, trial, and long-term use of amplification systems, audiologists will begin to close the gap between the number of hearing-impaired individuals who *could* benefit from amplification and the number who *do*.

REFERENCES

COMBS, A. (1986). *Hearing loss help*. Santa Maria, CA: Alpenglow Press.

COMPTON, C. L. (1989). *Assistive devices: Doorways to independence*. Washington, DC: Gallaudet University Press.

COX, R. M., & GILMORE, C. (1990). Development of the profile of hearing aid performance (PHAP). *Journal of Speech and Hearing Research, 33*, 343–357.

DAVIES, J. W., & MUELLER, H. G. (1987). Hearing aid selection. In H. G. Mueller & V. C. Geoffrey (Eds.), *Communication disorders in aging: Assessment and management*. Washington, DC: Gallaudet University Press.

DEPARTMENT OF JUSTICE. (1991a, July 26). 28 CFR Part 35 Nondiscrimination on the basis of disability in state and local government services: Final rule. *Federal Register, 56*(144), 35694–35723.

DEPARTMENT OF JUSTICE. (1991b, July 26). 28 CFR Part 36 Nondiscrimination on the basis of disability by public accommodations and in commercial facilities: Final rule. *Federal Register, 56*(144), 35544–35604.

EQUAL EMPLOYMENT OPPORTUNITY COMMISSION. (1991, July 26). 29 CFR Part 1630 Equal employment opportunity for individuals with disabilities: Final rule. *Federal Register, 56*(144), 35726–35755.

FEDERAL COMMUNICATIONS COMMISSION. (1991, August 1). 47 CFR Parts 0 and 64 Telecommunications services for hearing and speech disabled: Final rule. *Federal Register, 56*(148), 36729–36733.

FEIN, D. J. (1984). On aging. *Asha, 26*, 8, 25.

FINO, M. S., BESS, F. H., LICHTENSTEIN, M. J., & LOGAN, S. A. (1992). Factors differentiating elderly hearing aid wearers vs. non-wearers. *Hearing Instruments, 43*(2), 6, 8–10.

FRANKS, J. R., & BECKMANN, N. J. (1985). Rejection of hearing aids: Attitudes of a geriatric sample. *Ear and Hearing, 6*(3), 161–166.

GALLUP, F. (1980). *A survey concerning hearing problems and hearing aids in the United States*. Washington, DC: Hearing Industries Association.

GARSTECKI, D. C. (1988) Considerations for use of assistive devices by hearing-impaired adults. *Journal of the Academy of Rehabilitative Audiology, 21*, 153–157.

GARSTECKI, D. C. (1990). Hearing health knowledge of aging adults. *Journal of the Academy of Rehabilitative Audiology, 23*, 79–88.

GOLDSTEIN, D. P. (1984). Hearing impairment, hearing aids, and audiology. *Asha, 26*(9), 24–38.

GOOZNER, M. (1990, July 22). Workplace doors opening to disabled. *Chicago Tribune* (Business Section), pp. 1–2.

JOHNSON, C., & DANHAUER, J. (1982). Attitudes towards severely hearing-impaired geriatrics wearing hearing aids. *Journal of Speech and Hearing Disorders, 47,* 433–438.

KOCHKIN, S. (1991). Hearing professional's views on market expansion: Part 1. Why don't people buy hearing instruments? *Hearing Instruments, 42*(12), 6, 8.

LIBBY, E. R. (1990). Asking the non-buyer "why?" *Hearing Instruments, 41*(11), 26.

MADELL, J. R., PFEFFER, E. B., ROSS, M., & CHELLAPPA, M. (1991). Hearing aid returns at a community hearing and speech agency. *Hearing Journal, 44*(4), 18–23.

MARRER, J., & GARSTECKI, D. C. (1985). *Community-clinic management of hearing-impaired aging adults.* Paper presented at the Illinois Speech-Language-Hearing Convention, Chicago.

MORGAN, C. M. (1990). The over 50 population and their attitude toward health care. *Hearing Instruments, 43,* 8–9.

MUELLER, H. G., & GRIMES, A. M. (1987). Amplification systems for the hearing-impaired. In J. G. Alpiner & P. A. McCarthy (Eds.), *Rehabilitative audiology: Children and adults,* pp. 115–160. Baltimore: Williams & Wilkins.

NEWMAN, C. W., & WEINSTEIN, B. (1988). The HHIE as a measure of hearing aid benefit. *Ear and Hearing, 9*(2), 81–85.

PALMER, C. (1992). Assistive devices in the audiology practice. *American Journal of Audiology, 1, 2,* 37–57.

PALMER, C., GARSTECKI, D. C., & RAUTERKUS, M. (1990). *An interactive product locator for the selection of assistive devices.* Paper presented at the Annual Convention of the American Speech-Language-Hearing Association, Seattle.

PASCOE, D. P. (1990). Post-fitting and rehabilitative management of the adult hearing aid user. In R. E. Sandlin (Ed.), *Handbook of hearing aid amplification: Vol. 2. Clinical considerations and fitting practices,* pp. 61–86. Boston: College-Hill Press.

REBER, C. K. (1989). Motivation and the aging adult. *Hearing Instruments, 40*(4), 13–14, 16, 60.

REZEN, S., & HAUSMAN, C. (1985). *Coping with hearing loss.* New York: Dembner Books.

RIES, P. W. (1982). Hearing ability of persons by sociodemographic and health characteristics: United States. *Vital and Health Statistics,* Series 10, no. 140, DHHS Publication No. (PHS) 82-1568. Washington, DC: U.S. Government Printing Office.

SHEWAN, C. M. (1990). The prevalence of hearing impairment. *Asha, 32*(2), 62.

SHIMON, D. A. (1992). *Coping with hearing loss and hearing aids.* San Diego: Singular Publishing Group.

SKAFTE, M. D. (1992). Why hearing instruments cost what they do. Are hearing instruments too expensive? Are their prices truly excessive? *Hearing Instruments, 43*(2), 23–25.

SMEDLEY, T. C., & SCHOW, R. L. (1990). Frustrations with hearing aid use: Candid observations from the elderly. *Hearing Journal, 43*(6), 21–27.

STEPHENS, S. D. G., & GOLDSTEIN, D. P. (1983). Auditory rehabilitation for the elderly. In R. Hinchcliffe (Ed.), *Hearing and balance in the elderly* (pp. 201–226). London: Churchill Livingstone.

UNITED STATES ARCHITECTURAL AND TRANSPORTATION BARRIERS COMPLIANCE BOARD. (1991, July 26). Americans with disabilities act (ADA): Accessibility guidelines for buildings and facilities. *Federal Register, 56,* 144, 35455–35542.

WALDEN, B., DEMOREST, M., & HEPLER, E. (1984). Hearing aid performance inventory (HAPI). *Journal of Speech and Hearing Research, 27,* 49–56.

WEINSTEIN, B. E. (1991). Hearing aids at my age: Why bother? *Asha, 33*(12), 38–40.

APPENDIX 9–1
POSTFITTING ADJUSTMENT TO HEARING AID USE

A series of three, 90-minute postfitting sessions for small groups of new hearing aid users and their spouses, family members, or friends is intended to provide an extended hearing aid orientation-rehabilitation experience for those interested in information and discussion of matters relating to:

1. Hearing aid use
2. Hearing aid care and maintenance
3. Enhancement of hearing aid use with assistive listening devices
4. Improved access to employment settings, public accommodations, and telecommunication services

Topics for Week 1:

1. Experience with hearing aid use after 1 week. Participants discuss concerns related to hearing aid use that may not have been fully addressed or understood (or remembered) during the hearing aid fitting. Successes and failures in hearing aid use are shared. Problems noted during this discussion may suggest topics to be emphasized in subsequent sessions.

2. Reintroduction to hearing aids. General, brief review of the range of hearing aid styles and configurations. Microphone, amplifier, receiver, earmold, battery, external control, and special feature options (e.g., vents, tone controls) are identified and described.

3. Why your particular system is best for you. Brief, but personalized discussion of the hearing-loss characteristics (e.g., audiogram data) and personal amplification needs and preferences of each participant.

4. Earmold/hearing aid insertion and removal (as indicated). Earmold/hearing insertion and removal problems are addressed with individuals indicating a need for such information and/or demonstration.

5. Volume and tone control adjustment (as needed). Volume and tone control adjustment problems are addressed with individuals indicating a need for such information.

6. Batteries. Introduction to common battery sizes, numbers, and markings; battery substitution; common materials and their performance characteristics; battery life and factors that prolong and reduce battery drainage; how and where to purchase batteries; battery care, storage, and disposal; battery safety; and, general battery management.

7. Acoustic feedback. Acoustic feedback is defined. Instances in which it is likely to occur are explained: improper earmold/hearing aid seating, excessive volume control setting, cerumen-plugged ear canal, broken earhook and/or earmold tubing, loose fitting earmold and/or hearing aid, as well as improper positioning of telephone receivers. Procedures for remedying these problems are described and demonstrated.

8. Trouble-shooting an aid that sounds "funny." What to do when amplified sound is changed from usual is addressed in this portion of the program. Problems relating to battery power, microphone-telephone switch settings, aid power output settings, debris in the controls, internal malfunction, and earmold fitting are reviewed and remedies are discussed and demonstrated.

9. Aided listening strategies (general). Strategies for the new hearing aid user to apply to enhance success in interpersonal communication are reviewed and demonstrated. Emphasis is directed toward "stage-managing" difficult communication situations, developing appropriate assertiveness in modifying the communication behavior of others, developing strategies for verifying unclear information, developing strategies for positioning oneself for optimal listening, reading facial expression and body language, and the like.

10. Assistive device needs assessment. Participants are surveyed in regard to interest in or need for information relating to management of telephone communication (amplification and/or decoding devices), television amplification (or captioning devices), personal communication (for listening at a distance or in noise), and environmental alerting and warning needs. This is accomplished using assistive device locator software or questionnaires.

11. Hearing aid benefit survey (pretest). Participants are asked to complete one of several possible standardized questionnaires to evaluate hearing aid benefit to identify additional problems to address in the postfitting series, to determine the need for more extensive intervention after the scheduled series, and to discover ways in which the postfitting series might be modified and improved in the future.

> Handout materials
> Listings of area theaters, houses of worship, and public meeting places with special accommodations and/or amplifying devices for hearing-impaired persons.

Topics for Week 2:

1. Experience with hearing aid use after 2 weeks. Again, this introductory exercise provides an opportunity for participants to discuss their successes and failures in hearing aid use after 2 weeks' trial.

2. Tips for using the telephone with your new hearing aid. Strategies for using the hearing aid microphone and the telephone, the hearing aid telecoil and the telephone, the hearing aid and a telephone receiver equipped with an electromagnetic coupler, the hearing aid and a pocket amplifier or FM receiver or infrared receiver attached to the telephone and coupled to the ear using a neckloop, and the hearing aid and an infrared transmitter attached to the telephone with an infrared receiver-neckloop coupling system are reviewed and demonstrated in this portion of the program.

3. Hearing aid use in employment settings (as indicated). Addresses problems relating to hearing aid use on the job that may typically involve telephone, individual, and small-group communication in quiet and noisy settings. The unique problems of program participants are discussed. Information concerning federal regulations applying to access to employment for hearing-disabled individuals under the Americans with Disabilities Act is reviewed.

4. Cerumen management. Advice regarding self-use of cerumenolytic agents is provided and options for professional management of cerumen-related problems are discussed. Procedures for removing cerumen from the ears of hearing aid users are described, and procedures for removing cerumen from earmolds, tubing, and hearing aids are demonstrated.

5. Earmold care and maintenance. Points to address in visual inspection of earmolds and tubing are discussed. Procedures used to troubleshoot and repair earmold and tubing problems are demonstrated.

6. Trouble-shooting "dead" hearing aids. What to do when hearing aids stop working is covered in this portion of the program. Incorrect control or switch settings, battery position, battery power, plugged earmolds, plugged tubing, plugged sound ports, broken wires, plugged ear canals, changes in hearing sensitivity, and related factors are reviewed, and suggestions for resolving common problems are discussed and demonstrated.

7. Repair management. This topic clarifies which hearing aid troubleshooting and repair problems can and should be managed by the user, which should be referred to the audiologist-dispenser, and which problems the audiologist-dispenser are likely to refer to the manufacturer for resolution.

8. Assistive listening devices (direct audio input-BTE hearing aids and pocket amplifiers). The range of direct audio input options for BTE hearing aid users and of pocket amplifiers for all hearing-impaired individuals is presented and demonstrated. Advantages and limitations in their use are discussed. Factors to consider in selection and use are highlighted.

9. Hearing aid use in places of exhibition, entertainment, or public gathering. Addresses problems relating to hearing aid use in noisy public settings that may involve use of group or room amplification systems. The unique problems of program participants are discussed. Information concerning federal regulations applying to provision of access to places of exhibition, entertainment, or public gathering for hearing-disabled individuals under the Americans with Disabilities Act is reviewed.

Handout materials
Listings of area, state, regional, and national organizations concerned with problems relating to hearing loss.

Topics for Week 3:

1. Experience with hearing aid use after 3 weeks. Again, this introductory exercise provides an opportunity for participants to discuss their successes and failures in hearing aid use after 3 weeks' trial.

2. Aided listening in noise (strategies, problems, and concerns). The nature of noise as an acoustic masker, the concept of signal-to-noise ratio, strategies for minimizing the effect of noise on message understanding, impact of binaural amplification, noise suppression hearing aid circuitry, and assistive devices to enhance hearing aid use in noise are reviewed and demonstrated.

Problems relating to hearing aid use in noisy, public settings that may involve use of group or room amplification systems and problems relating to hearing aid use in telephone communication, including use of telephone amplifiers, text telephones, and telecommunication relay services are reviewed. Unique problems of program participants are discussed. Information concerning federal regulations applying to provision of access to stations for public transportation, recreation, exercise, and education and for access to telecommunications for hearing-disabled individuals under the Americans with Disabilities Act is reviewed.

3. Trouble-shooting hearing aids with moisture problems. What to do when hearing aids suffer from moisture problems is covered in this portion of the program. Potential problems relating to water accidents, sweating, and humidity are reviewed, and suggestions for their resolution are discussed and demonstrated.

4. Assistive listening devices (telephone and television amplifiers, multiple-use devices). The range of telephone and television amplifiers and multiple-use devices is presented and demonstrated. Advantages and limitations are discussed, and factors to consider in selection and use are highlighted.

5. Assistive listening devices (alerting and warning systems). The range of alerting and warning systems is presented and demonstrated. Advantages and limitations in their use are discussed. Factors to consider in selection and use are highlighted.

6. Aided listening strategies (anticipatory). Strategies for the hearing aid user to apply in anticipating problems in interpersonal communication are reviewed and demonstrated. Emphasis is placed on wearing hearing aids and eyeglasses; closing the speaker-listener gap; moving to quieter versus noisier areas; avoiding rooms with poor acoustics; anticipating vocabulary and dialogue from current events, the situation, or people in the environment; anticipating environmental problems; and considering ways to be appropriately assertive.

7. Aided listening strategies (repair). Strategies for the hearing aid user to apply in resolving problems that may occur in interpersonal communication are reviewed and demonstrated. Emphasis is directed toward identification of the most efficient and effective repair strategies to use in problem situations.

8. Warranties and insurance policies. Hearing aid and assistive device warranties are explained. Usual warranty terms and coverage are explained. Differences between warranties and insurance policies are described. Owner responsibilities for in-warranty and out-of-warranty repairs are clarified. Loaner aids and their advantages and disadvantages are discussed.

9. Federal and state regulations. Legal conditions applying to the hearing aid delivery system and consumer rights in dealing with problems in the fitting and purchase of hearing aids are reviewed.

10. Hearing aid benefit survey (posttest). Participants are asked to complete a resurvey of self-perceived hearing aid benefit in order to identify the need for more extensive intervention after the scheduled series and to identify ways in which the series might be modified and improved to address issues important to future new hearing aid users.

11. Hearing loss management program options (adult aural rehabilitation program, community speechreading classes, hearing-impaired consumer/self-help groups). Those who demonstrate an interest or need for extended rehabilitative service and/or peer socialization or more information regarding self-management of hearing loss are apprised of what is available in their community and how to obtain more information regarding enrollment in such programs.

> Handout materials
> Brochure on music for the hearing impaired
> Membership application to Self Help for Hard of Hearing People (SHHH)
> Listing of ALD distributors and ordering information
> Explanation of how to find otologists (otolaryngologists), audiologists, hearing aid dispensers, and hearing aid services

APPENDIX 9–2
HEARING AID USE AND REPAIR*

Identify your hearing aid style from the descriptions that follow. Then refer to care, use, and trouble-shooting hints for your particular aids below.

Hearing Aid Styles

a—*Behind-the-Ear* (BTE). Shrimp-shaped unit worn behind the ear and coupled to the ear by an earmold and tubing.

b—*In-the-Canal* (ITC). Finger-tip-shaped unit worn down the ear canal.

c—*Custom-Ear* (CE). One-piece unit filling the outer ear and opening to the ear canal.

d—*Eyeglass*. Built into an eyeglass frame (temple portion) and coupled to the ear by an earmold and tubing.

e—*Body*. Pocket-worn unit with a wire connecting it to a receiver and earmold.

Hearing Aid Care and Maintenance

a b c d e Keep your *hearing aids clean*. Use a *dry* tissue and *soft*-bristled toothbrush, pipe cleaner, or a wax loop to remove ear wax and debris from the hearing aid's outside casing. The microphone opening must be kept free of ear wax and debris at all times. Do *not* insert sharp objects, such as needles or pins, into the microphone opening or any other openings in the hearing aid case unless advised to do so by your dispenser.

a b c d e Keep your *hearing aids dry*. Sweat, humidity, and water accidents may cause your hearing aids to malfunction and could result in permanent damage. For routine care, use a drying agent available from your dispenser. In the event of a water accident, return your hearing aids to your dispenser for a drying agent, repair, or replacement.

a d e Keep your *earmolds clean*. The earmold opening must be kept free of ear wax and debris in order for hearing aids to function properly. If the earmold requires cleaning, detach it from the hearing aid and wash it with warm water and mild soap. Use a toothbrush to clean the outside and a pipe stem cleaner or wax loop to remove debris from difficult-to-reach surfaces. Rinse, then blow any remaining water or soap out of the earmold tubing and let dry before reattaching to the hearing aid. Do *not* use excessive heat, such as from a hair dryer or oven, for drying purposes, as heat may damage the earmold tubing.

a d Keep your *earmold tubing fresh*. When earmold tubing becomes discolored or brittle, have it replaced by your dispenser.

a b c d e Manage *batteries* properly. Keep the batteries fresh. Do *not* maintain more than a 6-month supply. Do *not* mix old and new batteries. Carry batteries only in a container, not loose. Store batteries in a cool, dry place. Remove the battery when hearing aids are not being used. Always carry a spare.

---

*Prepared with the assistance of P. Fiebig, lecturer, clinical supervisor, and director of clinical services in audiology, Northwestern University.

Remember, batteries may be harmful if swallowed. Keep them out of reach of children and pets.

If Your Hearing Aids Whistle

a d e   Check to see if your earmolds are seated properly. If not, remove and reinsert.

b c   Check to see if your hearing aids are seated properly. If not, remove and reinsert.

a b c d e   You may have excessive ear wax. Have your physician, or your dispenser, check your ear canals and remove excessive ear wax.

a d   Your tubing may have a hole in it. Have your dispenser check for cracks, splits, or holes in the earmold tubing and replace the tubing if necessary.

a b c d e   With continuous whistling, return the aids to your dispenser. They may need to be refitted to your ears or they may need to be repaired.

NOTE: It is normal for most hearing aids to whistle when the microphone opening is covered by a hat or hand or when the aids are turned on, but not in the ear. Whistling poses a problem when it occurs at unexpected times (e.g., when turning one's head or when bending one's head down), or when it occurs before reaching an optimal volume setting.

If Amplified Sound Cuts Off and On

a b c d e   Electrical contacts may be dirty. Move all controls and switches on and off (back and forth) to note occurrence of problem. Return hearing aids to the dispenser for repair.

a b c d e   Battery contacts may be dirty, corroded, loose, or broken. Battery surfaces may be dirty. If dirty or corroded, try cleaning battery contacts and battery surfaces with a pencil eraser. If battery contacts are loose or broken, return hearing aids to the dispenser for repair.

a d e   Moisture may be in the hearing aid, earmold, tubing, or battery compartment. You may even see droplets in the earmold or tubing. When this occurs, remove the earmold and tubing and clean and dry as indicated above. Dry the battery contacts and the battery. Use a drying agent to remove moisture from the hearing aid case. See your dispenser for a drying agent and instructions in its use.

b c   Moisture may be in the hearing aid case or battery compartment. Dry the battery contacts and the battery. Use a drying agent to remove moisture from the hearing aid case. See your dispenser for a drying agent and instructions in its use. This should definitely be the course of action when the symptoms worsen near the end of the day.

a d   You may be bending the earmold tubing when you insert the earmold or turn your head. Check appearance of tubing while wearing the hearing aid and note signal consistency when turning your head.

a d   Check dampers placed in the tubing to see they are not plugging the tubing. Return to hearing aid dispenser if this appears to be the problem.

a b c d e You may have a defective battery. Replace with a new battery.

If Your Hearing Aids Do Not Work at All

a b c d e Be sure that you are using the recommended battery.

a b c d e Check to see that the battery is inserted correctly into the hearing aid, according to the manufacturer's instruction booklet.

a b c d e Battery contacts may be dirty, corroded, loose, or broken. Battery surfaces may be dirty. If dirty or corroded, try cleaning battery contacts and battery surfaces with a pencil eraser. If battery contacts are loose or broken, return hearing aids to the dispenser for repair.

a b c d e The battery may be weak or dead. Test the battery or try a fresh battery. Try one from a different package to be certain. You may have purchased a defective batch of batteries.

a b c d e Check the battery door. Be sure it is closed completely when the hearing aid is in use.

a b c d e Check earmold and/or the receiver opening to see that it is free from ear wax and debris.

a b c d e If your hearing aids have a "T" switch, check that the microphone switch is on "M" for everyday listening and on "M" or "T" (telephone) for telephone listening.

a d Check to see that earmold tubing is not bent, crimped, or plugged with moisture.

e Check the cord leading from the hearing aid to the receiver and cord connectors for breaks.

a b c d e Use the hearing aid at room temperature with batteries at room temperature.

chapter ten

Helping People Cope with Hearing Loss

Samuel Trychin

The success of group intervention depends on the same counseling skills audiologists have already found necessary in providing emotional support for patients and families. In this Chapter, Dr. Trychin presents an approach to working with communication difficulties that can be a powerful adjunct to the individual services more typically offered to hard-of-hearing adults and their families. Dr. Trychin suggests positive ways of leading groups that will enable individuals to find their own solutions to residual communication problems and the stress these problems inevitably add to life.

> All experience is an arch to build upon.
> Henry Brooks Adams
> *The Education of Henry Adams*

INTRODUCTION

Audiologists who work with hard of hearing people and their families in group aural rehabilitation settings will find a wide variety of reported concerns and problems related to hearing loss. This chapter is a synopsis of a program for hard-of-hearing people and their hearing family members that I have been conducting for the past 6 years to help address these concerns and problems. I have focused efforts on trying to understand the psychosocial ramifications of hearing loss and attempting to develop strategies and procedures that help in reducing the psychological and interpersonal distress related to hearing loss. Because much of this distress results directly from communication problems, my approach has been to find ways to help people prevent or minimize those problems.

Audiologists may find it particularly helpful when working with hard-of-hearing adults and their families to remember that how people perceive communication problems (i.e., their meaning or significance to the people involved) is a very important factor to consider. For example, some hard-of-hearing people believe that, due to their hearing loss, they are a burden on other people, and this belief leads them to withdraw from social contact and also probably leads to depression. As another example, many people believe that hearing aids correct hearing problems to the same degree that glasses correct visual problems. It is difficult for people holding this belief to understand why a person wearing hearing aids does not understand what is being said, and it does not occur to them to think about doing anything else to remedy the situation. So, included in the programs I conduct are some ways to help people separate fact from fiction pertaining to hearing loss, and methods for helping hearing-impaired people develop a more realistic appraisal of themselves and their hearing problem (Trychin & Wright, 1988).

This program is strongly cognitive-behavioral in its orientation and procedures, but also includes behavior therapy concepts and procedures related to stress management (Trychin, 1986a, 1986b, 1987c). (See Dr. Clark's discussion in Chapter 1 for a review of cognitive and behavioral counseling theory.) It also emphasizes delivering accurate information about hearing loss and assistive and alerting devices (Bally & Trychin, 1989).

BACKGROUND OF THE COPING STRATEGIES PROGRAM

I am a psychologist by training and have been wearing hearing aids since 1953. From 1981 to 1985, I taught a variety of courses at Gallaudet University on topics related to stress management. Hearing, hard-of-hearing, and deaf graduate students, staff members, and teachers were enrolled in these classes. I began to see marked differences in the problems and concerns reported by the hearing, hard-of-hearing, and deaf people in these classes.

In the fall of 1984, I went to see Rocky Stone at the national office of Self Help for Hard of Hearing People (SHHH), and we agreed that I would conduct a stress management class for staff and volunteers at the SHHH office starting in January 1985. By 1986, it was apparent that there is a great demand for such classes, and I was enabled to devote full time to teaching them. Since then, I have taught more than 60 such classes in 21 states including Hawaii.

The course requires about 45 hours to cover the main material, and I teach it in one of two formats—an intensive 45-hour class that meets for 5 or 7 days for 7 to 9 hours per day, or a 15-week class that meets for 3-hour sessions once a week. The 15-week class has the advantages of being less exhausting for participants and allowing time for homework assignments to be completed between sessions. I limit the number of participants to 12 in the 45-hour classes in order to provide each person full opportunity to participate in every discussion.

Maintaining Focus

Although the content discussed during class sessions is highly personal and often elicits strong emotional responses, we make every effort to keep an educational focus and to avoid becoming a therapy group. One effective way to accomplish this is to establish a problem-solving orientation and keep the focus on problem-solving techniques. Adhering to a "What can be done about it?" and "Here's what I've tried that works" response to problems that participants raise helps to avoid lapsing into a mutual-sympathy group. Providing a variety of concrete, alternative strategies for dealing with communication problems maintains the focus on problem solving. Keeping the discussion focused on communication problems that are related to hearing loss is essential in maintaining an educational orientation. It is not always easy to distinguish between those problems that are due to hearing loss, those that are exacerbated by hearing loss, and those that are unrelated to hearing loss. But discussing this distinction can help keep people from blaming all their problems on hearing loss.

Another tactic that aids in keeping the group focused on problem solving is to clearly state and write down the goals and objectives of the class at the outset. There are a number of things that can be accomplished through these classes. One thing that many people report at the end of the class is that they are more accepting of their hearing loss or the hearing loss of their spouse or other family members. They report being more optimistic about being able to cope with hearing loss, and there is often an elevation of mood. These are all desired outcomes, and I believe that they are a result of achieving a number of objectives.

Course Objectives

The first objective is to teach participants to identify those situations in which they experience communication problems. Then they are taught to pinpoint the specific causes of the communication difficulties in those situations. Doing this helps people define the parameters of their communication problems, and affords greater objectivity when considering alternative solutions. Another objective is to teach participants to identify their patterns of response when they encounter communication problems. When they are able to do that, they are in a position to identify those responses that serve to make the communication situation worse and those that improve it. Anxiety, anger, depression, bluffing, dominating conversations, or withdrawing does not improve communication. Learning effective communication behavior can, however, significantly improve the communication situation.

A very important objective is to provide an opportunity for participants to practice effective communication behavior and to receive feedback about how well they are doing. One of the strengths of the group format is that it creates many opportunities for observing participants' communication behavior. Effective communication behavior can then be reinforced and faulty behavior can be corrected. In the same way, the class sessions provide ample opportunity for participants to get hands-on experience with a variety of assistive listening devices. Once they experience the benefits of these devices, they are more open to the consideration of acquiring them for use outside of the class sessions.

Another objective is to provide participants with information about their own hearing loss and about hearing loss in general. This serves to correct unrealistic expectations about what can be heard in a variety of listening situations. Sometimes, people have unreasonably high expectations about what they will be able to understand in certain situations and they often suffer disappointment as a result. More often, though, people have unreasonably low expectations about what they can understand and unnecessarily forgo many pleasurable experiences as a result. By altering the communication environment, participants often learn that they can, in fact, understand most of what is said, provided certain conditions prevail.

Achieving these objectives allows participants to anticipate communication problems before they occur. This objective is the culmination of all those preceding and provides participants with a means of preventing or reducing the frequency and severity of communication problems. Based on the experiences of group members, communication problems likely to occur in specific situations such as those that occur at family gatherings at holidays, in restaurants, or during business meetings are identified and listed. Specific actions that can be done to prevent or reduce these problems are then discussed and listed. This strategy allows people to be proactive and achieve a large measure of control over the communication problems they experience.

Obviously, there is much going on during the group sessions, and conscious effort is required by the group facilitator to keep the members on task in order to achieve the objectives and goals. The following rules are very helpful in keeping the group on track and achieving a smooth and orderly flow of events.

Group Rules

No bluffing. Encouraging people to raise their hands immediately when they fail to understand what is being said strengthens a necessary communication skill and ensures that all participants are understanding what is going on.

One person speaks at a time. This rule cuts down background noise and confusion and helps participants learn to focus attention on what is being said at any given time.

Whoever talks must use the microphone. We always use an induction loop system, and when several people are using the telecoil switch on their hearing aids, they cannot hear what is being said when the speaker does not use the microphone. This practice also serves to slow the communication process sufficiently so that the hard-of-hearing people can keep up, helps other participants identify who is speaking, and reduces inappropriate cross-talk.

We treat each other gently and with respect.   This rule enables us to identify and alter interchanges among participants that serve to put people off. If someone is offended by what or how something was said, we stop the interchange and say something like, "Could you say that in a way that the person will want to hear what you are saying?" Especially in intensive group sessions in which people are tired at the end of the day, it is important to minimize irritated, blaming, or sarcastic remarks. This rule goes a long way toward helping participants recognize aspects of their own communication behavior that may be turning other people off.

Leader Rules

Obviously, as in everything else, when conducting groups people have their own style and methods of doing things. Group leaders will differ in what they see as important or trivial. Still, a few of the things that we have learned may be helpful within the context of achieving the objectives discussed previously.

Do not preach.   Very few people can sit and pay attention for long when they are not actively involved in what is going on. Lecturing to people will put them to sleep very quickly, particularly if sessions are long. Even worse, they may not really be interested in what you are saying or, similarly, you may not be addressing what they want to discuss.

Ask questions.   Find out at the beginning what they are concerned about. Make a list of the issues they want to discuss, and cover those issues in subsequent sessions. If you know what you want them to know, you can either tell them, or ask the questions that will draw the response from them. When it comes from them, it is theirs, and they will remember it. Asking questions also keeps them involved in the process and will help keep participants alert. By asking questions we have the opportunity to learn something new. It is wise to remember that they, not we, are the experts in their lives.

Be prepared.   When you involve the participants in discussion and draw the material from them, you have to know what it is you want them to know. Being prepared also allows you to clearly see when discussion is being sidetracked from the topic at hand.

Make sure that everyone in the group is understanding most of what is being said even if you have to do a lot of writing on a chalkboard or newsprint.   There are few things worse than a hard-of-hearing person going to a session about coping with hearing loss and not understanding what is being said. This may be the final failure that results in the person giving up altogether.

Do not embarrass people. Even when a comment is off the point or wrong, avoid responses that may make the person feel or look foolish. Inadvertently embarrassing one group member often has the effect of dampening the other members' motivation to speak out.

Do not allow one or two people to hog the floor. If someone is allowed to dominate discussion, the advantages of the group format are reduced, and some members are likely to drop out.

Have people take turns in responding. One way to control the fact that some people are reluctant to say anything and others may want to talk incessantly is to have people take turns in responding. A time limit can help people organize their thoughts and get to the point, which is most helpful to hard-of-hearing people anyway.

Do not get caught in arguments about who or what is right or wrong. If someone does not agree with something you have to say, listen carefully to the reasons; it is another way to learn something. If there is a stalemate, leave it to a "Well, I see your point there, but we'll have to agree to disagree. Very little in life is black or white." Remember, you could win the argument, but lose the group.

Do not get caught trying to be an expert in the experience of hearing loss if you are not hard-of-hearing. You are an expert in many things related to hearing loss but, unless you have a hearing loss yourself, you cannot know how hard-of-hearing people and their hearing family members react to hearing loss.

Provide feedback about the communication behavior that occurs in the class sessions. This is one of the most valuable things you can do as a group facilitator, and when you have done it well, group members will begin to do it, too. I use play money, and whenever someone displays good communication behavior, I give him or her some money. Then I ask the participants what I gave the money for. They have to identify the behavior, and this procedure brings it to their conscious attention. I also use a humorous rubber figure whose eyes, ears, and tongue pop out when squeezed to signal incorrect communication behavior. It looks funny, and people usually laugh. I always use the latter on myself whenever I talk too fast, forget to use the microphone, or talk while facing the chalkboard. It is very important that people learn that feedback about communication behavior does not mean criticism; the goal of providing feedback is to develop the realization that when people talk in a particular way, communication problems are likely. When they talk in a different way, communication problems are less likely. Morality—good versus bad—is not involved at all.

Following these guidelines when conducting classes can help people who may never have conducted such classes before to avoid making costly mistakes. Audiologists can provide a much-needed service in their communities by making these kinds of classes available to hard-of-hearing people and their families and friends. Many audiologists do offer aural rehabilitation services, often on an individual basis. Based on my experience, I believe that the group format is much more efficient, addresses a wider variety of issues, and produces positive changes that are greater in number, more enduring, and occur much more rapidly. One reason for this, I believe, is that the group format is much less threatening to participants and, therefore, they are less defensive and more open to change. This may largely be due to the fact that group participants see that many of the problems they experience are shared by other people in similar circumstances. The problems are seen as "our" problems and as something that goes along with hearing loss. Many people report that they no longer feel that there is something wrong with them as individuals.

Participants in the group format also get innumerable, helpful suggestions from other people who they see as being in the same boat and, thus, having credibility. When people in the class raise a problem or concern they have been experiencing, others in the class may recognize for the first time that they are also experiencing that problem, or that the problem, such as depression, relates to their hearing loss. There is also a social ambience that develops as the people meet to share problems and experiences and the resultant mood persists long after the class is over. Because of these factors, I try, whenever possible, to see that people enroll in such a group rather than seeing them individually.

PROBLEM SITUATIONS FREQUENTLY REPORTED BY HARD-OF-HEARING PEOPLE AND THEIR HEARING FAMILY MEMBERS

Hearing loss is a communication disorder and, as such, affects everyone in the communication loop. Those people who interact most frequently with the hard-of-hearing person will probably be affected most by communication breakdowns. Hearing spouses are probably affected more than other family members. Those who interact most frequently with the hard-of-hearing person also have more opportunity to contribute to communication problems. It is my belief that full understanding of the effects of hearing loss can be achieved only by examining its effects on both listener and speaker. For this reason, I strongly encourage hearing family members and friends to participate in classes along with the hard-of-hearing person. It is very likely that those hard-of-hearing participants who are accompanied by hearing family members achieve the best results. This would be expected when communication problems are viewed as a function of both speaker and listener behavior. In fact, I have seen many situations in which the best solution to communication problems would be for the hearing spouse to get speech therapy.

When the hearing spouse does not know what to do to improve communication and the hard-of-hearing person cannot pinpoint what needs to be changed, anger, recrimination, and distancing are likely to ensue. When both sides have been educated about how to pinpoint the causes of communication problems and what to do to reduce them, successful resolution of such problems is more likely. The first step is to identify the range of situations that are likely to produce difficulty for hard-of-hearing people as a group.

Uncertainty about whether they have understood what has been said is a major source of anxiety for many hard-of-hearing people. There are four possibilities in communication situations: (1) Listeners know they have understood what has been said, (2) listeners know they did not understand what has been said, (3) listeners are not sure they understood what has been said, and (4) listeners think they understood what has been said but, in fact, did not understand correctly. Typically, situation 4 results in the worst problems and situation 3 the next worst for hard-of-hearing people. In situation 2 or 3 the hard-of-hearing person obviously can ask for clarification of what has been said. However, the typical response is to ask for one repetition and often to not pursue it further for fear of irritating the speaker.

Being excluded from conversations is a common experience for hard-of-hearing people, even in their own families. Hearing people often talk past them or about them without including them in the discussion. In a similar way, statements like "It wasn't important," "I'll tell you later," or "Never mind" in response to a query about what has just been said can have a devastating effect on hard-of-hearing people and lead them to believe that they are not important enough to be included.

Negative reactions from speakers can produce major discomfort in hard-of-hearing people. When the speaker feels irritation, anger, or frustration due to communication difficulties and having to repeat, the hard-of-hearing person may detect signs of these feelings and refrain from asking for further clarification of what has been said. Many hard-of-hearing people are very sensitive to such signs and will resort to bluffing (pretending to understand) when they appear. Some hard-of-hearing people have developed such a dread of asking people to repeat that they refrain from doing it altogether.

Difficulties using the telephone can cost the hard-of-hearing person a job, lead to feelings of isolation, or create major hassles in getting information from banks, stores, airlines, and so on. Irritation and arguments frequently result from having a family member make telephone calls for the hard-of-hearing person because the family member may not relay sufficient information or may resent making the call.

Missing out on valued sources of personal enjoyment due to one's hearing loss is a frequent complaint. Going to the opera, listening to music at home, or going to the theater or movies may no longer be feasible or possible for many hard-of-hearing people. Such losses may be difficult to replace through other activities and may contribute to depression.

As professionals working with hard-of-hearing people and their families, we are all aware of a number of other difficult communication situations. These may include difficulties that arise when the speaker fails to get the listener's attention before talking, when conversing within a group with multiple conversations, when topic transitions are omitted or missed, when conversing in a moving automobile, or simply when listening in the presence of competing noises or environmental sounds. At the beginning of a recent workshop, I asked all participants to tell us an issue, problem, or concern related to hearing loss that they would like to see discussed. Among the topics requested are situations listed above and others that are troublesome for hard-of-hearing people and their families. Table 10–1 lists the topics this particular group wanted to discuss.

Within the topics in Table 10–1 are items raised by hard-of-hearing people and items raised by hearing family members. In addition to the items listed in Table 10–1, there are four major complaints frequently voiced by hearing family members (Trychin, 1988b). The most frequently reported complaint is the frustration resulting from not knowing when hard-of-hearing people have understood and when they have not. A second major complaint relates to the confusion caused by the fact that the hard-of-hearing person seems to understand quite well sometimes and not at all at other times. The third frequently reported complaint by hearing family members is loneliness resulting from reduction in the spontaneity of verbal interactions at home, reduction in shared activities (e.g., going to movies, plays, restaurants, or entertaining friends), and loss of intimacy, sexual and nonsexual, in the relationship. A fourth complaint often voiced by hearing family members is that the hard-of-hearing person is too dependent on them. This dependency usually takes the form of relying on the hearing family member(s) to act as an interpreter and repeat whatever other people are saying. Serving as a "walking hearing aid" becomes tiresome very quickly.

These, then, are the kinds of problems that the hard-of-hearing and hearing family members in our classes want to deal with. The same issues arise in class after class and in different geographic areas, indicating that the problems

TABLE 10–1 Frequently Reported Issues, Concerns, and Problems

How to deal with being avoided by co-workers
How to raise confidence or self-esteem
How to be more assertive
How to deal with my own and others' irritation and frustration
How can the family cope with the hard-of-hearing person
How to survive at family gatherings such as holiday dinners
What to do in noisy situations
What to do so I do not have to repeat so often
Where to meet other hard-of-hearing people in my community
How to understand when there are multiple conversations
How to survive when going out to restaurants, and so on
How to tell other people what to do so I can understand them
How to get someone to stop talking from the other room
How to keep someone from turning the television up so loud
What to do to help someone be less dependent on me
How to deal with the isolation I feel at work
How to keep from losing friends
How to keep from feeling dumb or incompetent
How to know whether I understood
How to deal with the anger I feel because of my hearing problems

and concerns of hard-of-hearing people and their families, as a group, are highly predictable. Audiologists may find it useful to uncover their patients' and patients' families personal issues of concern in an effort to yield more fruitful discussions and extend the scope of their services.

An issue of great importance needs to be addressed at this point. Among the 1,000 plus people I have seen in these classes, probably more than 90% of the hard-of-hearing people already have hearing aids, and most of them have been using them for years. Yet these hearing aid users are experiencing the communication problems cited above. This indicates that hearing aids alone do not prevent or resolve communication problems for many of the people who use them. Advertisements that indicate otherwise are, for many people, incorrect and may lead to disappointment for unwary buyers. Perhaps, this accounts for some of those people whose hearing aids reside in the bureau drawer.

FREQUENTLY REPORTED RESPONSES
TO COMMUNICATION PROBLEMS

How people respond to communication problems influences the communication circumstance itself. Some reactions serve to improve the situation by resolving the difficulty and preventing or reducing further communication problems. Other responses have the effect of making the situation worse and increasing the likelihood of further communication difficulties. When the speaker says something and the listener fails to understand what has been said, both people will respond in some way.

If listeners indicate that they have not understood and offer a concrete suggestion for resolving the difficulty (e.g., "I need you to face me when you speak"), chances are good that the problem will be resolved. If, on the other hand, listeners bluff, pretending to have understood, there is no way to clear up the misunderstanding, and the likelihood of further communication problems is probably increased. If speakers show irritation at being asked to repeat, listeners may well become anxious or annoyed, and such emotional states can serve to render further communication difficult. Therefore, it is important to ascertain how people typically respond when communication problems occur and to determine what will be the likely effect of these responses on ensuing communication.

Table 10–2 shows the kinds of responses frequently reported by participants (hard-of-hearing *and* hearing people) in our classes when asked the question "What happens, i.e., what do you experience or what do you do, when communication problems occur?" (Trychin, 1991, pp. 25–41).

The responses in Table 10–2 are the kinds of responses that often serve to make situations worse. If hard-of-hearing people bluff, for example, they will become increasingly lost as the conversation continues and run the risk of being discovered by the speaker, who in turn may become angry and choose to terminate the discussion. Bluffing also deprives the listener of the opportunity to practice effective communication behavior, such as informing speakers that they need to

TABLE 10–2   Frequently Reported Responses to Communication Problems

Frustration	Withdrawal
Headaches	Embarrassment
Muscle tension	Fatigue
Anger	Inability to concentrate
Stomach problems	Difficulty thinking
Anxiety	Guilt
Depression	Bluffing
Domination of conversations	Loss of appetite
Crying	Sleep problems
Irritability	Situation avoidance
Low self-esteem	

slow down. A hard-of-hearing person who has developed a habit of bluffing also frequently loses the opportunity to practice paying attention to the speaker. Paying attention is a skill that deteriorates with lack of practice. Hard-of-hearing people are at risk for losing the ability to pay attention, and lack of attention may be a greater factor in many misunderstandings than the hearing loss itself.

If the person develops a headache, the pain will at least partially distract attention away from the speaker and probably result in decreased understanding of what the speaker is saying. If listeners try to dominate the conversation in an attempt to reduce the chance of misunderstanding what the other person might say, they lose the opportunity to practice effective communication behavior, as well as the opportunity to practice paying attention, and may lose friends as well. If listeners become tired from straining to hear what is said, they will find it more difficult to pay attention and will understand less of what is being said.

People also report adaptive responses that serve to improve the situation such as informing others about what they can do to be better understood. I make every effort to reinforce these adaptive responses whenever they are mentioned or occur during sessions.

As groups, hard-of-hearing people and the hearing people who relate to them report highly predictable responses; but there are many differences in how individuals respond. Understanding the effects of hearing loss in each individual case requires information about that person's audiological status, current family and work situation, and the coping methods used. In particular, it is important to pinpoint exactly what happens in current situations that produce communication problems for the individual (i.e., what the person does, thinks, and feels). In dealing with any issue related to hearing loss it is necessary to know why the people involved do or do not do the things that could be helpful for them.

We know, for example, that most of the people who could benefit from hearing aids do not have them and that some of those who do have them do not use them. One could resort to the concept of denial as a way of explaining this. But there are many other reasons why people fail to acquire or use hearing aids, and we have uncovered more than 25 of these reasons so far (Trychin, 1990). Table 10–3 presents a sample of these reasons. It is likely that the steps taken to help a

TABLE 10–3 Some Reasons Why People Do Not Acquire or Use Hearing Aids

Attracts unwanted attention
Other priorities, that is, health or relationship problems
Lack of money
Transportation problems
Fine or gross motor coordination problems
Overstimulation, that is, hears unwanted sounds
Afraid of physicians and other health professionals
Do not know how to operate a hearing aid
Pain in ear canal
Family resistance
Requires time to adjust to aided sounds
Too high expectations of what hearing aids can do
Too low expectations of what hearing aids can do
Previous bad experience with a hearing aid dispenser

person acquire or use hearing aids will be somewhat different for each reason, and that each individual will need to be seen and handled differently.

IDENTIFYING THE CAUSES OF COMMUNICATION PROBLEMS

Many hard-of-hearing people I have worked with had the belief that the communication problems they experienced were solely the result of their hearing loss. This misconception often leads to the erroneous belief "Because I have a hearing loss, communication is 100% my responsibility." This belief then leads to guilty feelings if the speaker has to put out more effort to be understood and contributes to the reluctance of many hard-of-hearing people to inform speakers about how to communicate so that they can be understood.

There are many factors that contribute to misunderstandings other than degree or type of hearing loss, and they can frequently be reduced or eliminated (Trychin, 1991, pp. 17–21). These causes of communication problems fall into three categories—speaker factors, environmental factors, and listener factors. Examples of each are presented in Table 10–4.

Teaching people to identify the causes of communication problems helps them to view these experiences more objectively and to understand that communication is the responsibility of the speaker as well as the listener, and that it is to the benefit of both to optimize the environmental conditions. Once the cause(s) of a communication breakdown are identified, solutions become evident. The hard-of-hearing person then has something concrete to do to deal with the problem, and that is the essence of coping behavior: expending effort to solve a problem.

When hearing people who relate to hard-of-hearing people can identify the causes of communication problems, they are much less apt to be mystified by them and much less likely to make statements such as "She can hear me when she wants to." Instead, for example, the hearing wife is more apt to realize that the hard-of-hearing husband understands better in the morning than in the evening

TABLE 10–4 Sample of Causes of Communication Problems

SPEAKER FACTORS	ENVIRONMENTAL FACTORS	LISTENER FACTORS
Voice loudness	Background noise	Level of hearing loss
Rate of speech	Poor lighting conditions	Type of hearing loss
Clarity of speech	Poor acoustics	Improper use of hearing aids
Lack of or conflicting facial expression	Interfering objects	Failure to pay attention
Lack of or conflicting body language	Visual distractions	Emotionality
Foreign accents/dialects	Lack of use of visual aids	Distracting sensations
Facing away from listener	Unavailability of ALDs	Distracting thoughts
Objects in mouth	Distance from sound source	Poor speechreading skill
Distracting mannerisms	Poor angle of vision	Bothersome tinnitus
Emotionality, that is, angry, upset, and so on	Inadequate room ventilation	Unrealistic expectations
		Fatigue

because he is less tired then. Hearing family members are then also better able to pinpoint their own contribution to communication problems and make appropriate corrections, such as facing the hard-of-hearing person before talking.

COPING WITH ENVIRONMENTAL BARRIERS

Once people are able to identify environmental conditions that interfere with understanding what is being said, they are in a better position to deal with them, and there are several ways of doing so. A direct approach is to find ways to alter the environment by adjusting lighting, reducing background noise, and removing obstacles and distractions. This is easy to accomplish in one's home or office, but many people are reluctant to ask for such changes in other situations. When to do so is always a judgment call. If there is loud background music at a party where people are standing around talking, there will probably be little resistance to asking the host to turn the music down. If, on the other hand, most people are dancing, such a request might well be denied.

Another way to deal with interfering environmental conditions is to position oneself in the best possible place in that setting. If loud music is coming over a stereo speaker 3 feet from where we are holding a conversation, I could ask you to step over to the other side of the room with me in order to hear you better. We could move to a spot where I could see your face more clearly. These things seem obvious, but some people are very reluctant to make these types of request and suffer needless communication hassles.

Our concern is that too many hard-of-hearing people never make attempts to modify environmental conditions, or positioning, even in situations where it would be appropriate and helpful. Talking about this in class and having participants cite examples of instances in which they have been successful in seeking environmental change can "give permission" to others to try it. Some people may need further assistance and practice in being assertive in this regard.

To assist in positioning it is also helpful to anticipate what is likely to cause problems for hard-of-hearing people in a given situation and plan ways to minimize such problems. At lectures, for example, this will require arriving early or having a seat reserved in advance, both of which involve some planning. Hard-of-hearing people need to learn not to walk unprepared into situations, but to anticipate and plan strategies for minimizing communication problems.

When dealing with environmental barriers to understanding, hard-of-hearing people may need to alter their expectations. In some situations it isn't possible to alter the environment or choose one's location within it. If the situation is such that there is little possibility of understanding what is being said, it is probably better to accept that fact and relax rather than to struggle to hear and become upset. The danger is that some people set their expectations too low in many situations and miss out on much that they could hear if they adopted either or both of the strategies discussed above. Some others set their expectations of what they can hear too high and are constantly disappointed.

USING ASSISTIVE LISTENING DEVICES

Of all the various coping strategies we cover in our classes, the one that can have the most dramatic and instantaneous result is having people try assistive listening devices (ALDs). Many people are amazed at what they can hear when using ALDs, and their use brings some people to tears with the realization that they do not really have to exist in a world of virtual silence. However, as Flexer (1991) points out, if audiologists fail to introduce the variety of technologies that hard-of-hearing people need to access varied listening environments, then those with hearing loss are forced to function with unnecessary barriers. A discussion of the limitations of hearing aids can stimulate interest in trying ALDs. Once people experience the benefits of frequency-modulated (FM), hard-wired, and/or infrared systems, they often become more optimistic about their ability to overcome communication problems in a variety of situations.

Another topic related to ALDs that requires discussion is the function of telecoil switches on hearing aids. Unfortunately, many people are not aware that telecoils are useful beyond their telephone function. Given their usefulness, it is a shame that so many people have hearing aids without telecoil switches. In work and educational settings, using an ALD together with a telecoil switch on a hearing aid can make the difference between success and failure for some people.

In my experience people need to practice using ALDs within different settings in order to fully understand their benefits. Merely talking about them or displaying them is insufficient to demonstrate what they are able to do for people with hearing loss. Even when they have experienced the positive results of using ALDs, however, some people are reluctant to purchase them. Their use in public certainly attracts more attention than wearing hearing aids, and some people would rather not hear than be the focus of unwanted attention. It is likely that many of the reasons that people do not acquire or wear hearing aids cited previously in Table 10–3 also pertain to ALDs. Allowing people to role-play situations, such as using an ALD in a restaurant while other diners are staring at it, can help them overcome embarrassment about its use.

MODIFYING COMMUNICATION BEHAVIOR

As indicated previously, speaker and listener behaviors often contribute to communication difficulties. Most often, hard-of-hearing people are unable to correct faulty communication behavior on the part of the speaker. Frequently, they will say things like, "Huh?" "What?" "I'm sorry." "Would you repeat that?" "I didn't get what you said." or "Excuse me; I have a hearing loss." All of these responses are wrong in the sense that they provide the speaker with no information about what to do to correct the communication problem. These responses need to be replaced by those that clearly inform speakers about what they need to do to be understood.

Speaker Guidelines

There are numbers of guidelines or rules for effective speaker communication behavior that, if followed, can prevent or reduce communication problems (Trychin & Boone, 1987; Trychin, 1991, pp. 88–91). A list of specific guidelines for speaker communication behavior is presented in Appendix 10–1 and may be photocopied for use as class or individual handouts. When discussing speaker guidelines with hearing family members or others interacting with the hard-of-hearing person, the following considerations regarding a speaker's communication behavior should be stressed.

Speakers need to know that getting the hard-of-hearing person's attention before speaking will prevent a great many communication problems and result in their having to repeat less. But it is equally important for them to consider how to get the person's attention. A jab in the back, a loud, "Hey," and intruding into the individual's "personal space" are examples of attention-getting behaviors that are likely to result in that person becoming irritated and not caring to listen to what is being said. Approaching from several feet away and gently waving a hand to attract attention is much more preferable. Another important consideration is when to get the person's attention. If the hard-of-hearing individual is engaged in an activity that might cause a problem if interrupted, such as taking something hot out of the oven, it is probably better to wait until that activity is finished. In this regard it is wise to reinforce the fact that hard-of-hearing people ordinarily cannot do two things at one time when one of them involves trying to understand what someone else is saying.

When speakers alter their communication behavior as outlined in Appendix 10–1, the communication problems are reduced to a manageable level and speakers feel less frustrated and irritated. Unfortunately, not many people are aware of such guidelines and are caught in a seemingly endless chain of hassles whenever they talk to the hard-of-hearing person. It happens all too frequently that hearing family members may attempt to avoid communication problems and the need to repeat by refraining from talking to the hard-of-hearing person. They sometimes do this by ignoring the hard-of-hearing person and speaking instead to a hearing family member who happens to be present. "How is Uncle John doing?" directed at Aunt Mary while John sits 2 feet away is one example. People need to be told to direct their questions and comments about the hard-of-hearing person to that person. Otherwise, the hard-of-hearing person becomes, at best, a marginal member in any group situation even in the family. Many complain that they do not belong anywhere—not in the deaf world and not in the hearing world.

Listener Guidelines

Sometimes, hard-of-hearing people themselves fail to recognize that aspects of their behavior contribute to or cause communication problems. There are numbers of specific things that hard-of-hearing people can do to prevent or reduce communication problems (Trychin & Boone, 1987; Trychin, 1991, pp. 92–97). A list of specific guidelines for hard of hearing listeners to follow in communication situations is presented in Appendix 10–2. Again, when providing the guidelines within the appendices, it is helpful to stress the following information.

Informing others of a hearing loss. A very important consideration has to do with informing other people about one's hearing loss. Some hard-of-hearing people make it a habit to do this right away when they first meet people, and others never do it. Still others wait until they are having trouble understanding what is being said. It is always a judgment call whether or when to inform other people about the hearing loss, but not doing so usually means that the person also does not inform the speaker about what to do to be understood (thus increasing the probability of communication failures). A second problem with not informing others about one's hearing loss is that they, not knowing about the listener's hearing loss, may resort to other explanations of an off-the-wall response. For example:

SPEAKER:	"My mother died last week."
HARD-OF-HEARING PERSON (NOT UNDERSTANDING AND BLUFFING, SMILES):	"Oh, that's nice."

How can such a response be interpreted if the speaker does not know that the other person has a hearing loss and has misunderstood? Most frequently, such *gaffes* are interpreted as signs of low intelligence, "mental" problems, insensitivity, rudeness, and so on. The risk of failing to inform others about one's hearing loss is the increase in occurrence of such misinterpretations and the possibility of damaged relationships.

Another issue in this regard is how the person introduces his or her hearing loss. Usually, as a matter of fact, positive statement of the loss is sufficient. "I have a hearing loss, and I'll let you know if I don't understand something you say." This is better than being apologetic or prophesying problems as in, "Gee, I have this awful problem understanding, I hope you won't be upset and walk away." Those people who have never made a practice of informing others of their hearing loss often need help in formulating and practicing a simple, direct statement. They may also profit from homework assignments that allow them to practice informing others in situations that are graded in difficulty from least to most threatening.

Hard-of-hearing people often make the erroneous assumption that once someone has been informed of their hearing loss, that person will remember forevermore. They also may believe that once they have informed the other person about how to best talk to them, that person will remember to do it on all ensuing occasions. Life is just not that simple. Communication behavior is complex and unconscious (in the sense that people are usually more concerned about what they are saying than about how they are saying it). For these reasons, it is hard for people to change their communication behavior. If I have been talking fast for 50 years, learning to slow down to accommodate my spouse's recent hearing loss won't happen overnight. Additionally, if my spouse is the only person who fails to understand me when I talk fast, and I get away with it with many other people during the day, it will be difficult for me to learn to slow down when talking to her.

What usually happens is that, when reminded, speakers will modify their communication behavior, for example, by talking more slowly for a minute or two and then will forget and lapse back into their habitual way of talking too fast. If the hard-of-hearing person has to constantly interrupt speakers to remind them of helpful ways to speak, frustration and irritation are likely to arise in both people. It is often helpful for the people involved to agree on hand signals to serve as reminders for speakers to slow down, speak a little louder or more softly, or remove a hand from in front of their faces. These signals remind people without the necessity of interrupting verbally.

It is helpful in reducing negative emotional reactions to point out to hard-of-hearing people and hearing family members that we are all human beings and, as such, we forget, and we forget often. Hard-of-hearing people sometimes harbor anger toward hearing people because they hold the faulty assumption that because these people know about the hearing loss, they should always adapt their communication behavior to accommodate the hard-of-hearing person. Understanding that people simply forget and that hard-of-hearing people have a responsibility to remind them, as unobtrusively as possible, can go a long way toward alleviating anger.

Improving attention. Hard-of-hearing people also often become angry when accused of not paying attention. Unfortunately, the accusation is frequently correct. Paying attention is a skill and, as with other skills, practice is required to maintain it at a functional level. Anything the hard-of-hearing person does that interferes with or prevents the practicing of this skill (bluffing, withdrawing, controlling conversations, etc.) will result in its erosion. Furthermore, it is difficult to pay attention in situations in which one does not understand much of what is being said. There is a natural tendency to drift off into one's own thoughts. So hard-of-hearing people are at risk for losing the ability to pay attention, and this fact may account for a great deal of the misunderstandings that occur. In such cases it is not the hearing loss per se that produces the misunderstanding, but the lack of attention to the speaker. If situations are arranged so that hard-of-hearing people understand most of what is being said, they are likely to pay better attention, and a positive cycle is established. The following case illustrates how inattention can develop and how devastating it can be.

I was conducting a 7-day coping strategies course, and 12 participants had registered. The evening before the first class there was a general orientation to the facility in which the course was being held. We had placed an auditory loop around three rows of chairs for the people in our class and anyone else who might be wearing a hearing aid with a "T" switch. I sat in the fourth row, and an elderly couple came in and sat in front of me in the third row. After every statement made by the speaker, the elderly hard-of-hearing man would lean over to his hearing wife and ask, "What did he say?" She would repeat every statement to him. After about 5 minutes of observing this, I leaned forward and asked if he had a "T" switch on his hearing aid. He answered affirmatively, and I told him that if he would turn it on, he could hear directly from the loop system. He said, "My 'T' switch is on."

I separated this couple during our class sessions, with him sitting at one end of a long table and her sitting at the other end. We also used an auditory loop during our sessions. At the end of the first day, I asked him how much he had understood. He shook his head in despair and responded, "Only about five percent." At the end of the seventh day, I repeated the same question, and his response was, "About ninety-five percent. When I think of how low I had sunk, I get goose bumps on my flesh. I want to thank you one and all." Had his hearing improved that much during one week? What had happened was that he had learned to pay attention again. His wife was also much relieved to get out of her role as a "walking hearing aid."

This is an example of a dependency habit that was so overlearned that it overrode direct information input. This elderly gentleman had become so dependent upon his wife for spoken information that he no longer received it directly from its source. This example indicates the extent to which inattention can be a factor in communication problems.

Another reason that hard-of-hearing people may have difficulty paying attention is fatigue. Long discussions requiring sustained visual attention are very tiring for hard-of-hearing people. Arranging the environment in ways that facilitate understanding as discussed previously will alleviate some of the strain and allow for less frequent breaks, but there should be at least one break every hour when communication demands are high, as in business meetings.

Providing feedback to speakers. Along with making a real effort to pay attention, hard-of-hearing people need to learn to inform speakers whether they have understood what has been said. This addresses the complaint that many hearing people express that they frequently do not know whether they are being understood. A nod or thumbs-up signal can serve to inform hearing people that they have been understood. However, for important information that can produce major problems if misunderstood, verbal feedback is best. Who, what, when, and where should always be repeated aloud so that the speaker knows the information has been correctly received. Also, it is important to request a clarification of the specific item that was missed as in, "Did you say July 30th?" In that way the speaker doesn't have to repeat everything that was said.

If something said has not been understood, speakers need to be prompted about what specifically to do so that they will be understood. "Huh?" "What?" "Please repeat that," and the like are ineffective in informing speakers about what to do to be understood. Statements such as "Please raise the volume of your voice," "Please face me when you talk to me," "Could you paraphrase that for me? I seem to be missing one of the main words," or "I need you to slow down a little" are much more effective because they provide information about what to do.

It is important that hard-of-hearing people learn to tell speakers when they are doing well. "Your voice volume and speed are just right; I'm understanding just about everything you're saying" provides important information to the speaker about how to best communicate. It is also a nice verbal "pat on the back" and is appreciated as such. It is always possible to find something that the speaker is doing well and to find ways to reinforce that behavior as a way of strengthening the relationship. No one likes to hear only about what is wrong.

It can be useful to remind hard-of-hearing people that other people also have rights and that there needs to be a balance in situations so that the needs of the hard-of-hearing person are weighed against those of the hearing people. If, for example, a hard-of-hearing person is not understanding what is being said in a group discussion, should the person interrupt the others and ask for a repeat following every statement missed? There are no hard-and-fast rules to apply, and it always requires judgment to arrive at a decision about how frequently to interrupt to ask for a repeat. Much depends on the importance of the information being conveyed.

Another issue for consideration involves when to interrupt speakers to inform them that one has not understood. A good rule is to let the speaker know as soon as it becomes clear that one has not understood. Waiting until the speaker has continued further will require a lengthier repetition, which may produce frustration and irritation on the part of the speaker.

A third issue is how to interrupt. Hand signals or signs can be preferable to verbally interrupting because they can prompt speakers to alter their communication behavior without stopping the flow of conversation. A hand with the palm turned upward moving in an upward direction can be used to signal the speaker to increase voice volume. A woman in one of our groups taped signs on a ping-pong paddle. One side said, "Please slow down." The other side said, "Thank you."

This simple device helped me to alter my communication behavior in an unobtrusive and polite way. Agreement about the use of such signal systems should be worked out with the people involved at the outset of the particular communication situation.

When there has been a misunderstanding, the easiest situation to deal with occurs when hard-of-hearing people know they have not understood. More difficult to deal with are those times hard-of-hearing people think they have understood but did not. The following is an example of the latter situation.

I was traveling in a car from the Los Angeles airport to Riverside, California, with four other people. The woman sitting to my right in the back seat of the car lived in the area we were passing through. I had never met her before, and to be sociable and to make conversation, I asked her about the name of the large tower we were passing. In response she said, "It's not very far." I responded by saying that she had misunderstood my question and repeated my query about the name of the structure we had passed. She responded more loudly and with some irritation, "It's not very far." At that point I was becoming frustrated and irritated, but was determined to clear up the misunderstanding. I was absolutely convinced that she had misunderstood what I was asking. I repeated my question for the third time, asking the name of the structure we had passed "back there." Obviously annoyed, she responded, "It's Knottsberry Farm." If one says aloud "Knottsberry Farm and "not very far" the reason for the confusion becomes apparent.

In this example I was absolutely convinced that I was "right" and she was "wrong." This is a trivial example, and we have both had several good laughs over it, but think about the many situations in which such a misunderstanding might have serious social, employment, financial, legal, or medical consequences.

Often, such a misunderstanding as in the preceding example is not apparent until later when the person shows up at the wrong place or at the wrong time or hasn't completed a task that had been assigned. To prevent this it is essential that hard-of-hearing people provide feedback about what they understood the speaker to have said. A simple summary of key points is often sufficient: "Party, next Saturday, at Bill's house, eight o'clock. OK, I'll be there." The time and effort required to repeat key points is usually insignificant compared to what might happen if there has been a significant misunderstanding.

How hard-of-hearing people provide feedback or request changes in communication behavior is very important. One of the things I discovered early in working with hard-of-hearing people and their families is that some of them knew what to do, but did it in such a way as to turn other people off. Issuing demands ("You'd better speak up!") instead of making requests is a turn off. Tone of voice, facial expression, and other body language can have as much effect on other people as the particular words spoken. Interactions that serve to make other people angry, anxious, or guilty are not likely to result in cooperation and understanding. Most often, people are not aware of the negative effects of their own behavior on other people and need help in identifying such behavior and learning how to change it (Trychin, 1987a, 1987b).

Furthermore, some families do not have much success resolving any problems or disputes including communication issues. In these families almost any attempt at resolving a problem someone is experiencing results in argument and hurt feelings. In such a family, the hard-of-hearing person may feel hopeless about getting someone to change behavior (e.g., getting the hearing husband to stop talking from the next room), and may have given up on asking for any change. Such families may need to develop problem-solving skills before they can begin to resolve communication problems related to hearing loss (Forgatch & Trychin, 1988a, 1988b).

Audiologists can provide a much-needed service to hard-of-hearing people and their families by finding ways to inform them about the issues discussed in this section and by acquainting them with the guidelines listed in the appendices. My experience indicates that the vast majority of these people do not have this information and do not know where to turn for help in dealing with the communication problems they encounter daily. As a result, they are forced to deal with these frustrating encounters in a reactive, nonproductive fashion that too often results in damaged relationships.

TEACHING GROUPS TO ANTICIPATE PROBLEMS AND PLAN SOLUTIONS

Helping people learn to anticipate problem situations is, as indicated previously, a major goal of a good coping program. In order to be able to anticipate, it is helpful for people to (a) know the situations that are likely to cause communication problems, (b) be able to identify the specific causes of communication difficulties in those situations, (c) refrain from behaviors that are likely to create or exacerbate communication problems, and (d) be able to do those things that are likely to prevent or reduce communication problems.

If the likely causes of communication problems in a given situation are known, the person can plan strategies for avoiding or reducing them. For example, people who have difficulty understanding waiters in restaurants can get the menu and a list of specials before going to the table and know exactly what to order when the waiter arrives. This will not eliminate all questions (we have all had the experience of ordering black coffee only to be asked, "Cream and sugar?"), but it will reduce their number. Given any situation, people can generate a list of possible things to do to prevent or reduce communication problems. I have used a problem-solving format that I call "The 15 Things Method" with great success (Trychin, 1991).

This method is a brainstorming procedure designed to elicit a large number of suggestions or possible solutions for specific problems. First, the problem is clearly stated. "I have difficulty in social situations" is too vague. A better statement would be "I have difficulty understanding people at parties where there is a lot of conversation noise and loud music playing." When everyone clearly understands the nature of the problem situation, each participant, in turn, is asked to suggest a possible solution. We keep going around the room that way until all suggestions have been given. All suggestions are written down. Censoring is not permitted at this point; that is, statements such as "That's silly," "That won't work," "I already tried that," "He'd never agree to that," and so on, are not allowed. Such censoring punishes the person who made the suggestion and may inhibit the flow of ideas.

People are encouraged to say whatever ideas come to mind. Sometimes the one that seems the most far out when mentioned turns out to be the best alternative. We do not let the process stop until at least 15 suggestions have been listed. When the list of ideas has been completed, we give the list to the person who raised the problem. That person can then ask the group questions in order to clarify certain points. The person then selects those suggestions that feel most comfortable and tries them out. In subsequent sessions the person informs the class about what worked and what did not work and gets further suggestions if necessary.

In one session The 15 Things Method for the problem situation "going out to eat in a restaurant without getting all stressed out and losing my appetite" yielded helpful suggestions, including (a) to call ahead to make a reservation for a time that is before or after the busiest (and noisiest) hours, (b) to reserve a table in a quiet and adequately lighted area—explain the requirements to the person taking the reservation, (c) when arriving at the restaurant, to ask to see the menu and a listing of any specials of the day before going to the table, and (d) to inform the server that you have a hearing loss and what you need him or her to do (speak at a moderate pace, keep face unobstructed, etc.) so that you will understand.

This process of anticipating and planning helps people focus on the specifics of situations that cause them problems and engenders a problem-solving orientation that is helpful in keeping emotional reactivity in check. It is also useful in teaching them to develop strategies for preventing or reducing communication problems and to employ more adaptive ways of responding when they do occur.

STRESS MANAGEMENT

This section is included in order to indicate how the information discussed previously can be brought to bear on a specific problem area. Stress is ubiquitous these days, and hard-of-hearing people and their families seem to have more than their fair share of it. From the perspective of this chapter, stress reactions are of major importance because they serve to increase the probability of occurrence and severity of communication problems. The variety of psychological, physiological, and social manifestations of stress (or more accurately, distress) negatively influence the person's ability to pay attention to what is being said and often have a detrimental influence on relationships. For example, one of the effects of anxiety is that sufferers can experience difficulty thinking and/or focusing attention.

Increased muscle tension resulting in pain in the neck or shoulders or headaches competes for attention with whatever is going on in the environment. Anxious people can be irritable and short with others, causing them to want to terminate the interaction. When these things happen, people may blame hearing loss for the breakdown in communication, when in reality it may be due to the anxiety reactions.

Anxiety reactions may create a cycle in which communication problems produce anxiety, the anxiety contributes to further communication problems, which, in turn, cause increased anxiety. The major goal in such cases is to help the people involved find ways to break the cycle and, ultimately, to prevent its occurrence.

Reducing Distress through Improved Communication

Helping people prevent, reduce, or better manage the distress related to communication difficulties may be approached by arranging the listening situation so that communication problems are prevented and/or reduced as discussed earlier, using assistive and alerting devices to intervene directly to make improvements in the communication situation, or by following the guidelines for effective communication behavior listed in the appendices of this chapter. Reducing the number of communication problems experienced in these ways can have an immediate, positive effect on mood, self-esteem, and morale and may be sufficient to enable the people involved to adjust to the hearing loss and get on with their lives.

Reducing Distress by Modifying Beliefs

A second way to proceed in reducing distress stemming from communication problems related to hearing loss is helping people identify and change unrealistic beliefs (Trychin & Wright, 1988). Some generally held, culturally determined beliefs can lead to undue distress for hard-of-hearing people and those who interact with them. Those males, for example, who believe that admitting to any infirmity or that asking for help is a sign of weakness may not disclose their hearing loss, acquire hearing aids, or ask others to alter their communication behavior. The result is that the number of communication problems experienced, and the distress related to them, will be much higher than they need be. Some women hold the unrealistic, culturally determined belief that a "good woman" takes care of other people. A woman having such a belief may encourage dependency in a hard-of-hearing spouse by intervening in all communication with other people. This results in an undue burden for her and prevents the spouse from engaging in effective communication behavior that might otherwise reduce the number of communication problems experienced.

Certain beliefs more closely related to hearing loss also produce distress reactions in many hard-of-hearing people. One is, "Because I have the hearing loss, resolution of communication problems is 100% my responsibility." Those holding this erroneous assumption place themselves under needless psychological pressure and its resulting physical tension. In addition, this belief prevents one from requesting others to modify their communication behavior, resulting in communication problems multiplying instead of being resolved.

Another unrealistic belief held by some hard-of-hearing people is that they will automatically be rejected if others find out they have a hearing problem. This belief leads people to attempt to hide the fact of their hearing loss and resort to bluffing to cover it up. Bluffing leads to anxiety that one may be discovered at any moment, and to the anxiety that stems from not really knowing what is being said. A related, dysfunctional belief increasing distress is that it is a terrible thing to misunderstand what someone is saying and that this is a sign of general incompetence.

It is frequently the case that these kinds of beliefs produce greater distress than the communication situations themselves. Helping people identify and alter these kinds of beliefs is an effective way of preventing distress reactions. A review of cognitive therapy and how it may be applied to help modify nonconstructive beliefs is presented by Dr. Clark in Chapter 1.

In many instances hard-of-hearing people and their family members hold dysfunctional beliefs, faulty assumptions, and unrealistic expectations because they do not have adequate or correct information about hearing loss. Many with whom I have worked had never before met another hard-of-hearing person. Such people function in an information vacuum that lends itself to the development of inaccurate and maladaptive ideas. An effective way to rectify this is to encourage them to join both the national organization Self Help for Hard of Hearing People (address given in Appendix 10–3) and its local chapter in their area. This consumer organization offers a wide variety of useful information about hearing loss and provides opportunities to meet other people sharing similar experiences.

Reducing Distress Reactions

A third way to proceed in managing distress is to work on reducing the distress reactions themselves. For example, many people experience a great deal of physical tension when communication problems arise. This increased tension may result in neck or shoulder pain or headaches that distract the person's attention. Relaxation training provides people with a method for reducing physical tension and serves to remove a major source of the discomfort associated with communication problems. In addition, relaxation is an effective procedure for preventing the buildup of the fatigue that is so frequently reported. It also provides a sense of self-control that can increase self-esteem. Increased self-esteem, in turn, can have the benefit of allowing the person to take the risk of requesting speakers to change some aspect of their communication behavior, such as saying, "Please face me when you speak."

Another example of dealing directly with distress responses is helping people to resist withdrawing from difficult communication situations. Physically withdrawing, terminating a discussion, or "tuning out" are frequently reported responses to the distress resulting from communication breakdowns. Avoiding or withdrawing from these situations prevents the development of effective communication skills and contributes to the deterioration of the ability to pay attention. Providing constructive alternatives to withdrawing, such as teaching the various methods for preventing or reducing communication problems discussed previously, is an effective procedure for dealing with the tendency to escape from difficult situations.

CONCLUSION

I have found that an effective way to help people overcome the negative psychosocial consequences of hearing loss is to help them find ways to prevent or reduce the communication problems resulting from that hearing loss. I have also found that an efficient way to achieve this is to include the hearing members of the family in the process and to focus attention on their problems that stem from relating to someone with a hearing loss. My experience indicates that a group format with an educational orientation including both hard-of-hearing people and the hearing people who frequently relate to them provides fairly rapid, beneficial changes in behavior, mood, and beliefs.

A major area for direct intervention involves the communication situation itself, including properties of the physical environment in which the communication occurs, the use of assistive listening devices, speaker behavior, and aspects of listener behavior. I have attempted to point out the specific changes that can be made in each of these areas to prevent or reduce communication problems. I have also indicated that changing behavior, even simple behavior, is difficult and requires practice with feedback. Just telling people what they ought to do is frequently not enough—especially when dealing with communication behaviors.

Another area of concern is what the people involved believe about hearing loss, its attendant communication problems, and the person who has it. There are many faulty assumptions and beliefs about hearing loss, hearing aids, and people who are hard of hearing that are held by both hearing and hard-of-hearing people. These faulty cognitions often need correction before lasting behavior change will occur.

Ultimately, audiologists would like to see hard-of-hearing people, and the hearing people to whom they frequently relate, able to pinpoint the specific causes of their communication problems, anticipate those problems in upcoming situations, and plan strategies for preventing or reducing those problems. When that happens, they function more effectively and feel better about themselves.

Audiologists are in a unique position to help their hard-of-hearing patients and family members identify and prevent or reduce many of the hearing-loss-related problems they experience on a daily basis. Providing such service in one or two individual consultations may not be as efficient or effective as meeting with a group of people over an extended period of time.

REFERENCES

BALLY, S., & TRYCHIN, S. (Eds.). (1989). *A newcomer's guide to an old problem: Hearing loss*. Washington, DC: Gallaudet University Press.

FLEXER, C. (1991). Access to communication environments through assistive listening devices. *Hearsay, 6*(1), 9–14.

FORGATCH, M., & TRYCHIN, S. (1988a). *Getting along* (manual). Washington, DC: Gallaudet University Press.

FORGATCH, M., & TRYCHIN, S. (1988b). *Getting along* (videotape). Washington, DC: Gallaudet University Press.

TRYCHIN, S. (1986a). *Relaxation training for hard of hearing people: Trainee's manual*. Washington, DC: Gallaudet University Press.

TRYCHIN, S. (1986b). *Relaxation training for hard of hearing people* (videotapes). Washington DC: Gallaudet University Press.

TRYCHIN, S. (1987a). *Did I do that?* (manual). Washington, DC: Gallaudet University Press.

TRYCHIN, S. (1987b). *Did I do that?* (videotape). Washington, DC: Gallaudet University Press.

TRYCHIN, S. (1987c). *Relaxation training for hard of hearing people: Practitioner's manual*. Washington, DC: Gallaudet University Press.

TRYCHIN, S. (1990, April/May). Why people don't acquire and/or wear hearing aids. *Shhh*, pp. 13–16.

TRYCHIN, S. (1991). *Manual for mental health professionals: Part 2. Psychosocial challenges faced by hard of hearing people*. Washington, DC: Gallaudet University Press.

TRYCHIN, S., & BOONE, M. (1987). *Communication rules for hard of hearing people* (manual). Washington, DC: Gallaudet University Press.

TRYCHIN, S., & WRIGHT, F. (1988). *Is that what you think?* Washington, DC: Gallaudet University Press.

APPENDIX 10–1
COMMUNICATION GUIDELINES FOR SPEAKING
TO PEOPLE WITH HEARING LOSS*

1. Be sure to get the hard-of-hearing person's attention before you speak. Saying the person's name and waiting for an acknowledgment before beginning can greatly decrease your need for repetitions. Similarly, keep in mind that the individual with a hearing loss may not hear the soft sounds of someone entering the room. Calling the person's name as you are approaching or knocking on the door (even if it is open) is a gentle means of alerting the individual that someone is coming.

2. The speaker should never speak directly into the ears of someone with a hearing loss, since this, of course, makes it impossible for the listener to make use of visual cues. Research has shown that the addition of visual cues can raise the intelligibility of received speech by approximately 20%.

3. Do not put obstacles in front of your face and always speak without anything in your mouth. Pipes, cigarettes, pencils, eyeglass frames, chewing gum, and so on, are distracting to those with hearing loss who may be using visual cues from the speaker's lips and face.

4. Speak clearly and decrease your speech to a slow-normal rate to allow the listener to "catch up." Pausing between sentences can also be helpful.

5. Do not hesitate to ask the listener if you are speaking at an effective level. Typically it is helpful to speak slightly louder than normal, *but do not shout.* Too much loudness can actually distort the speech signal in an ear with hearing loss.

6. Use facial expressions and gestures to supplement what you are saying. Facial expressions do not mean overarticulation. Overarticulation not only distorts the sounds of speech, but also the speaker's face, making the use of visual cues more difficult. Everyone reads lips (known today as 'speech reading'). Some do this more proficiently than others, but we all do it, either consciously or subconsciously. Facial expressions and gestures help clarify the message seen on the lips. To maximize these nonverbal signals, be sure there is adequate lighting on your face. Remember that for the hard of hearing, face-to-face communication is a must, with an optimal distance for communication exchange between 3 to 6 feet.

7. Alert the listener with a hearing loss that the subject is shifting when changing topics during group or individual conversations. A statement such as the following can be helpful: "We're talking about last night's Red's game, Tom."

8. If the person with a hearing loss does not appear to understand what is being said, try rephrasing the statement rather than simply repeating the misunderstood words. Quite often the same one or two words in the sentence will continue to be missed during each repetition. Rephrasing eliminates many frustrations. This is extremely important, but much too often overlooked.

---

*Compiled by Samuel Trychin, John Greer Clark, and Marjorie Boone.

9. Avoid conversation if the television or radio is playing, or if the dishwasher is running, and so on. If you are talking with a person who has a hearing loss, invite that person to move with you to the other side of the room where it might be less noisy.

10. Talk to hard-of-hearing people, not about them. Too often hearing family members may avoid the need to repeat by talking around the person with a hearing loss. "How is Uncle John doing?" may be directed to Aunt Mary while John is 2 feet away. In such instances, the hard-of-hearing person becomes, at best, a marginal member in any group situation.

11. Communication with a hard-of-hearing person can be difficult at times. If you can follow these guidelines and remain patient, positive, and relaxed, you will find the benefits worthwhile. When you become impatient, negative, and tense, communication will become more difficult.

12. When in doubt, ask the hard-of-hearing person for suggestions about ways to improve communication.

APPENDIX 10–2
COMMUNICATION GUIDELINES FOR PEOPLE
WITH HEARING LOSS*

1. Dimly lit and noisy areas can create difficult listening situations even for those with normal hearing. For those with hearing loss such areas can greatly increase the listening difficulties encountered. Whenever possible, if you find yourself in a poorly lit or noisy area, invite your communication partner to an area more appropriate for conversing.

2. With a little preplanning it is often possible to anticipate difficult listening situations and thereby lessen their impact. As an example, if going out for dinner make reservations for a less busy (noisy) time and tell the host you would like a seat in a well-lit area away from high-traffic areas. Similarly, arriving early to a meeting or lecture will allow you to select a seat that may allow you to hear better.

3. When you misunderstand what has been said, do not simply ask for a repetition. Tell the speaker you have a hearing loss and what is helpful to you (i.e., "Please face me when you talk, and speak slightly slower and a little louder").

4. When hearing is difficult, it is easy to allow the mind to wander. Practice paying close attention to the speaker at all times. Paying close attention can sometimes be exhausting. Therefore arrange for frequent breaks if discussions or meetings are expected to run long.

5. Although you may have had no formal training in speech reading (lip reading), research has demonstrated that the addition of visual cues to what the ear hears can increase understanding as much as 20%. Always strive for a clear, unobstructed view of the speaker's face. An optimal distance for communication exchange is 3 to 6 feet.

6. Important instructions, information, or key words such as addresses, telephone numbers, measurements, dollar figures, and so on, should always be written out to avoid confusion.

7. Let others know when you do or do not understand what has been said. Keep in mind that "Huh?" "What?" "Please repeat that" are all ineffective in that they do not tell the speaker what would be helpful. Statements such as "Please raise the volume of your voice," "Please face me when you talk to me," or "I need you to slow down a little" are all much more effective.

8. Try not to interrupt too often. How frequently to interrupt calls for a great deal of judgment, but always try to be as unobtrusive as possible. Sometimes a prearranged hand signal for the speaker to slow down, speak up, or to move a hand from in front of the face, and so on, can be useful.

9. Provide feedback to those who talk with you to let them know how well they are doing. No one likes to hear only about what is wrong. "Your voice volume and

---

*Compiled by Samuel Trychin, John Greer Clark, and Marjorie Boone.

speed are just right; I'm understanding everything you are saying" provides a nice verbal "pat on the back" as well as important information to the speaker about how best to communicate.

10. Do not bluff! Bluffing robs you of opportunities to practice good communication skills. The risk of not informing others about your hearing loss is an increase in the occurrence of misinterpretations and the possibility of damaged relationships.

11. Set realistic goals about what you can expect to understand. If you are in a nearly impossible listening situation, it may be best to relax and ride it out. More manageable listening settings will be forthcoming.

12. Remember that hearing aids have limitations. Often the use of additional assistive listening devices can turn an impossible listening situation into one that is possible.

APPENDIX 10–3

The following manuals and videotapes were developed as part of the Living with Hearing Loss Program and address the various facets of coping with hearing loss. Information about accessing the mental health manuals can be obtained from Dr. Trychin. Information on all other material may be obtained from Dr. Trychin, 6 Tower Road, Severna Park, MD 21146, or from Self Help for Hard of Hearing People (SHHH), 7800 Wisconsin Avenue, Bethesda, MD 20814.

BALLY, S., & TRYCHIN, S. (Eds). (1989). *A newcomer's guide to an old problem: Hearing loss.* Washington, DC: Gallaudet University Press.

FORGATCH, M., & TRYCHIN, S. (1988). *Getting along* (manual). Washington, DC: Gallaudet University Press.

FORGATCH, M., & TRYCHIN, S. (1988). *Getting along* (videotape). Washington, DC: Gallaudet University Press.

TRYCHIN, S. (1986). *Relaxation training for hard of hearing people: Trainee's manual.* Washington, DC: Gallaudet University Press.

TRYCHIN, S. (1986). *Relaxation training for hard of hearing people* (audiotapes). Washington, DC: Gallaudet University Press.

TRYCHIN, S. (1986). *Relaxation training for hard of hearing people* (videotapes). Washington, DC: Gallaudet University Press.

TRYCHIN, S. (1986). *Stress management video series for deaf people: Trainee's manual.* Washington, DC: Gallaudet University Press.

TRYCHIN, S. (1986). *Stress management video series for deaf people* (videotapes). Washington, DC: Gallaudet University Press.

TRYCHIN, S. (1987). *Communication rules for hard of hearing people* (videotape). Washington, DC: Gallaudet University Press.

TRYCHIN, S. (1987). *Did I do that?* (manual). Washington, DC: Gallaudet University Press.

TRYCHIN, S. (1987). *Did I do that?* (videotape). Washington, DC: Gallaudet University Press.

TRYCHIN, S. (1987). *Relaxation training for hard of hearing people: Practitioner's manual.* Washington, DC: Gallaudet University Press.

TRYCHIN, S. (1987). *Stress management video series for deaf people: Practitioner's manual.* Washington, DC: Gallaudet University Press.

TRYCHIN, S. (1988). *So that's the problem!* Washington, DC: Gallaudet University Press.

TRYCHIN, S. (1990). *Speak out: Tips on speaking in public for individuals with a hearing loss.* Washington, DC: Gallaudet University Press.

TRYCHIN, S. (1991). *Manual for mental health professionals: Part 2. Psychosocial challenges faced by hard of hearing people.* Washington, DC: Gallaudet University Press.

TRYCHIN, S., & BONVILLIAN, B. (1991). *Actions speak louder: Tips for putting on skits relating to hearing loss.* Washington, DC: Gallaudet University Press.

TRYCHIN, S., & BOONE, M. (1987). *Communication rules for hard of hearing people* (manual). Washington, DC: Gallaudet University Press.

TRYCHIN, S., & BUSACCO, D. (1991). *Manual for mental health professionals: Part 1. Making services accessible to hard of hearing people.* Washington, DC: Gallaudet University Press.

TRYCHIN, S., & WRIGHT, F. (1988). *Is that what you think!* Washington, DC: Gallaudet University Press.

chapter eleven

Counseling Geriatric Patients and Their Families

Jerome G. Alpiner

The focus of this final chapter brings to full circle the chronological perspective of the patients with whom audiologists work and, at the same time, demonstrates from a counseling perspective that the care given to older patients is only a different stage of the same journey: the continued effort to find ways of giving more complete care to those with hearing loss. In this chapter, Dr. Alpiner presents the counseling needs of our elderly through a discussion of the impact of hearing loss on this population. Through Dr. Alpiner's discussion of the assessment of problem areas confronting the elderly, audiologists can better plan strategies for counseling elderly patients and their families.

"One more try," he asked. "We are not quite done."
"What is the use of trying?"
"It is a thing which people do."

Merlyn to an aging Arthur
in T. H. White's
The Book of Merlyn

INTRODUCTION

A number of years ago, my family went camping in the Colorado Rockies. We met an older gentleman at our favorite campsite and we nicknamed him the Mushroom Man, since his favorite activity was showing us which mushrooms were edible. We visited with him on many occasions during that time period. When we moved from Colorado, my daughter continued to stay in touch with the Mushroom Man as a pen pal. Recently, she called me to say that the gentleman, age 90 now, wanted to move from his retirement trailer in Arizona to Colorado to be close to her, since he had no family and she was the only person to ever keep in touch with him. She wanted to know what I thought about this elderly gentleman living with her family. My initial reaction was negative. "What in the world do you think you are doing taking in someone with so many potential problems?" I was reminded that a considerable portion of my career was devoted to working with seniors. Apparently, the major difficulty for the Mushroom Man was hearing loss; otherwise, he was very physically fit.

My thoughts began to reflect on attitudes of society. If *I* felt this way, what about the vast majority of persons in this country who know little about the aging process? This personal experience has helped me to organize my own thoughts about the needs of the older population and how we may effectively help these individuals. This chapter is about counseling older patients with hearing loss and their families. In reality, we counsel patients who are people, not problems. Problems affect people, of course, but our treatment must focus on feelings and attitudes of these persons.

EXTENT OF HEARING LOSS

Of all of the chronic conditions affecting the noninstitutionalized elderly, hearing loss is the third most prevalent condition, exceeded only by arthritis and hypertension (Feller, 1981). Various estimates indicate the extent of hearing loss in the United States. About 30% of individuals outside of nursing homes have impaired hearing (Margolis, Levy, & Sherman, 1981), while as many as 90% of nursing home residents may have impaired hearing (Chafee, 1967). Williams (1986) has estimated that 60% of persons over the age of 65, and as many as 90% of persons age 80 over have some degree of hearing impairment; 55% of adults with hearing loss severe enough to inhibit communication are age 65 or older. In terms of numbers of people, Mulrow et al., (1990) have indicated that over 18 million elderly persons suffer from some form of hearing loss, and this number will approach 25 million in the 1990s.

The bottom line indicates that there are millions of older adults with hearing loss who also possess various concomitant problems caused by sensory deprivation. Audiologists, therefore, have a responsibility to determine what problems exist secondary to hearing loss and how we may help. We could assume that our counseling role commences after hearing aids are fit, except that only 18%–20% of elderly hearing-impaired persons use hearing aids (Weinstein, 1990). Instead, counseling should include efforts toward amplification for those who can benefit from it. When we discuss counseling, from an audiological view, it is important to note that our efforts are directed to more than talking about hearing. We need to ask ourselves about the areas of everyday living that are affected by hearing loss. We want to know what the effects of hearing loss are on an individual's feelings, attitudes, self-esteem, communication ability, and relationships with families, friends, and associates (Wylde, 1982).

A PROFILE OF THE GERIATRIC CLIENT

The problem of defining what is meant by the term *older people* becomes apparent from even a cursory inspection of the literature (Robertson-Tchabo, 1985). Homogeneity is not a characteristic of the group of individuals called elderly. Perhaps the chronological designation of age is the most consistent aspect of aging. Very often, age 65 is designated as the beginning of old age, for medical-legal purposes, not always for actual human function. I have seen 80-year-old patients who look like they are in their 50s and 60s, and sometimes, patients in their 50s and 60s who look like they are in their 80s.

There is, however, an association between advancing age and an increased incidence of disease and disability (McCarthy, 1993). Those persons with acute disease experience more days of restricted activity than do younger individuals (Ries, 1979). Chronic disease increases with age, and most persons over the age of 65 have some chronic condition, even though it is usually not disabling (Atchley, 1988).

It is advisable to consider each individual according to specific problems and the effects of these problems on everyday living. We can then evaluate needs for counseling on this basis rather than on a generalization that all older people exhibit the same difficulties. Some students have asked, with this approach, how the older population differs from any other age group. The question is a reasonable one. It is necessary to emphasize that there are some general differences. A large percentage of elderly persons are no longer gainfully employed, many are single by virtue of the death of a spouse, health problems do exist and can restrict activities, some have to live alone, some are confined to nursing homes, transportation limitations restrict mobility, and for some the future offers little hope.

A psychological-social model (Figure 11–1) was developed to view geriatric patients according to their own situations (Alpiner, 1979). The reason for this model was to demonstrate that not all older citizens undergo the same social and emotional difficulties. Some individuals find that being older can be fun and challenging. The key to these feelings seems to relate to the ability to remain active, with participation in the activities afforded by the community (Alpiner, 1979).

It appears that there are four significant factors that may ultimately lead to the emergence of different attitudes: communicative status, physiological problems, environmental constraints, and economic limitations. Their collective interaction leads to psychological interactions that occur in an individual. It is a time of sorting out and processing; it may be a time of confusion and frustration. These interactions ultimately lead to a psychological set. At this stage a person begins to develop a means by which the self is viewed as well as how others view the individual. The attitude that eventually emerges may be acceptance, rejection, or uncertainty. The patient may choose to enter the mainstream in society or perhaps

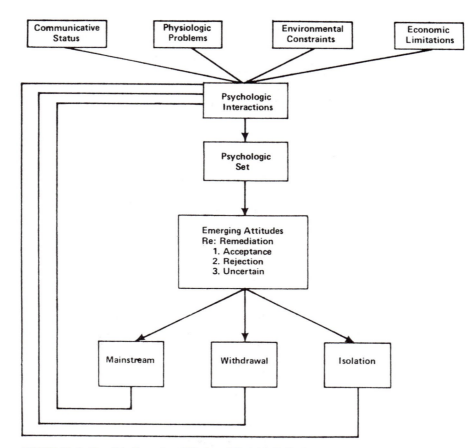

FIGURE 11–1 Possible Emerging Attitudes of Geriatric Patients

choose withdrawal or isolation. The audiologist needs to be aware of all of these factors and how the rehabilitation process may be affected. This model permits us to assess the individual according to needs rather than age.

The American Association of Retired Persons (1990) provides some general information regarding the profile of older Americans. This information may help us to better understand the differences in this population as we plan our counseling strategies. The median income of older persons in 1989 was $13,107 for males and $7,655 for females. Households containing families headed by persons over age 65 reported a median income in 1989 of $23,179 for whites, $19,310 for Hispanics, and $15,766 for African Americans. The major source of income for older couples and individuals in 1988 was Social Security (39%), followed by asset income (25%), earnings (17%), public and private pensions (17%), and all other sources (3%). The poverty rate for persons over age 65 was 11.4%. Another 8% were classified as "near poor." All of this information becomes relevant when we consider how closely income will influence health care provisions such as the purchase of hearing aids and rehabilitative audiology services.

In 1988 about 12% of the older population were still in the labor force. About half of the workers over age 65 in 1989 were employed part time. About 25% were self-employed, compared to 8% for younger workers. The median level of education was 12.1 years in 1988. African Americans and Hispanics had less schooling than whites. In 1988, 29% of older persons assessed their health as fair or poor compared to 7% for persons under age 65.

Most older persons have at least one chronic condition and many have multiple conditions. The most frequently occurring conditions for the elderly in 1988 were arthritis (49%), hypertension (37%), hearing impairment (32%), heart disease (30%), and tinnitus (8%).

The majority (67%) of older persons lived in a family setting in 1989. A 1984 study found that four of every five older persons had living children. Of these, two-thirds (66%) lived within 30 minutes of their children. Six out of ten (62%) had at least weekly visits with their children and three-fourths (76%) talked on the phone at least weekly with their children. Adult children of older Americans may play a significant role in our counseling efforts. Hearing loss can be considered a family affair, and rehabilitative efforts have an opportunity to be more successful when significant others are available to help.

Change appears to be a way of life for persons of all ages. For the elderly, there may be an increasing number of changes that affect lifestyle on a permanent basis. Ronch (1982) indicates changes that may occur more frequently with the older age group. Family members, spouses, and peers become seriously ill or die. Work no longer occupies personal time. Recreational activities become limited due to physical health and transportation problems.

Efforts to keep persons in the mainstream of society appear to be a logical goal. Communication, obviously, is a requisite for anyone who wishes to be part of everyday living activities.

CONCOMITANT PROBLEMS AFFECTING THE ELDERLY

We see about 1,200 audiology patients a year at the Veterans Administration (VA) Medical Center in Sioux Falls. The vast majority of patients are age 65 and over. About 85% are outpatients, and the remainder are either in the center's extended-care unit or other inpatient wards. If fitting hearing aids were the only rehabilitative task, our responsibility would be rather an easy one. There are many patients who exhibit concomitant problems that increase the complexity of the rehabilitative process. The impact of significant hearing loss results in a number of psychological/social characteristics such as depression, irritability, avoidance, withdrawal, rejection, and negativism (Alpiner, 1978). A study by Herbst (1983) indicates that hearing loss appears to be associated with poor general health, reduced interpersonal communication, and depression. While hearing impairment may not be the cause of these problems, the important consideration is to emphasize that hearing loss is not the individual's only problem. It is not, therefore, a simple matter of treating only the hearing loss. It is very common to encounter patients who want to talk about other problems that affect their total lives. It is important that audiologists take some time to listen.

Other physical problems exist and may affect hearing rehabilitation. Some of the major problems that audiologists need to consider are changes in vision and touch, and chronic health conditions. These problems need not be a deterrent to hearing rehabilitation as long as their effects are understood. Vision, for example, is one area that is crucial if we advocate a bisensory approach to better hearing and understanding. We know that, with amplification, vision contributes significantly to understanding auditory stimuli. It is imperative, therefore, that visual examinations be administered to patients.

Changes in touch can be significant when we realize how miniaturized hearing aids are compared to only several years ago. Axelrod and Cohen (1961) reported that light touch on both the palm and the thumb may be considerably decreased in older subjects. We observe difficulty for a number of older patients when trying to manipulate the small volume control on hearing aids or trying to change batteries with the small battery door that needs to be opened. Vision and touch play a role in inserting the battery properly with the "plus" side facing the proper battery contact. The battery can be both difficult to handle and the "plus" sign impossible to see.

Some older persons may feel that the effort to wear hearing aids is too much of an overload for them and that they prefer to be left alone. This is often true when there are no family members or significant others to assist in the helping process. It is sometimes difficult to decide whether amplification should be recommended. Consider the situation in which no one is available, including hospital staff. Should we fit hearing aids, let the patient then go to struggle alone, and learn later that the hearing aids have found a place in a dresser drawer? Who is supposed to assume responsibility for this patient and probably thousands of others in this country? There are many elderly persons who do not present these kinds of problems. Our goal here, however, is to determine how we may help those individuals who require a variety of solutions for problems that may range from easy to difficult.

RESPONSIBILITIES FOR THE COUNSELING PROCESS

Since most seniors are in relatively good health, audiologists can make a significant contribution to mainstreaming through their work with those persons who have hearing loss. After all, there are not many activities in which one can participate without the ability to hear well and to speak effectively.

The absence of adequate communication can be portrayed by the commentary of a 79-year-old internist (Lipkin & Williams, 1986). This physician states:

> the degree of disability shown by hearing impaired people varies greatly depending on factors intrinsic in the particular person . . . some older people simply withdraw . . . some demand that people around them modify their speech . . . some become frustrated and angry . . . some acknowledge the infirmity, others conceal or deny it . . . some accept the need to help themselves . . . some use every possible help to continue meaningful work . . . others just give up . . . some mourn the loss of a considerable part of life's pleasures . . . as with most handicaps, attitudes are a major determinant of the degree of impairment of the quality of life. (p. 400)

Hearing aids were recommended for this physician. He indicated that there were no other suggestions by the otologist or the audiologist. It was emphasized that the experiences of many persons have been similarly disappointing. Little or no attention was paid to the psychological considerations that are so important in adapting to disability. No other information was provided to this physician about help for his communication problems.

While no audiologist will diminish the importance of the diagnostic and hearing aid aspects of the profession, the need continues, as it has for many years, to think about people's problems related to hearing loss. As Lowe (1992) so aptly states:

> while the equipment gets more complex, and next year's screen will be in six colors instead of four, we must insure that tomorrow's audiologists will be people-oriented and skilled at personal interaction with their clients. To do that requires rigorous training in the art of rehabilitation. Such a concept does not appear to be a high priority issue in our training programs however, and has not been for far too long. Perhaps it is time for the pendulum to swing a bit. (p. 21)

Counseling has always been an integral component in rehabilitative audiology. The audiologist has confined the counseling effort to problems manifested by hearing loss. A concern about counseling has been that audiologists' counseling efforts may exceed training and qualifications. Wylde (1982) has discussed boundaries for counseling for the audiologist. Five aspects are considered:

1. The counseling process should be related to assisting the patient to improve communication and alleviating problems caused by the loss of hearing sensitivity.
2. The counseling process should be guided by the individual and family members.
3. The counseling process should be supportive of individual and family members.
4. The counseling process should center on the course of action best suited for the individual.
5. The counseling process should not enter the realm of the clinical psychologist or psychiatrist.

Audiologists are the experts when dealing with hearing problems. The fifth boundary is the one that needs some clarification. Wylde (1987) states that the fifth boundary is one that allows audiologists to stay within the confines of the profession. Individuals who experience emotional and psychological difficulties beyond our "comfort zone" should be referred for counseling with a mental health professional. While comfort zone is a rather nebulous definition, it is one that audiologists need to define for themselves. If a patient presents an emotional demeanor with which we are uncomfortable because it appears to be extreme, or abnormal, then it may very well be abnormal and a referral to a psychologist, or psychiatrist is in order. Dr. Clark provides further discussion in Chapter 1 on the means of making effective counseling referrals.

When counseling older patients, it is expected that the audiologist will have expertise in both normal and abnormal processes of hearing. This is part of the usual training program for audiologists. In addition, the audiologist who counsels older patients should have knowledge and expertise in geriatric processes. Let us now proceed to deal with those aspects of counseling that will assist audiologists in better meeting all the communication needs of hearing-impaired older patients.

ASSESSMENT OF COUNSELING NEEDS

A primary objective of rehabilitative audiology is to improve the hearing-impaired person's communication ability to the maximum extent possible so that they may function better in the roles of everyday living. In order to plan strategies for counseling patients, we need to determine the problem areas that need attention. The routine audiological test battery offers information on the type and degree of hearing impairment, but is limited in providing information about the effects of the deficit on communication function.

We have a protocol at our hospital that includes hearing aid orientation and enables us to obtain both pre- and postrehabilitation information about patients who use amplification. The following procedures are performed:

1. The hearing aids are checked for operation, and the ear canals are checked for cerumen.
2. The patient is asked how the aids perform; the hearing aids' adjustments are checked.
3. The hearing aid survey form is completed (Appendix 11–1).
4. The Alpiner-Meline Aural Rehabilitation (AMAR) Scale is completed (Appendix 11–2).

During approximately the past 30 years, a variety of assessment scales of communication function have been developed. Our protocol is only one way to assess communication. It is important to try to evaluate individuals according to their unique living situations, while remembering that not all assessment tools can apply to all individuals and all items within a given instrument may not be appropriate.

Mr. Quinn, a 65-year-old semiretired male, was seen for a hearing aid evaluation. Previous audiometric evaluation had indicated the presence of a moderate to severe high-frequency sensorineural hearing loss bilaterally with fair discrimination ability (70%–80%). Binaural amplification was recommended.

The patient and his wife were counseled about the realistic expectations of hearing aids. Mr. Quinn and his spouse appeared to understand that amplification would not restore hearing to completely normal levels, and that environmental noise may continue to interfere with the understanding of all conversation. They were counseled regarding the role that auditory, visual, and tactile channels plays in effective communication and the resultant deficit or communication breakdown that occurs whenever the integrity of one or more of the sensory receptors is compromised. In order to identify potential communication problems that may be unaddressed by traditional audiometric procedures, the AMAR Screening Scale was administered. Part I of the screening scale explores an individual's attitude toward hearing loss. The items attempt to examine how often hearing loss influences an individual's perceptions and the reactions of significant others toward hearing loss in three communication areas: social, emotional, and vocational. Mr. Quinn indicated all nine items in Part I on the attitude of hearing loss as problem areas.

Mr. Quinn expressed emotional feelings of isolation and frustration, indicating that the hearing loss has affected life in general. He also expressed that he had social problems such as avoiding others. He reported that others were not tolerant of his hearing loss and that it interfered in his relationship with his wife. Items related to vocational performance indicated embarrassment, and an attempt to hide his hearing loss from co-workers. He reported stress in his part-time employment because of the hearing loss and the inability to perform optimally. Mr. Quinn's perceived hearing handicap was significant based on his responses.

It is especially important to note that Mr. Quinn's wife, who took Form B of the AMAR scale, reported responses inconsistent with those of her spouse. She indicated that his hearing loss did not affect his relationships with her, that it did not affect his life in general, and that it did not interfere with his job performance.

Without some type of assessment tool to evaluate the concomitant problems of hearing loss, these divergent perceptions would not have surfaced and we would have no structured base from which to begin counseling.

While it is possible to "jump" into aural rehabilitation directly from a scale such as the AMAR, a complete aural rehabilitation needs assessment may be accomplished. A number of assessment scales are available for use with the elderly to accomplish this purpose if it is felt necessary. One of the major assessment scales for the elderly is the Hearing Handicap Inventory for the Elderly (HHIE) (Ventry & Weinstein, 1982). This assessment tool evaluates the social and emotional effects of hearing in the noninstitutionalized older person (Appendix 11–3), and can be administered either face to face with the audiologist or in a paper-and-pencil format (Newman & Weinstein, 1989).

The Denver Scale of Communication Function for Senior Citizens Living in Retirement Centers (DSSC) (Zarnoch & Alpiner, 1977; Appendix 11–4) was designed for presentation through individual interview with retirement center residents. Clinical experience indicates that some self-scoring scales are not feasible for some persons in extended-care facilities. Residents seem to understand the task better when they are interviewed by the audiologist and allowed to respond verbally. The DSSC consists of seven major question categories that cover the following general areas of communication: family, emotional, other persons, general communication, self-concept, group situations, and rehabilitation. Included under each of the main questions is a "Probe Effect" and an "Exploration Effect." The Probe Effect determines the specific problem areas related to the general question and the Exploration Effect tries to determine how applicable the general question is to the individual client. For example, question 1 asks, "Do you have trouble communicating with your family because of your hearing problem?" The probe questions that follow, then determine if there are specific areas related to the family that are creating problems for the individual. The exploration questions help to determine the full impact of the problem, if one does exist. There may not be a family, or they may live so far away that the patient never sees them. In those cases, the question would be irrelevant and could be eliminated from future therapy goals. The scale does not attempt to compare one individual's performance with another, but rather to evaluate patients' impressions of their communication performance prior to and following any rehabilitative procedures. A scoring form is utilized to help in the interpretation of the responses. For each category, appropriate scoring boxes are included for the main questions and probe effects. A "+" or "−" is placed in each of the boxes to indicate a response of yes or no. Adjacent to the score boxes is a section for writing the responses to the exploration effects. Finally, there are two additional boxes for each category, labeled as "Problem" or "No Problem." After examining all of the responses in a particular category, one of the boxes should be checked depending on the clinician's final decision on whether a client's responses indicate a problem area.

As indicated previously there are a number of other assessment tools that may be used. The intent of this chapter is to focus on counseling with procedures that may be utilized to maximize this process. For a further discussion on assessment scales, the reader is referred to Alpiner and McCarthy (1993).

DEFINING AREAS FOR THE COUNSELING PROCESS

It is all too easy to take at face value patients' declaration that they have no difficulties (Erdman, 1992). According to Erdman, stoic patients who maintain an "everything-is-just-fine" attitude are a significant reason practitioners end up treating the pathology rather than the patient. Assessment scales can help to avoid this situation.

What are some of the problems with which patients are confronted? In reviewing several hundred patient records at the VA Medical Center, some consistency does seem to occur regarding problem areas.

Logistical Problems

Obviously, we have to deal with logistical problems that can result in frustration for the patient. These difficulties cannot be minimized; they are important to the patient who wants to hear well. Routine clinical monitoring reveals some of these problems so they can be addressed successfully:

1. Cerumen blocking the receiver of the hearing aid
2. A dead battery
3. Hearing aids with malfunctioning microphones, volume controls, and receivers
4. Acoustic feedback
5. Hearing aids that fit too tightly
6. Background noise making it difficult to hear
7. Inability to manipulate controls and/or place hearing aids in the ears appropriately

Hearing Handicap Problems

Hearing loss refers to reduced sensitivity to sound; hearing handicap is not synonymous with loss, but rather is defined as the effect of the hearing loss on an individuals's life (Voeks, Gallagher, & Langer, 1990). There are several ways in which we can view the problems resulting in hearing handicap. These include family, emotional (self), social-vocational, specific situation, and communication breakdown. Table 11–1 outlines some of the problems that occur in each of these categories.

The above aspects of communication in Table 11–1 are not intended to be all inclusive. Further, we need to be cognizant of the fact that many of these situations can be interrelated, as difficulties rarely occur in isolation. For example, difficulty hearing in social situations may be related to inappropriate amplification, causes a person to become frustrated and to withdraw from communication. There are so many factors that need to be considered that it is important to structure our information gathering in order to permit counseling to focus on the proper problem issues, and in the proper sequence. It is our responsibility to use those assessment tools and procedures that best meet the needs of each individual patient. We should not be reluctant to modify our procedures. Wylde (1987) reminds us that it is important to remember that each hearing-impaired adult is an individual with different communicative demands and needs. Each person brings to us a different developmental, social, psychological, and oto-audiological profile.

THE COUNSELING PROCESS

Bess et al. (1989) studied the impact of hearing impairment on 153 patients over the age of 65. Pure tone audiometry was conducted to determine hearing levels and functional health status was assessed using the Sickness Impact Profile (SIP)

TABLE 11–1   Problems Resulting from Hearing Handicap

FAMILY DIFFICULTIES
1. Acceptance of hearing loss
2. Participation in daily activities (decision making, communication, etc.)
3. Role of family members and/or care givers
EMOTIONAL (SELF) DIFFICULTIES
1. Withdrawal because of hearing loss
2. Frustration due to missing communication
3. Lack of interest or motivation
4. Inability to relax in communication situations
5. People seem to avoid
6. Negative feelings about life
SOCIAL-VOCATIONAL DIFFICULTIES
1. Social activities minimized
2. Les time spent with friends
3. Hesitant to meet new friends
4. Avoids group communication situations
5. Does not feel comfortable in communication situations
6. Unable to perform job adequately
7. Difficulty with employer and colleagues
8. Job causes feelings of stress
SPECIFIC SITUATION
1. Difficulty on telephone
2. Problems with television, radio, recordings
3. Difficulty at theater, religious services, movies
4. Social situation problems at parties, and so on
5. Difficulty hearing in automobiles, airplanes, and trains
6. Problems even with amplification devices
7. Lack of assertiveness in communication
COMMUNICATION BREAKDOWNS
1. Degree of hearing loss (loudness and clarity)
2. Visual aptitude in communication
3. Auditory aptitude in communication
4. Effects of background noise

(Bess et al. 1989). The SIP is a 136-item standardized questionnaire that assesses physical and psychosocial function. Three main scales are formed by combining 12 subscales: physical (ambulation, mobility, body care/movement), psychosocial (social interactions, communication, alertness, emotional), and overall (combining all 12 subscales). Results of the study demonstrate that poor hearing was associated with higher SIP scores and increased overall dysfunction. Progressive hearing impairment in elderly patients was associated with progressive physical and psychosocial dysfunction. Hearing loss appears to be an important determinant related to health status. It will be helpful to the counseling audiologist if health care is considered and efforts accomplished to allow for proper medical treatment. It is necessary to ensure that there are no unattended medical problems that might interfere with the counseling aspects of rehabilitative audiology.

Counseling the Patient

Frankel (1981) found that almost two-thirds of the respondents to her study indicated that they wanted to talk to someone about their hearing loss. The specific reasons for wanting to talk included trouble at home, trouble at work, interpersonal problems related to hearing loss, and the need for information about hearing aids and rehabilitation. Going through the logistical phase of counseling in the form of an orientation before hearing aids are fitted may circumvent or minimize problems that might be encountered after the fitting. We designed a booklet for first-time hearing aid users (Alpiner, Meline, & Holifield, 1990) that addresses many of the logistical counseling concerns outlined in Table 11–2.

Remember that hearing aids are regarded as the major component of rehabilitative audiology. Remember, too, that many elderly patients will need help for proper utilization of these devices. Many of the problems related to hearing loss cannot be resolved without some kind of amplification; we cannot counsel very easily if our patients cannot hear us. Erdman (1993) states that counseling is the cornerstone of rehabilitative audiology. The effectiveness of counseling determines the extent to which all other rehabilitative measures—from hearing aid use to speechreading—succeed or fail.

Patients, however, do not always come to us with open arms for counseling. There can be resistance for several reasons. Often the patient is still not convinced that help is needed, especially after hearing aids have been fit. The feeling can be one of "The hearing aid should do it all." In some cases that may be true, and that is a good reason for a rehabilitative audiology evaluation beyond audiometrics and

---

TABLE 11–2 Getting Ready for Hearing Aids

A. DISCUSSION ASPECTS
1. Why do you need hearing aids?
2. Individuals have communication difficulties in various environments. What about you? With family and friends, at work, in social gatherings, at recreational events, other situations.
3. Do you have difficulties related to loudness, clarity, frustration?
4. Do any of the following apply to you? You may think people mumble. You may think people avoid you. You don't understand all of the words. It may seem easier to stay home and avoid people.
5. Where do you have problems because of your hearing? Think for a moment. Let's name some of the problems.
6. Why do you have these problems?

B. INFORMATIONAL ASPECTS
1. Different kinds of hearing loss. Conductive hearing loss, sensorineural hearing loss, mixed hearing loss.

C. AMPLIFICATION ASPECTS
1. What do you know about hearing aids and how do you think they can help?
2. What are the different kinds of hearing aids?
3. Do you know about other kinds of assistive devices that can help?
4. What kind of hearing aid(s) are you going to get? Why are you getting this type?
5. Are you getting one or two hearing aids? Why are you getting one or two aids? What make and model are you getting?

Source: Alpiner, Meline, and Holifield (1990).

the "fit." Sometimes other problems take precedence over the desire for counseling: health, vocational, personal, economic. I believe that we will find most older persons will be willing to "give counseling a try." It must, however, be according to patient needs, not the audiologist's projection of needs. We should be expeditious, especially depending on who pays the professional fee for our services. There are not many funding sources to pay for aural rehabilitation.

When considering the older American, we will find ourselves planning goals for those who live independently as well as for those who live in retirement centers or extended-care facilities. The reason this is so important is that persons who are interested in improved communication need reasons to communicate. If a nursing home patient sleeps all day and is continually medicated for one reason or another, our chances for rehabilitative success are quite limited. The same situation may hold true for one who lives alone in a retirement center with no family and few friends and little need to talk to or listen to anyone. Assessment scales can be of assistance as we plan our counseling goals for each patient.

I recall a situation at an extended-care facility that caused me to think about patients' physical environments. This facility had a pay telephone at a height that would be satisfactory for an ambulatory person. In this case, however, a resident in a wheel chair wanted to make a telephone call and was unable to reach the telephone. This seemed like such an obvious situation for correction, but it was not obvious until the administrator of the nursing home was made aware of this situation. As a result of this experience, we designed a Physical Environment Check List, which has been helpful to us in evaluating environments in which individuals live and communicate (Appendix 11–5). We examined such areas as excessive noise from vending machines, traffic, heating and cooling systems, appliances, and so on. If noise levels were excessive, then the most adjusted person in the world would have difficulty hearing. We considered furniture arrangement: Were distances appropriate for people to see one another adequately and to hear efficiently?

Although we were evaluating this situation in an extended-care facility, it is entirely appropriate to do the same in a private residence. I recall the times patients have told me that the television set was all the way across the room from where they sit; I have heard a patient complain about the spouse who insists on running the dishwasher while trying to carry on a conversation. My suggestion is to check the environment in which the patient lives, regardless of where it is, and make it as conducive as possible for good communication. Appropriate action may necessitate the need to contact family members or significant others in the client's environment. It does not make much difference where a person lives when we consider that our mission is to make communication meaningful.

Many elderly patients will do well without extra counseling from the audiologist beyond routine hearing aid orientation. For those who do need our counseling assistance, where do we start? The importance of providing our full attention void of all distractions, a nonjudgmental listening posture, a respect for silent reflection, and a means of ensuring comprehension of what the patient intended is discussed in detail in Chapter 2.

Table 11–3 summarizes an early publication by Brammer (1973), which provides a series of stages for counseling within "helping relationships."

It is in the **entry** stage of the helping relationship that we allow the patient to talk about the problem(s). We may initiate the area of entry from the results of an assessment scale, a case history, and so on. Caruso (1985a) suggests some methods of problem identification that may be used for the entry stage: (a) Ask questions that lead the patient to state the problem, and (b) listen to what the patient is saying; do not interrupt.

In the **clarification** stage we help the patient define the specific problem and its effect on everyday living.

The **structure** stage is more matter-of-fact. We need to determine if this is a problem that we can handle with our level of training as well as the logistics involved in the process, such as fees for service, times for counseling, and so on.

TABLE 11–3   Eight Stages of the Helping Relationship

STAGE	GOALS
Entry	1. Open the avenue for assistance from the audiologist. 2. Lay the groundwork for trust. 3. Enable the patient to define his problems related to his hearing impairment.
Clarification	1. Define the client's specific problems as related to his/her hearing impairment. 2. Get a better feel for how the client sees his/her hearing impairment and its effect on his general life situation.
Structure	1. Determine if the audiologist has the skills necessary to meet the client's needs. 2. Identification of the agency and the type of help offered, the qualifications and limitations of the audiologist. 3. Acknowledgment of the time to be involved, any fees to be charged, and any restrictions to be imposed.
Relationship	A turning point in the process. The client and audiologist either continue to build the relationship through mutual agreement or the relationship is terminated by either party.
Exploration	1. The strategies for intervention are outlined. 2. The client's feelings are explored. 3. The alternatives of action are outlined.
Consolidation	1. The client will decide on a course of action. 2. The client's feelings are clarified. 3. The client will practice new skills.
Planning	1. Plans for termination and continuing alone are formulated. 2. Plans for referral are completed (agencies are contacted, applications completed).

Termination	1. Accomplishments are summarized.
	2. The helping relationship is ended through:
	  a. Termination
	  b. Referral
	  c. The promise of follow-up
	  d. The offer of "stand-by" help

Source: From L. Brammer as cited in Wylde (1982).

Relationship refers to an agreement between the audiologist and the patient as to whether to proceed in the counseling process. It is at this point where both parties must feel that there is a mutual relationship, one of trust and cooperation. If not, then the counseling relationship is terminated. The audiologist may recommend other professional persons to the patient for contact. This aspect is especially important if the audiologist feels that help is necessary.

In the **exploration** stage, the audiologist outlines and explains the goals to be worked toward in the relationship; these goals should be based on patient input. Both the audiologist and the patient should work together in establishing goals.

The **consolidation** stage permits the patient to elaborate feelings of concern and at the same time allow the audiologist to clarify issues that are being discussed in the counseling process.

The **planning** stage is one in which we work with patients to help them deal with the specific situations that have emerged in counseling. Solutions to problems are discussed as well as possible referrals to other sources if needed. At this point, the patient needs to have some insight on how to cope with the problems that have been discussed once counseling has been terminated.

In the **termination** stage, the solutions and strategies that have been formulated in counseling will be discussed. The patient will be informed that help will continue to be available if needed. It is essential that the patient know that our services are available for follow-up. We do not want to terminate the patient from counseling without this kind of reassurance.

We can return to the case of Mr. Quinn and determine how this particular model can be implemented. One of the problems stated was that hearing loss interfered with the relationship with his spouse. For the point of entry, the audiologist sets an appointment for both husband and wife. The husband and wife agree to discuss problems related to hearing loss. Mr. Quinn stresses that the inability to hear well in most situations is just one of frustration, since his wife expects him to go to movies, church, and other social activities. In the clarification stage, focus is on an inability to understand what people say. His wife seems not to be able to comprehend that the problem may be one of both loudness and clarity. The audiologist, in the structure stage, attempts to explain and illustrate this aspect of communication, hopefully creating some understanding and acceptance between husband and wife. In the relationship stage, both persons need to agree that they will work through this problem. (Of course, they may decide that this is not their wish and discontinue counseling.) The exploration stage allows for feelings to be expressed by both parties. For the consolidation stage, feelings are clarified and courses of action to overcome the problems of loudness, clarity, and the subsequent frustrations are discussed. Planning allows for more long range decisions in the counseling process, and ultimately the termination stage will complete remediation. The time line for this counseling process may be one session or it may be several sessions. It simply depends on how well the spouse deals with the situation and how capable the audiologist is in guiding the sessions. We need to look at counseling in terms of what outcomes we expect as part of our effort.

Counseling the Family

I believe that it is necessary that family members or significant others be part of the counseling process. It is not always possible for this situation to exist. Family members may live too far away, some may not want to be involved, or there may be no family members or friends. Intergenerational care giving is becoming a significant issue in this era of high health costs and fewer persons to help in rehabilitation. Research on family care giving has demonstrated the predominance of women, particularly wives and daughters, among the care providers for our nation's elderly (Young & Willmott, 1957; Crystal, 1982; Brody, 1981). Increased incidence of both psychological and somatic symptoms are possible for care givers. Bowers (1987) reports a study in which care givers ranged in age from 38 to 72 with their parents ranging in age from 62 to 97. We may say that care giving is the work of caring for an aging parent. For our purposes, we narrow the task in terms of activities for improving communication aspects that may include hearing aid orientation and patient instruction for an assertive attitude to hear better those in the environment. In a broader sense, questions about care giving may include the following:

1. How does one care for aging parents while preventing them from discovering that they are being cared for?
2. How does this goal influence interactions with other offspring, other relatives, or health care providers?
3. What strategies are used to respond to parents who perceive that they are being cared for?
4. Under what conditions are parents not upset about being cared for by offspring? How would this affect strategies for care giving?
5. How do adult children react when they have finally reared their own children only to find themselves in the role of now caring for their parents?

The importance of family counseling is contingent on the availability of adult children and their willingness to participate in the process. I have thought about some of my frustrations in fitting hearing aids on some senior citizens who simply will not be able to go it alone in managing the basic mechanics of hearing aid use. There are times when I say that monaural is better than binaural, since it is doubtful that the person can handle even one hearing aid.

If our expectations for success are based on family members or significant others being available to help, then it is a good idea to examine the status of the care givers. A number of studies have discussed the importance of geographical distance relative to parent–child interactions (Lee, 1980; Dewit, Wister, & Burch, 1988; Krout, 1988). In 1962, about 51% of elderly persons saw one of their children every day or two; by 1975 the figure declined to 43% and by 1984 only 34% saw one of their children at least every other day (Crimmins & Ingegneri, 1990). About 66% of older people live within 30 minutes of their children even though parent–child contacts may not be as often as desired.

For our purposes in family counseling, we need to evaluate the situation carefully and determine if care givers are available as needed. My own experience indicates that efforts have to be made to involve others in the process of counseling the patient who cannot cope alone. We must try to meet with those significant persons in the patients' domain and explain to them how important their help can be and how success may depend on their willingness to participate. There is no point in saying that help will require only a little effort or that there will be no frustration as a result of these efforts. I like to stress that the quality of life of the family member may be improved and that family assistance offers the best opportunity for success. The audiologist should realize that success will not occur 100% of the time. It should be realized, however, that we did not create these frustrating situations but rather inherited them. Obviously when all goes well we need to feel good about the situation for our own mental health. There are successes and these are the goals we wish to achieve.

In Chapter 6, Dr. Atkins discusses audiologists' needs to manage their own personal stress that may accompany failure of efforts at intervention with families.

CONCLUSION

Dr. Clark has discussed counseling theories in Chapter 1. The various aspects discussed in this chapter can be related to those theories depending on philosophical beliefs. There are numerous counseling approaches in the literature that may be adapted to our counseling with elderly patients. We should keep in mind Wylde's (1982) comments that there is not now, nor will there probably ever be, a description of the effects of hearing loss on the psychological and social well-being of hearing-impaired persons that will be directly applicable to the clients we meet on a day-to-day basis. The challenge of counseling is with the audiologist who deals with problems related to hearing impairment.

There are some helpful suggestions for audiologists as well as for family members communicating with persons who have hearing loss. A description of these suggestions may be found in Appendix 10–1 of Chapter 10. These suggestions are presented for a younger adult population. For many older persons, however, age may not be a factor in counseling "differently" from the way we would for any adult.

Patience is one of the greatest virtues in counseling many older persons. We cannot assume that an explanation need be repeated only one time. I believe that the need to be "extrapatient" is often a major difference in counseling senior citizens compared to other populations. Another major factor is to encourage the participation of significant others whether they are family members or friends. It is my impression that significant others can make a major contribution in enhancing motivation, which is necessary for successful counseling. We also should know that a major problem may not only be the frustration of not understanding. A broken battery door, for many, may be equally frustrating.

There are many factors that can be considered in the counseling process. The need for accuracy of information, empathetic understanding, the sharing of emotional concerns, and adjustment to hearing impairment are a few of these aspects (Erdman, 1993). With increased knowledge about the helping process, let counseling begin. Let us help the older population achieve a good quality of life and the ability to communicate in a world that demands listening and talking in order to exist.

REFERENCES

ALPINER, J. G. (Ed.). (1978). *Handbook of adult rehabilitative audiology.* Baltimore: Williams & Wilkins.

ALPINER, J. G. (1979). Psychological and social aspects of aging as related to hearing loss. In M. A. Henoch (Ed.), *Aural rehabilitation for the elderly.* New York: Grune & Stratton.

ALPINER, J. G., & MCCARTHY, P. (Eds.). (1993). *Rehabilitative audiology: Children and adults.* Baltimore: Williams & Wilkins.

ALPINER, J. G., MELINE, N. C., & COTTON, A. D. (1991). An aural rehabilitation screening scale: Self assessment, auditory aptitude, and visual aptitude. *Journal of the Academy of Rehabilitative Audiology, 24,* 75–83.

ALPINER, J. G., MELINE, N. C., & HOLIFIELD, M. (1990). *Getting ready for hearing aids.* Birmingham, AL: Department of Affairs Medical Center.

AMERICAN ASSOCIATION OF RETIRED PERSONS. (1990). *A profile of older Americans.* Washington, DC.

ATCHLEY, R. (1988). *Social forces and aging.* Belmont, CA: Wadsworth.

AXELROD, S., & COHEN, L. D. (1961). Senescence and embedded—figure performance in vision and touch. *Perceptual Psychophysiology, 12,* 283–288.

BESS, F., LICHTENSTEIN, J., LOGAN, S., BURGER, J., & NELSON, E. (1989). Hearing impairment as a determinant of function in the elderly. *Journal of the American Geriatrics Society, 37,* 123–128.

BOWERS, B. J. (1987). Intergenerational caregiving: Adult caregivers and their aging parents. *Advances in Nursing Science, 9,* 20–31.

BRAMMER, L. (1973). *The helping relationship: Process and skills.* Englewood Cliffs, NJ: Prentice Hall.

BRODY, E. (1981). Women in the middle and family help to older people. *Gerontologist, 21,* 471–480.

CARUSO, B. K. (1985a). How to sell the benefits of wearing hearing aids: Part 1. The concept. *Hearing Instruments, 36*(3), 8–11.

CARUSO, B. K. (1985b). How to sell the benefits of wearing hearing aids: Part 2. The benefits. *Hearing Instruments, 36*(4), 8–11.

CARUSO, B. K. (1985c). How to sell the benefits of wearing hearing aids: Part 3. The sales strategy. *Hearing Instruments, 36*(9), 14–15.

CHAFEE, C. E. (1967). Rehabilitation needs of nursing home patients. *Rehabilitation Literature, 28,* 377–382.

CRIMMINS, E. M., & INGEGNERI, D. G. (1990). Interaction and living arrangements of older parents and their children., *Research on Aging, 12,* 3–35.

CRYSTAL, S. (1982). *America's old age crisis.* New York: Basic Books.

DEWIT, D., WISTER, A., & BURCH, T. (1988). Physical distance and social contact between elders and their adult children. *Research on Aging, 10,* 56–80.

ERDMAN, S. A. (1993). Counseling hearing impaired adults. In J. Alpiner & P. McCarthy (Eds.), *Rehabilitative audiology: Children and adults,* pp. 374–413. Baltimore: Williams & Wilkins.

FELLER, B. A. (1981). Prevalence of selected impairments, U.S. 1977. *Vital and Health Statistics,* Series 10, No. 134, DHHS 81–1562. Washington, DC: U.S. Government Printing Office.

FRANKEL, B. J. (1981). *Adult onset hearing impairment: Social and psychological correlates of adjustment.* Doctoral dissertation. University of Western Ontario, London, Ontario.

HERBST, K. R. G. (1983). Psycho-social consequences of disorders of hearing in the elderly. In R. Hinchcliffe (Ed.), *Hearing and balance in the elderly,* pp. 174–200. Edinburgh: Churchill Livingstone.

KROUT, J. A. (1988). Rural versus urban differences in elderly parents contact with their children. *Gerontologist, 28*, 198–203.

LEE, G. (1980). Kinship in the seventies: A decade review of research and theory. *Journal of Marriage and the Family, 42*, 923–934 (1980).

LIPKIN, M., & WILLIAMS, M. E. (1986). Presbycusis and communication. *Journal of General Internal Medicine, 1*(6), 399–401.

LOWE, A. D. (1992). "Trust me" audiology: A threat to our future? *Audiology Today, 4*, 21.

MCCARTHY, P. A. (1993). Rehabilitation consideration with the geriatric population. In J. G. Alpiner & P. A. McCarthy (Eds.), *Rehabilitative audiology: Children and adults*, pp. 331–373. Baltimore Williams & Wilkins.

MARGOLIS, M., LEVY, B., & SHERMAN, F. T. (1981). Hearing disorders. In L. S. Libow & F. T. Sherman (Eds.), *The core of geriatric medicine*, pp. 186–206. St. Louis: Mosby.

MULROW, C. D., AGUILAR, C., ENDICOTT, J. E., TULEY, M. R., VELEZ, R., CHARLIP, W. S., RHODES, M. C., HILL, J. A., & DENINI, L. A. (1990). Quality of life changes and hearing impairment. *Annals of Internal Medicine, 113*, 188–194.

NEWMAN, C. W., & WEINSTEIN, B. E. (1989). Test–retest reliability of the hearing handicap inventory for the elderly using two administration approaches. *Ear and Hearing, 10*, 190–191.

RIES, P. W. (1979). Acute conditions: Incidence and associated disability: U.S., 1977–78. *Vital and Health Statistics*, Series 10, No. 132. Washington, DC: U.S. Government Printing Office.

ROBERTSON-TCHABO, E. (1984). Psychological changes with aging. In L. Jacobs-Condit (Ed.) *Gerontology and communication disorders*, pp. 73–130. Rockville, MD: American Speech-Language-Hearing Association.

RONCH, J. L. (1982). Who are these aging persons? In R. Hull (Ed.), *Rehabilitative audiology*, pp. 185–213. New York: Grune & Stratton.

VENTRY, I., & WEINSTEIN, B. (1982). The hearing handicap inventory for the elderly: A new tool. *Ear and Hearing, 3*, 128–134.

VOEKS, S., GALLAGHER, C., & LANGER, E. (1990). Hearing loss in the nursing home. *Journal of the American Geriatrics Society, 38*, 141–145.

WEINSTEIN, B. E. (1990). Evaluation and management of the hearing impaired elderly. *Geriatrics, 45*, 75, 79–80, 83.

WILLIAMS, P. (1986). *Hearing impairment and elderly people—Background paper*. Washington, DC: Congress of the United States, Office of Technology Assessment.

WYLDE, M. A. (1982). The remediation process: Psychologic and counseling aspect. In J. G. Alpiner (Ed.), *Handbook of adult rehabilitative audiology*. Baltimore: Williams & Wilkins.

WYLDE, M. A. (1987). Psychological and counseling aspects of the adult remediation process. In J. G. Alpiner and P. A. McCarthy (Eds.), *Rehabilitative Audiology: Children and Adults*. Baltimore: Williams & Wilkins, 343–369.

YOUNG, M., & WILLMOTT, P. (1957). *Family and Kinship in East London*. London: Routledge & Kegan Paul.

ZARNOCH, J. M., & ALPINER, J. G. (1977). *The Denver Scale of Communication Function for Senior Citizens Living in Retirement Centers*. Unpublished study.

APPENDIX 11–1
HEARING AID SURVEY FORM

Name: _____   New/Experienced: _____
SS #: _____   ITE/BTE/OTHER: _____
Phone #: _____   Monaural/Binaural: _____
Work #: _____   Date Issued: _____
Date: _____   Audiologist: _____

1. I am satisfied with the benefit of my new hearing aid(s).   Yes   No   ?
   Comments:

2. I wear my new hearing aid(s) at least six hours a day.   Yes   No   ?
   Comments:

3. I wear my hearing aid(s) every day.   Yes   No   ?
   Comments:

4. My new hearing aid(s) are comfortable.   Yes   No   ?
   Comments:

5. The batteries for my hearing aid(s) last about two weeks.   Yes   No   ?
   Comments:

6. I can use my hearing aid(s) successfully with the telephone.   Yes   No   ?
   Comments:

7. I can turn the volume of my heaing aid(s) up as loud as I need to with-   Yes   No   ?
   out any problems.
   Comments:

8. I can wear my hearing aid(s) without excessive whistling when I eat,   Yes   No   ?
   walk, talk, or smile.
   Comments:

9. I know how to operate my new hearing aid(s).   Yes   No   ?
   Comments:

*10. I know how to get my hearing aid(s) repaired.   Yes   No   ?
   Comments:

*11. I received printed materials with my hearing aid and found them very helpful.   Yes   No   ?
Comments:

12. I hear well with my hearing aid(s) at a distance, in the presence of background noise, and when I cannot see the speaker's face.   Yes   No   ?
Comments:

13. My family understands my hearing loss and is very supportive of me.   Yes   No   ?
Comments:

*14. I was pleased with the service(s) provided by the Audiology Section.   Yes   No   ?
Comments:

15. Do you feel like you need any help with your hearing aid(s) now?   Yes   No   ?
Comments:

16. I am interested in attending a group meeting to learn how to get better help from my hearing aid(s).   Yes   No   ?
Comments:

Respondent: _____ Patient: _____ Other: _____

Source: Reprinted by permission from J. G. Alpiner, VA Medical Center, Birmingham, Alabama (1990).

APPENDIX 11–2
ALPINER-MELINE AURAL REHABILITATION SCREENING SCALE

Name: _____

Birthday: _____ Age: _____ SSN: _____

Hearing aid status:
(Circle one) NONE ITE BODY BONE EYEGLASS MONAURAL BINAURAL

Number of years of hearing aid use: _____

Occupation: _____

Audiologist: _____ Date of screening: _____

PART I: SELF-ASSESSMENT OF HEARING HANDICAP

(Choose One)   A = Always   U = Usually   S = Sometimes   R = Rarely   N = Never

1. I feel like I am isolated from things because of my hearing loss.   A U S R N   + −
2. I feel very frustrated when I cannot understand a conversation.   A U S R N   + −
3. My hearing loss has affected my life.   A U S R N   + −
4. I tend to avoid people because of my hearing loss.   A U S R N   + −
5. People in general are tolerant of my hearing loss.   A U S R N   + −
6. My hearing loss has affected my relationship with my spouse.   A U S R N   + −
7. I try to hide my hearing loss from my co-workers.   A U S R N   + −
8. My hearing loss has interfered with job performance.   A U S R N   + −
9. I feel more pressure at work because of my hearing loss.   A U S R N   + −

PART I PROBLEMS _____

PART II: VISUAL APTITUDE

---

1. Good morning. . . . . + −
2. How old are you? . . . . + −
3. I live in (state of residence). . . . . + −
4. I only have a dollar. . . . . + −
5. There is somebody at the door. . . . . + −

PART II PROBLEMS _____

PART III: AUDITORY APTITUDE

---

1. FEW   CHEW . . . . + −
2. FIT   KIT . . . . + −
3. THIN   FIN . . . . + −
4. THUMB   SUM . . . . + −
5. TIE   THIGH . . . . + −
6. KICK   TICK . . . . + −

PART III PROBLEMS _____

00–10 Problems = NO NEED
11–13 Problems = QUESTIONABLE NEED
14–20 Problems = ABSOLUTE NEED

TOTAL
AMAR PROBLEMS _____

Source: Jerome G. Alpiner, Ph.D., Nannette C. Meline, M.S., Amy D. Cotton, M.C.D. VA Medical Center, Birmingham, Ala. (1990).

APPENDIX 11–3
THE HEARING HANDICAP INVENTORY FOR THE ELDERLY

Instructions: The purpose of this scale is to identify the problems your hearing loss may be causing you. Answer *Yes, Sometimes,* or *No* for each question. *Do not skip a question if you avoid a situation because of your hearing problem.* If you use a hearing aid, please answer the way you hear *without* the aid.

		YES (4)	SOMETIMES (2)	NO (0)
S-1.	Does a hearing problem cause you to use the phone less often than you would like?			
E-2.	Does a hearing problem cause you to feel embarrassed when meeting new people?			
S-3.	Does a hearing problem cause you to avoid groups of people?			
E-4.	Does a hearing problem make you irritable?			
E-5.	Does a hearing problem cause you to feel frustrated when talking to members of your family?			
S-6.	Does a hearing problem cause you difficulty when attending a party?			
E-7.	Does a hearing problem cause you to feel "stupid" or "dumb"?			
S-8.	Do you have difficulty hearing when someone speaks in a whisper?			
E-9.	Do you feel handicapped by a hearing problem?			
S-10.	Does a hearing problem cause you difficulty when visiting friends, relatives, or neighbors?			
S-11.	Does a hearing problem cause you to attend religious services less often than you would like?			
E-12.	Does a hearing problem cause you to be nervous?			
S-13.	Does a hearing problem cause you to visit friends, relatives, or neighbors less often than you would like?			
E-14.	Does a hearing problem cause you to have arguments with family members?			
S-15.	Does a hearing problem cause you difficulty when listening to TV or radio?			
S-16.	Does a hearing problem cause you to go shopping less often than you would like?			

E-17.   Does any problem or difficulty with your hearing upset you at all?   _____   _____   _____

E-18.   Does a hearing problem cause you to want to be by yourself?   _____   _____   _____

S-19.   Does a hearing problem cause you to talk to family members less often than you would like?   _____   _____   _____

E-20.   Do you feel that any difficulty with your hearing limits or hampers your personal or social life?   _____   _____   _____

S-21.   Does a hearing problem cause you difficulty when in a restaurant with relatives or friends?   _____   _____   _____

E-22.   Does a hearing problem cause you to feel depressed?   _____   _____   _____

S-23.   Does a hearing problem cause you to listen to TV or radio less often than you would like?   _____   _____   _____

E-24.   Does a hearing problem cause you to feel uncomfortable when talking to friends?   _____   _____   _____

E-25.   Does a hearing problem cause you to feel left out when you are with a group of people?   _____   _____   _____

FOR CLINICIAN'S USE ONLY: Total Score: _____
Subtotal E: _____
Subtotal S: _____

Source: From Ventry and Weinstein (1982). Reprinted by permission.

APPENDIX 11–4
THE DENVER SCALE OF COMMUNICATION FUNCTION
FOR SENIOR CITIZENS LIVING IN RETIREMENT CENTERS

NAME: _____   DATE OF PRE-TEST: _____

ADDRESS: _____   DATE OF POST-TEST: _____

AGE: _____   EXAMINER: _____

SEX: _____

1. Do you have trouble communicating with your family because of your hearing problem? Yes ___ No ___

   Probe Effect I

   a. Does your family make decisions for you because of your hearing problem? Yes ___ No ___

   b. Does your family leave you out of discussions because of your hearing problem? Yes ___ No ___

   c. Does your family get angry or annoyed with you because of your hearing problem? Yes ___ No ___

   Exploration Effect

   a. Do you have a family? Yes ___ No ___

   b. How often does your family visit you? _____

   c. How far away does your family live? In a city ___ Other ___

   d. How often do you visit your family? _____

2. Do you get upset when you cannot hear or understand what is being said? Yes ___ No ___

   Probe Effect I (to be used only if person responds yes)

   a. Do your friends know you get upset? Yes ___ No ___

   b. Does your family know you get upset? Yes ___ No ___

   c. Does the staff know you get upset? Yes ___ No ___

   Probe Effect II (to be used only if person responds no)

   a. Do your friends realize you are not upset? Yes ___ No ___

   b. Does your family realize you are not upset? Yes ___ No ___

   c. Does the staff realize you are not upset? Yes ___ No ___

   Exploration Effect (to be used only if person responds yes)

   a. How does your behavior change when you become upset? _____

3. Do you think your family, your friends, and the staff understand what it is like to have a hearing problem? Yes ___ No ___

   Probe Effect

   a. Do they avoid you because of your hearing problem? Yes ___ No ___

   b. Do they leave you out of discussions? Yes ___ No ___

   c. Do they hesitate to ask you to socialize with them? Yes ___ No ___

   Exploration Effect

   a. Family? Yes ___ No ___

   b. Friends? Yes ___ No ___

   c. Staff? Yes ___ No ___

4. Do you avoid communicating with other people because of your hearing problem? Yes ___ No ___

   Probe Effect

   a. Do you communicate with people during meal times? Yes ___ No ___

   b. Do you communicate with your roommate(s)? Yes ___ No ___

   c. Do you communicate during the social activities in the home? Yes ___ No ___

   d. Do you communicate with visiting family or friends? Yes ___ No ___

   e. Do you communicate with the staff? Yes ___ No ___

   Exploration Effect

   a. Is your roommate capable of communication? Yes ___ No ___

   b. What are the social acitivities of the home? _____

   c. Which ones do you attend? _____

5. Do you feel that you are a relaxed person? Yes ___ No ___
   Probe Effect
   a. Do you think you are an irritable person because of your hearing problem? Yes ___ No ___
   b. Do you think you are an irritable person because of your age? Yes ___ No ___
   c. Do you think you are an irritable person because you live in this home? Yes ___ No ___
   Exploration Effect
   Do you have to live in this home? Yes ___ No ___
6. Do you feel relaxed in group communicative situations? Yes ___ No ___
   Probe Effect
   a. Do you get nervous when you have to ask people to repeat what they have said if you have not understood them? Yes ___ No ___
   b. Do you feel nervous if you have to tell a person that you have a hearing problem? Yes ___ No ___
   Exploration Effect
   a. Do you watch facial expressions? Yes ___ No ___
   b. Do you watch gestures? Yes ___ No ___
   c. Do you think you are a good listener? Yes ___ No ___ Why?
   d. Do you have a hearing aid? Yes ___ No ___
   e. Do you wear your aid? Yes ___ No ___
7. Do you think you need help in overcoming your hearing problem? Yes ___ No ___
   Exploration Effect I
   a. A person can improve communication ability by using lipreading (or speechreading), which means watching the speaker's lips, facial expressions, and gestures when speaking to you.
   b. Do you agree with that definition of lipreading?
   Probe Effect
   a. If lipreading training was available, would you attend? Yes ___ No ___
   b. Do you think this home provides adequate activities to make you want to communicate? Yes ___ No ___
   Exploration Effect II
   a. Is your vision adequate? Yes ___ No ___
   b. Are you able to get around unassisted? Yes ___ No ___

Source: From Zarnock and Alpiner (1977). Reprinted by permission.

APPENDIX 11–5

THE DENVER SCALE OF COMMUNICATION FUNCTION FOR SENIOR CITIZENS LIVING IN RETIREMENT CENTERS

by
Janet M. Zarnoch, M.A., and Jerome G. Alpiner, Ph.D.

NAME: _____

ADDRESS: _____

AGE: _____

DATE OF PRE-TEST: _____

DATE OF POST-TEST: _____

EXAMINER: _____   SEX: _____

_____ Initial evaluation

_____ Final evaluation

CATEGORY	MAIN QUESTION	PROBE EFFECTS	EXPLORATION EFFECTS	PROBLEM	NO PROBLEM
Family	1 + □ – □	a □ b □ c □	a. _____ b. _____ c. _____ d. _____		
Emotional	2 + □ – □	I a □ b □ c □ II a □ b □ c □	a. _____		
Other persons	3 + □ – □	a □ b □ c □	a. _____ b. _____ c. _____		

General communication	4	+ ☐ − ☐	a ☐ b ☐ c ☐ d ☐	a. _____
				b. _____
			e ☐	c. _____
Self-concept	5	+ ☐ − ☐	a ☐ b ☐ c ☐	a. _____
Group situations	6	+ ☐ − ☐	a ☐ b ☐ c ☐	a. _____
				b. _____
				c. _____
				d. _____
				e. _____
Rehabilitation	7	+ ☐ − ☐	a ☐ b ☐	Ia. _____
				b. _____
				IIa. _____
				b. _____

Key + = Person responded yes to question
    − = Person responded no to question

Additional client comments:

1. _____
2. _____
3. _____
4. _____
5. _____
6. _____
7. _____

Physical Environment Check List

AREA	NOISE LEVEL	OBSTRUCTIONS	INTERNAL CORRECTION	EXTERNAL CORRECTION
1. Lounge no. _____				
2. Lounge no. _____				
3. Lounge no. _____				
4. Dining area no. _____				
5. Dining area no. _____				
6. Outdoor area no. _____				
7. Hallway area no. _____				
8. Hallway area no. _____				
9. Hallway area no. _____				
10. Hallway area no. _____				
11. Telephone area no. _____				
12. Telephone area no. _____				
13. Personal room				
14. Kitchen				
15. Living room				
16. Dining room				
17. Family room				
18. Patio area				
19. Recreation room				
20. Basement area				
21. Other: _____				
22. TV viewing				

Physical Environment Check List: Obstruction Code

1. Excessive ambient noise from: _____
   a. Vending machines
   b. Intercom system
   c. Cleaning apparatus
   d. Traffic
   e. Staff activity
   f. Kitchen activity
   g. Heating and cooling systems
   h. Television or radio
   i. Appliances
   j. Other _____
2. Personal safety
   a. Stairways
   b. Lighting
   c. Floor covering
   d. Wheelchair mobility
   e. Hand rails for walking
   f. Telephone and electric switch access
   g. Other _____
3. Furniture arrangement
   a. Conducive to communication (placement)
   b. Accessible for television and radio
   c. Levels of furniture (for tuning in at eye level)
   d. Shades or curtains for controlling light
   e. Communication areas separate from game areas and television/radio areas.
4. Other (specify)
   a.
   b.
   c.
   d.
   e.

dB Level

Index